Airway Management

Airway Management

Editor

Geetanjali S Verma
DNB (Anesthesiology) MNAMS EDAIC
Registrar
Department of Anaesthetics
North Cumbria University Hospitals
Carlisle, UK

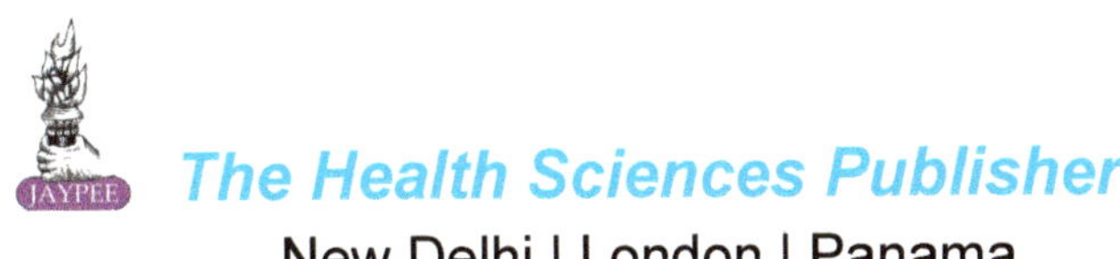

New Delhi | London | Panama

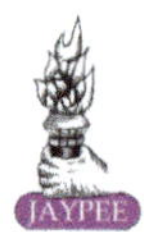

Jaypee Brothers Medical Publishers (P) Ltd

Headquarters

Jaypee Brothers Medical Publishers (P) Ltd
4838/24, Ansari Road, Daryaganj
New Delhi 110 002, India
Phone: +91-11-43574357
Fax: +91-11-43574314
Email: jaypee@jaypeebrothers.com

Overseas Offices

J.P. Medical Ltd
83 Victoria Street, London
SW1H 0HW (UK)
Phone: +44 20 3170 8910
Fax: +44 (0)20 3008 6180
Email: info@jpmedpub.com

Jaypee-Highlights Medical Publishers Inc
City of Knowledge, Bld. 235, 2nd Floor, Clayton
Panama City, Panama
Phone: +1 507-301-0496
Fax: +1 507-301-0499
Email: cservice@jphmedical.com

Jaypee Brothers Medical Publishers (P) Ltd
17/1-B Babar Road, Block-B, Shaymali
Mohammadpur, Dhaka-1207
Bangladesh
Mobile: +08801912003485
Email: jaypeedhaka@gmail.com

Jaypee Brothers Medical Publishers (P) Ltd
Bhotahity, Kathmandu, Nepal
Phone +977-9741283608
Email: kathmandu@jaypeebrothers.com

Website: www.jaypeebrothers.com
Website: www.jaypeedigital.com

Airway Management

First Edition: **2019**

ISBN: 978-93-5270-170-4

Dedicated to

My Family and
The first word of thanks to the Almighty for presenting me
with the beautiful opportunities in my life and
for having given me patience and
strength to make every chance a success.

Contributors

Deva Evu Subhas
MD DA DNB (Anesthesiology)
Consultant (Anesthesiology)
CSI Kalyani Multispecialty Hospital
Chennai, Tamil Nadu, India
E-mail: deva.subhas@gmail.com

Supraja Nagaiah
MD DNB (Anesthesiology)
Consultant (Anesthesiology)
CSI Kalyani Multispecialty Hospital
Chennai, Tamil Nadu, India
E-mail: supraja.nagaiah@gmail.com

Geetanjali S Verma
DNB (Anesthesiology) MNAMS EDAIC
Registrar
Department of Anaesthetics
North Cumbria University Hospitals
Carlisle, UK
E-mail: geetanjali0512@gmail.com

Preface

This book has been my dream, not only because it has seen a lot of hard work and sweat, but also because the topic forms the basis of the approach to any emergency situation. Whether the guidelines change from A-B-C to C-A-B in life-saving measures, A (airway) will always remain the priority at all times. The significance of 'A' cannot be further justified when the field of Anesthesia itself begins with the same alphabet.

The knowledge of the airway is tested in every examination—MCQs, written examinations, OSCE/viva, in all parts of the world. Whether one is preparing for MD/DNB/Anesthesia superspecialty in India or FRCA/EDAIC/EDIC in the European subcontinent to USMLE and Anesthesia examinations in USA/Canada, the topic of the airway is always touched upon.

Airway as a topic may seem small but it needs vast knowledge of all spheres—anatomy, physiology, pharmacology and instruments. We find it difficult to gain all the information in a single book as most books on airway have been written and published outside Asia. This is thus my effort to compile all details that we need to know pertaining to the airway in a single book, accessible to all and useful to not only students of Anesthesia but also to all those practicing in the field.

A sincere effort has been taken to update the latest topics and guidelines in the book and I have tried to present it in the simplest form.

I hope you enjoy reading the book and it proves useful in everyday practice.

Geetanjali S Verma

Acknowledgments

This book would have never been possible if it were not for my family. My parents (Sushil and Ranjana) have always been the supporting pillars in my life, guiding and encouraging me to excel in my field. My brother (Shantanu) has been my inspiration and always taught me to fight and believe in myself. I would have never come this far if it was not for their love and support at all times. Also, I would thank the editors, the contributors (my mentor-friends) and Jaypee Brothers Medical Publishers, New Delhi, India who helped me turn my dream into reality.

I especially appreciate the constant support and encouragement of Mr Jitendar P Vij (Group Chairman) and Mr Ankit Vij (Group President), Jaypee Brothers Medical Publishers (P) Ltd, New Delhi, India in publishing this book and also their associates particularly Ms Chetna Malhotra Vohra (Associate Director—Content Strategy) and Ms Nikita Chauhan (Development Editor) who have been prompt, efficient and most helpful.

Contents

1 Understanding the Basics

Geetanjali S Verma

ANATOMY

Geetanjali S Verma

The important anatomy to the airway consists of the relationship of pharynx to its surrounding structures, larynx and mobility of tissues.

THE PHARYNX

Extension: Sphenoid bone to C_6
12 to 15 cm long

It is widest at the level of the hyoid bone (5 cm) and narrowest at the level of the esophagus (1.5 cm), which is the most common site for obstruction after foreign body aspiration.

Lies parallel to vertebra, covered by anterior/longitudinal ligament and fascial layers beneath mucosa and constrictor muscles. The retropharyngeal space (between superficial buccopharyngeal fascia and prevertebral fascia) permits free movement of pharynx during deglutition. *Retropharngeal abscesses may infiltrate to superior mediastinum through here.*

Parts (Fig. 1)

- *Nasopharynx*: Extends from skull base to soft palate at caudal aspect of C1
- *Oropharynx*: Extension of nasopharynx to caudal aspect of C_3; also involves anterior 1/3 to posterior 2/3rd of tongue
- *Layngopharynx (hypopharynx)*: Merges with esophagus at C_6, where the cricopharyngeus encircles the esophagus to form its upper sphincter *(similar function of Sellick's maneuver in anesthetized patients).*

Nasopharynx

Anterioriorly opens into choanae, nasal passages, and nostrils (Fig. 2).

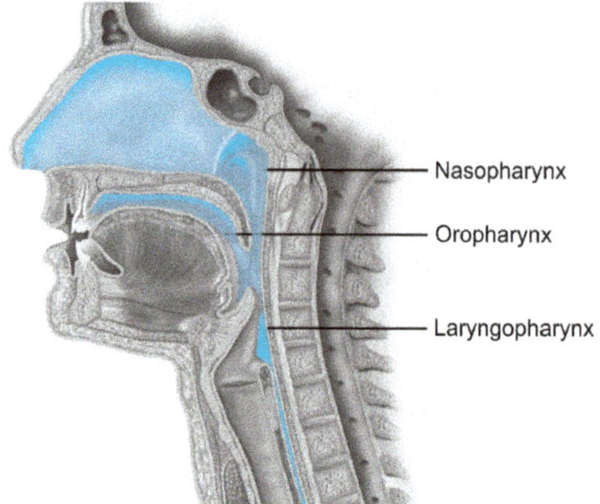

Fig. 1: Parts of pharynx.

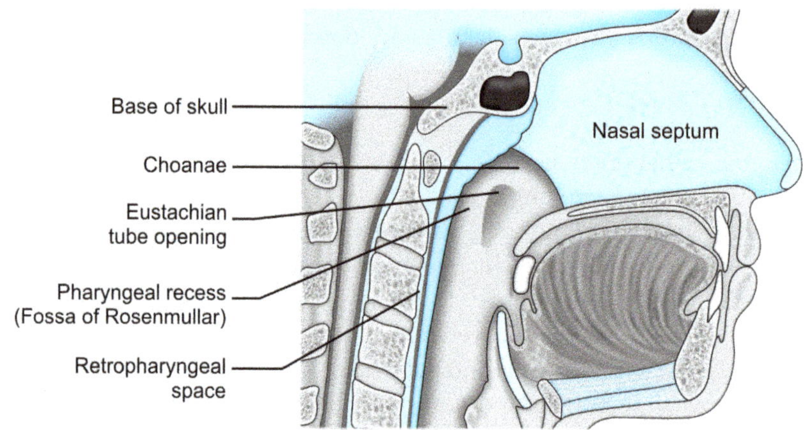

Fig. 2: Nasopharynx.

The nose: The nose is divided into two nasal fossae which extend uo to 10 to 14 cm from the nostrils to the nasopharynx. The two fossae are divided by a cartilaginous septum. The nasal septum is composed of the perpendicular plate of the ethmoid bone descending from the cribriform plate, septal cartilage, and the vomer.

Disruption of the cribriform plate (due to facial trauma/head injury) may allow direct communication with the anterior fossa. Use of positive-pressure mask ventilation in such conditions may lead to the entry of bacteria or foreign material, causing meningitis or sepsis. Also there is a probability of nasal airways, nasotracheal tubes, and nasogastric tubes being introduced into the subarachnoid space.

Functions of nose:
1. Smell
2. Humidification
3. Prevention of entry of dust/microorganisms.

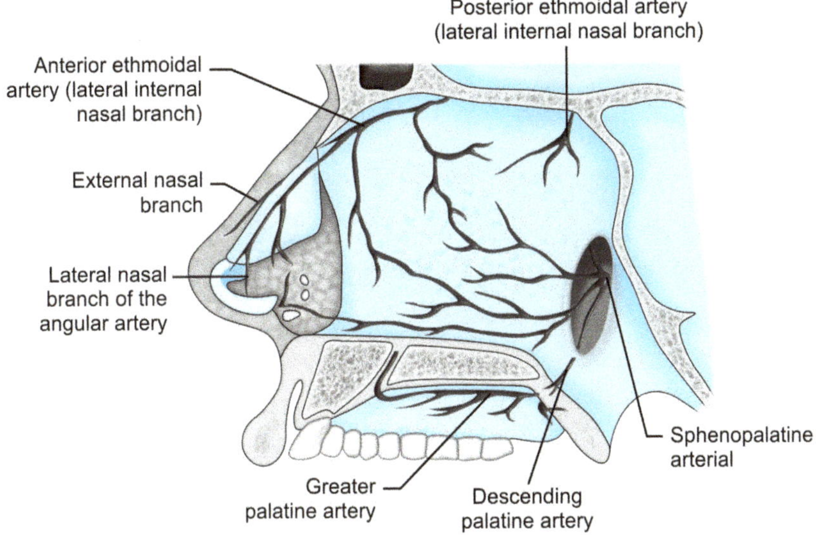

Fig. 3: Blood supply of nose.

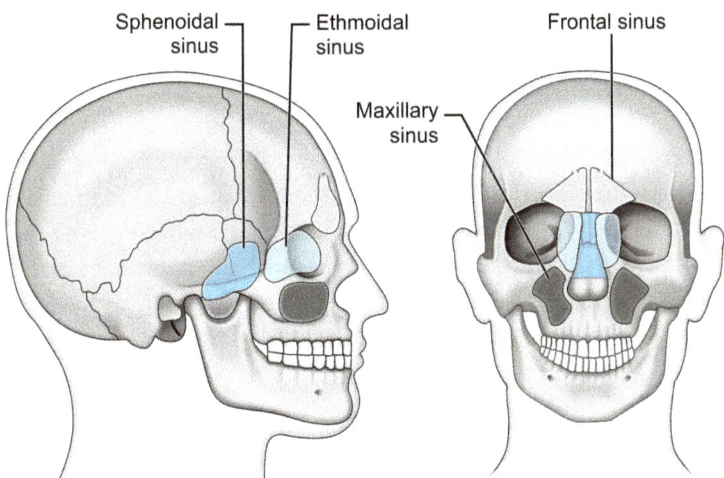

Fig. 4: Paranasal sinuses.

Blood Supply (Fig. 3)

1. Ethmoid branches of the ophthalmic artery
2. Sphenopalatine and greater palatine branches of the maxillary artery
3. Superior labial and lateral nasal branches of the facial artery.

Kiesselbach's plexus, where these vessels anastomose, is situated in Little's area on the anterior-inferior portion of the nasal septum—a source of significant epistaxis.

Paranasal sinuses: Sphenoid, ethmoid, maxillary, and frontal (Fig. 4).

These drain through apertures into the lateral wall of the nose.

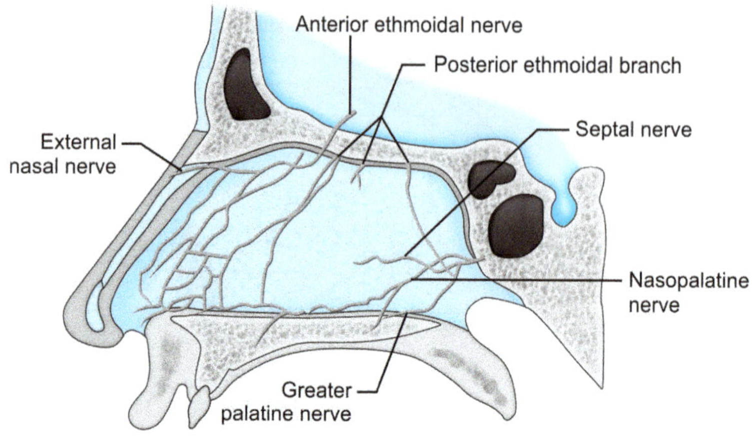

Fig. 5: Nerve supply of nose.

Prolonged nasotracheal intubation has most often been associated with infection of the maxillary sinus as its drainage is hindered by the location of the ostia superiorly in the sinus promoting a chronic infectious process.

Nerve supply (Fig. 5): The olfactory area consists of the middle and upper septum and the superior turbinate bone, located in the upper third of the nasal fossa. The olfactory cells have specialized hairlike processes (olfactory hair) innervated by the olfactory nerve.

The respiratory portion is located in the lower third of the nasal fossa.

Trigeminal nerve (1st 2 divisions) supplies the nonolfactory sensory area.

The parasympathetic autonomic nerves reach the mucosa from the facial nerve after relaying through the sphenopalatine ganglion, and sympathetic fibers are derived from the plexus surrounding the internal carotid artery through the vidian nerve.

Oropharynx

It starts below the soft palate, and extends to the superior edge of the epiglottis (Fig. 6).

Anterior wall is formed by the posterior third of the tongue.

During anesthesia or sedation with the patient in supine position, muscle relaxation + gravity = movement of base of the tongue toward the posterior oropharyngeal wall, causing airway obstruction. This is managed by use of oral airways or jaw lift.

The oropharynx opens to the oral cavity at the palatoglossal folds, marking the division between the anterior two-thirds and posterior one-third of the tongue. The palatoglossal folds make the fauces, which contain the tonsils.

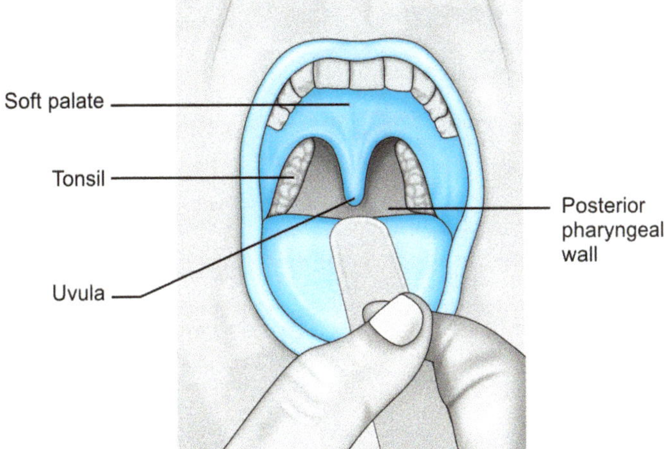

Fig. 6: Oropharynx.

Hypertrophied tonsils can cause a challenge during mask ventilation or intubation.

Anterior to the fauces is the oral cavity proper, separated from the vestibule by the teeth and gums. *Prominent or bucked maxillary teeth can interfere with laryngoscopy and intubation.*

Laryngopharynx

Lies opposite $C_{3\text{-}6}$ vertebrae

Consists of 3 paired and 3 unpaired cartilages, supporting muscles and membranes (Fig. 7).

Paired: Arytenoids, corniculate, cuneiform.

Unpaired: Epiglottis, thyroid, cricoid.

	Adult male larynx	*Adult female larynx*
Length	44	36
Transverse diameter	43	41
Sagittal diameter	36	26

CARTILAGES

Hyoid bone: U shaped, 2.5 cm wide, 1 cm thick, has greater and lesser horns (cornu).

It is attached to the styloid processes of the temporal bones by the stylohyoid ligament and to the thyroid cartilage by the thyrohyoid membrane and muscle. Intrinsic tongue muscles originate on the hyoid, and the pharyngeal constrictors are attached here.

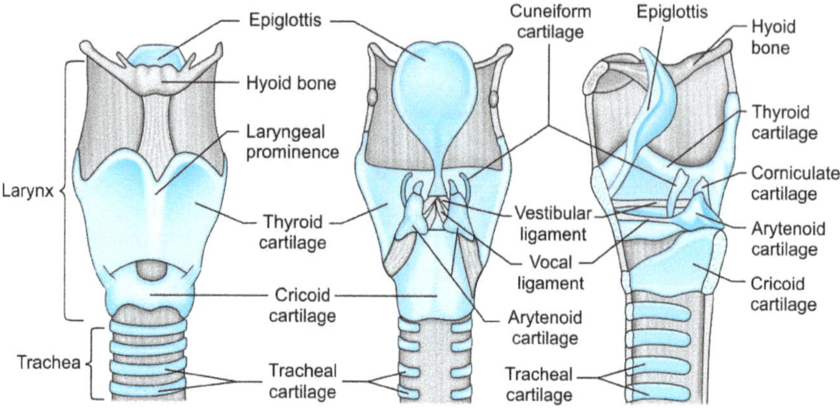

Fig. 7: Laryngopharynx.

Thyroid Cartilage

Named so for its shield-like shape (from embryologic midline fusion of the two distinct quadrilateral laminae). In females, the sides join at approximately 120 degrees, and in males is approx 90 degrees (Adam's apple). The thyroid notch lies in the midline at the top of the fusion site of the two laminae. On the inner side of this fusion line are attached the vestibular ligaments and, below them, the vocal ligaments. The superior (greater) and inferior (lesser) cornu of the thyroid are the slender posteriorly directed extensions of the edges of the lamina. The lateral thyrohyoid ligament attaches the superior cornu to the hyoid bone, and the cricoid cartilage articulates with the inferior cornu at the cricothyroid joint. The movements of this joint are rotatory and gliding, which leads to changes in the length of the vocal folds.

Cricoid Cartilage

The tracheal rings connect to the cricoid by ligaments and muscles and it attaches to the thyroid cartilage by the cricothyroid membrane (a site for percutaneous or sugical cricothyroidotomy).

The superior thyroid artery, the superior and inferior thyroid veins and the jugular veins were reported to traverse the membrane.

Arytenoid Cartilage

These are shaped like three-sided pyramids, and they lie in the posterior aspect of the larynx. The base of the arytenoid is concave and articulates by a true diarthrodial joint with the superior lateral aspect of the posterior lamina of the cricoid cartilage. The lateral extension of the arytenoid base is called the muscular process, where intrinsic laryngeal muscles, lateral and posterior cricoarytenoids originate. The medial extension of the arytenoid base is called the vocal process. Vocal ligaments, the bases of the true vocal folds, extend from the vocal process to the midline of the inner surface of the thyroid lamina. Broyles' ligament connects the vocal ligament to the thyroid cartilage and contains lymphatics and blood vessels (*acts as a source for extension of laryngeal cancer outside the larynx*).

Epiglottis

It is shaped like a leaf and is found between the larynx and the base of the tongue.

The upper border of the epiglottis is attached by its narrow tip to the midline of the thyroid cartilage by the thyroepiglottic ligament. The hyoepiglottic ligament connects the epiglottis to the back of the body of the hyoid bone. The mucous membrane that covers the anterior aspect of the epiglottis sweeps forward to the tongue as the median glossoepiglottic fold and to the pharynx as the paired lateral pharyngoepiglottic folds. The pouch-like areas found between the median and lateral folds are the valleculae (site of impaction of foreign body)

Cuneiform and Corniculate Cartilages

The epiglottis is connected to the arytenoid cartilages by the laterally placed aryepiglottic ligaments and folds. Two sets of paired fibroelastic cartilages are embedded in each aryepiglottic fold. The sesamoid cuneiform cartilage is roughly cylindrical and lies anterosuperior to the corniculate in the fold. The cuneiform may be seen laryngoscopically as a whitish elevation through the mucosa. The cuneiform and corniculate cartilages reinforce and support the aryepiglottic folds and may help the arytenoids move.

Laryngeal Cavity

Extends from the laryngeal inlet to the lower border of the cricoid cartilage. It consists of the superiorly placed vestibular folds (false cords), and vocal folds (true vocal cords). The space between the true cords is called the rima glottidis, or the glottis. The glottis is divided into two parts—anterior intermembranous section (situated between the two vocal folds) and posterior intercartilaginous part (which passes between the two arytenoid cartilages and the mucosa, stretching between them in the midline posteriorly, forming the posterior commissure of the larynx).

The area extending from the laryngeal inlet to the vestibular folds is known as the vestibule or supraglottic larynx. The laryngeal space from the free border of the cords to the cricoid cartilage is called the subglottic or infraglottic larynx.

The region between the vestibular folds and the glottis is termed the ventricle or the sinus. The ventricle may expand anterolaterally to a pouch-like area with many lubricating mucous glands called the laryngeal saccule. The pyriform sinus lies laterally to the aryepiglottic fold within the inner surface of the thyroid cartilage.

MUSCLES (FIG. 8)

Extrinsic Muscles of the Larynx

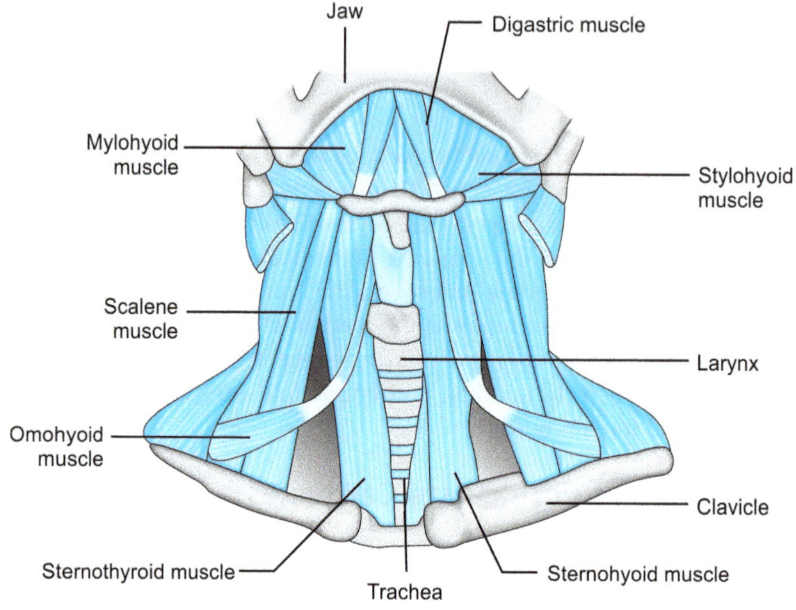

Fig. 8: Extrinsic muscles of larynx.

Muscle	*Function*	*Innervation*
Sternohyoid	Indirect depressor of the larynx	Cervical plexus Ansa hypoglossi C_1, C_2, C_3
Sternothyroid	Depresses the larynx Modifies the thyrohyoid and aryepiglottic folds	Same as above
Thyrohyoid	Same as above	Cervical plexus Hypoglossal nerve C_1, C_2
Thyroepiglottic	Mucosal inversion of aryepiglottic fold	Recurrent laryngeal nerve
Stylopharyngeus	Assists folding of thyroid cartilage	Glossopharyngeal
Inferior pharyngeal constrictor	Assists in swallowing	Vagus, pharyngeal plexus

Source: Benumof JL: Airway Management—Principles and Practice.

Intrinsic Musculature of the Larynx (Fig. 9)

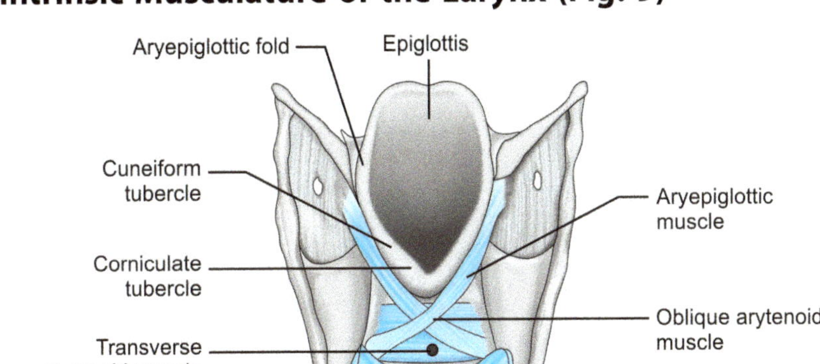

Fig. 9: Internal muscles of larynx.

Muscle	*Function*	*Innervation*
Posterior cricoarytenoid	Abductor of vocal cords	Recurrent laryngeal
Lateral cricoarytenoid	Adducts arytenoids closing glottis	Recurrent laryngeal
Transverse arytenoid	Adducts arytenoids	Recurrent laryngeal
Oblique arytenoid	Closes glottis	Recurrent laryngeal
Aryepiglottic	Closes glottis	Recurrent laryngeal
Vocalis	Relaxes the cords	Recurrent laryngeal
Thyroarytenoid	Relaxes tension cords	Recurrent laryngeal
Cricothyroid	Tensor of the cords	Superior laryngeal (external branch)

Source: Benumof JL: Airway Management—Principles and Practice.

BLOOD SUPPLY (FIG. 10)

The external carotid gives rise to the superior thyroid artery, which bifurcates, forming the superior laryngeal artery. This artery courses with the superior laryngeal nerve through the thyrohyoid membrane to supply the supraglottic region.

The inferior thyroid artery (from thyrocervical trunk), terminates as the inferior laryngeal artery. This vessel travels in the tracheoesophageal groove with the recurrent laryngeal nerve and supplies the infraglottic larynx. There are extensive connections with the ipsilateral superior laryngeal artery and

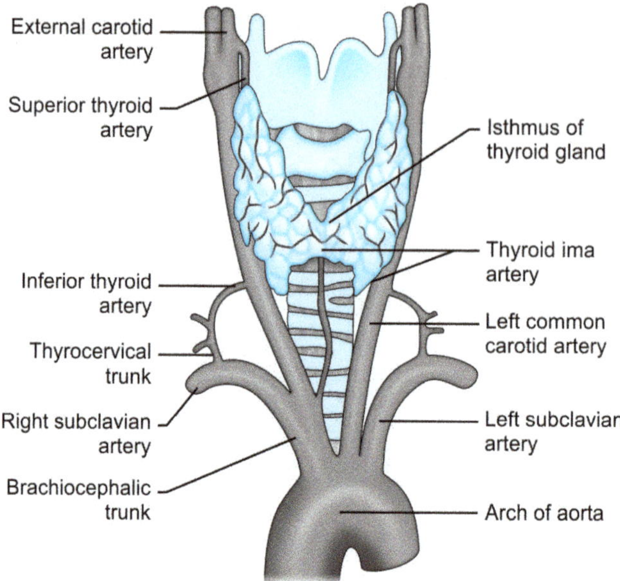

Fig. 10: Blood supply of larynx.

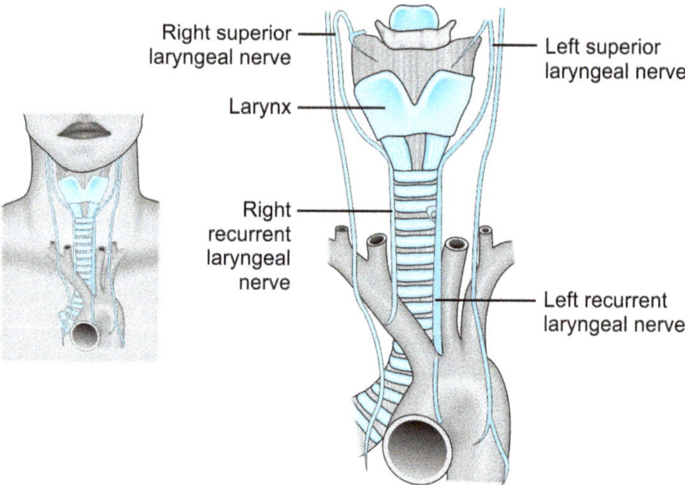

Fig. 11: Nerves innervating larynx.

across the midline. A small cricothyroid artery may branch from the superior thyroid and cross the cricothyroid membrane. It most commonly travels near the inferior border of the thyroid cartilage.

NERVES (FIG. 11)

The main nerves of the larynx are the recurrent laryngeal nerves and the internal and external branches of the superior laryngeal nerves (from vagus nerve). The external branch of the superior laryngeal nerve supplies motor innervation to the cricothyroid muscle. All other motor supply to the laryngeal musculature is provided by the recurrent laryngeal nerve.

The recurrent laryngeal nerve also provides sensory innervation to the larynx below the vocal cords.

VOCAL CORD PALSY

There is an intimate and important relationship between the nerves that supply the larynx and the vessels that supply the thyroid gland.

The external branch of the superior laryngeal nerve descends over the inferior constrictor muscle of the pharynx immediately deep to the superior thyroid artery and vein as these pass to the superior pole of the gland; at this site the nerve may be damaged in securing these vessels (Figs. 12A and B).

The glottic chink appears oblique during phonation. The aryepiglottic fold on the affected side appears shortened and the one on the normal side is lengthened. The cords may appear wavy. The symptoms include frequent throat clearing and difficulty in raising the vocal pitch. A total bilateral paralysis of vagus nerves affects the recurrent laryngeal nerves and the superior laryngeal nerves. In this condition, the cords assume the abducted, cadaveric position. The vocal cords are relaxed and appear wavy. A similar picture may be seen following the use of muscle relaxants.

The recurrent laryngeal nerve, as it ascends in the tracheoesophageal groove, is overlapped by the lateral lobe of the thyroid gland, and here comes into close relationship with the inferior thyroid artery as this passes medially, behind the common carotid artery, to the gland. The artery may cross posteriorly or anteriorly to the nerve, or the nerve may pass between the terminal branches of the artery. On the right side, there is an equal chance of locating the nerve in each of these three situations; on the left, the nerve is more likely to lie posterior to the artery.

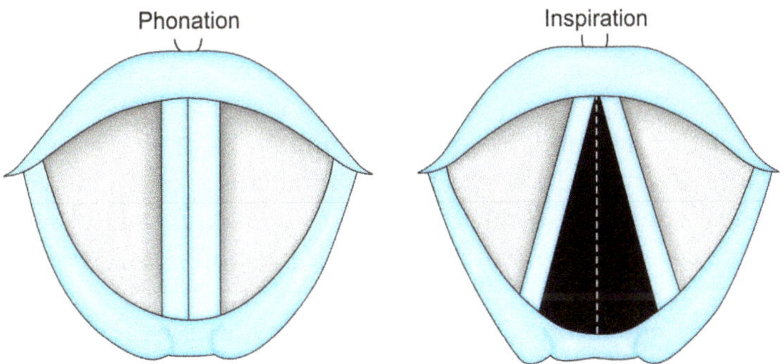

Fig. 12A: Position of vocal cords during phonation and inspiration.
Source: Hodder Headline PLC, London.

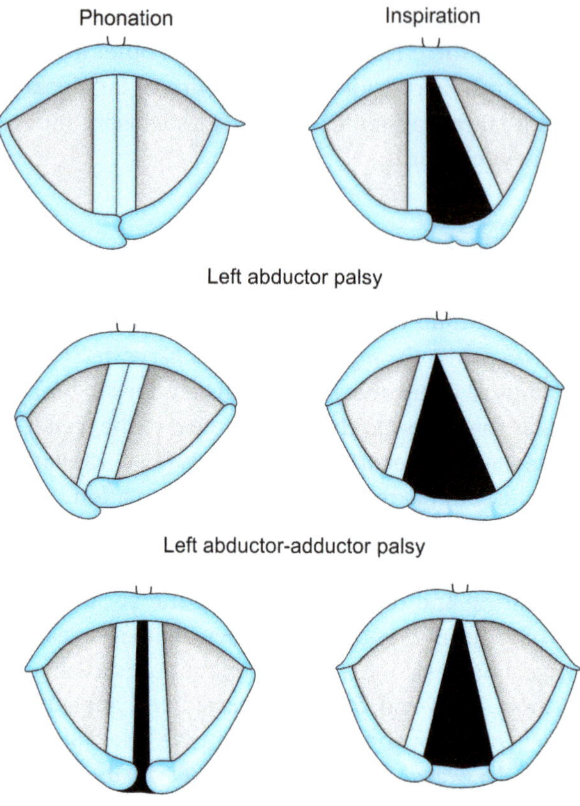

Fig. 12B: Diagrammatic representation of different types of vocal cord palsies. Note that in complete bilateral recurrent laryngeal palsy (bottom), vocal cords remain in the abducted position and the glottic opening is preserved.
Source: Hodder Headline PLC, London.

Injury to the recurrent nerve is an obvious hazard of thyroidectomy, especially since the nerve may be displaced from its normal anatomical location by a diseased thyroid gland. Recurrent laryngeal nerve paralysis may occur not only as a result of injury at thyroidectomy but also from involvement of the nerve by a malignant or occasionally benign enlargement of the thyroid gland, by enlarged lymph nodes or by cervical trauma. The recurrent laryngeal nerve carries both abductor and adductor fibers to the vocal cords. The abductor fibers are more vulnerable, and moderate trauma causes a pure abductor paralysis (Selmon's law). Severe trauma causes both abductor and adductor fibers to be affected. Pure adductor paralysis does not occur as a clinical entity. In the case of pure unilateral abductor palsy, both cords meet in the midline on phonation (since adduction is still possible on the affected side). However, only the normal cord abducts during inspiration.

In the case of complete unilateral palsy of the recurrent laryngeal nerve, both abductors and adductors are affected. On phonation, the unaffected cord crosses the midline to meet its paralyzed counterpart, appearing to lie in front of the affected cord. On inspiration, the unaffected cord moves to full abduction. When abductor fibers are damaged bilaterally (incomplete bilateral damage to the recurrent laryngeal nerve), the adductor fibers draw the cords toward each other and the glottic opening is reduced to a slit, resulting in severe respiratory distress. However, with a complete palsy, each vocal cord lies midway between abduction and adduction and a reasonable glottic opening exists. Thus, bilateral incomplete palsy is more dangerous than the complete variety.

TRACHEA

The trachea extends from its attachment to the lower end of the cricoid cartilage, at the level of the 6th cervical vertebra, to its termination at the bronchial bifurcation In the preserved dissecting-room cadaver, this is at the level of the 4th thoracic vertebra and the manubriosternal junction (the angle of Louis), but in the living subject in the erect position, the lower end of the trachea can be seen in oblique radiographs of the chest to extend to the level of the 5th, or in full inspiration the 6th, thoracic vertebra. In the adult, the trachea is 15 cm long, of which 5 cm lie above the suprasternal notch; this portion is somewhat greater (nearly 8 cm) when the neck is fully extended. The diameter of the trachea is correlated with the size of the subject; a good working rule is that it has the same diameter as the patient's index finger. The patency of the trachea is due to a series of 16–20 C-shaped cartilages joined vertically by fibroelastic tissue and closed posteriorly by the nonstriated trachealis muscle. The cartilage at the tracheal bifurcation is the keel-shaped carina, which is seen as a very obvious sagittal ridge when the trachea is inspected bronchoscopically. Should the sharp edge of the carina become flattened, this usually denotes enlargement of the hilar lymph nodes or gross distortion of the pulmonary anatomy by fibrosis, tumor or other pathology

Relations

The trachea lies exactly in the midline in the cervical part of its course but within the thorax it is deviated slightly to the right by the arch of the aorta. In the neck, it is covered anteriorly by the skin and by the superficial and deep fascia, through which the rings are easily felt. The 2nd to the 4th rings are covered by the isthmus of the thyroid where, along the upper border, branches of the superior thyroid artery join from either side. In the lower part of the neck, the edges of the sternohyoid and sternothyroid muscles overlap the trachea, which is here also covered by the inferior thyroid veins (as they stream downwards to the brachiocephalic veins), by the cross-communication between the anterior jugular veins and, when present, by the thyroidea ima artery, which ascends from the arch of the aorta or from the brachiocephalic artery. It is because of this close relationship with the brachiocephalic artery that erosion of the tracheal wall by a tracheostomy tube may cause sudden profuse hemorrhage. It is less common for the carotid artery to be involved in this way. On either side are the lateral lobes of the thyroid gland, which intervene between the trachea and the carotid sheath and its contents (the common carotid artery, the internal jugular vein and the vagus nerve). Posteriorly, the trachea rests on the esophagus, with the recurrent laryngeal nerves lying on either side in a groove between the two. The close relationship of the unsupported posterior tracheal wall and the esophagus is revealed during esophagoscopy. The thoracic part of the trachea descends through the superior mediastinum. Anteriorly, from above downwards, lie the inferior thyroid veins, the origins of the sternothyroid muscles from the back of the manubrium, the remains of the thymus, the brachiocephalic artery and the left common carotid arterya which separate the trachea from the left brachiocephalic vein and, lastly, the arch of the aorta. Posteriorly, as in its cervical course, the trachea lies throughout on the esophagus, with the left recurrent laryngeal nerve placed in a groove between the left borders of these two structures. On the right side, the trachea is in contact with the mediastinal pleura, except where it is separated by the azygos vein and the right vagus nerve. On the left, the left common carotid and left subclavian arteries, the aortic arch and the left vagus intervene between the trachea and the pleura; the altering relationships between the major arteries and the trachea are due to the diverging, somewhat spiral, course of the arteries from their aortic origins to the root of the neck. The large tracheobronchial lymph nodes lie at the sides of the trachea and in the angle between the two bronchi. In infants, these relationships are somewhat modified; the brachiocephalic artery is higher and crosses the trachea just as it descends behind the suprasternal notch. The left brachiocephalic vein may project upwards into the neck to form an anterior relation of the cervical trachea frightening encounter, if found tensely distended with blood when performing a tracheotomy on an asphyxiating baby. In children up to the age of 2 years, the thymus is large and lies in front of the lower part of the cervical trachea.

THE MAIN BRONCHUS

The trachea bifurcates in the supine cadaver at the level of the 4th thoracic vertebra into the right and left bronchi. In the erect position in full inspiration in life, the level of bifurcation is at T_6. The right main bronchus is shorter, wider and more vertically placed than the left: shorter because it gives off its upper lobe bronchus sooner (after a course of only 2.5 cm);

wider because it supplies the larger lung; and more vertically placed (at 25° to the vertical compared with 45° on the left) because the left bronchus has to extend laterally behind the aortic arch to reach its lung hilum. Thus, inhaled foreign bodies are more inclined to enter the wider and more vertical right bronchus than the narrower and more obliquely placed left. The right pulmonary artery is first below and then in front of the right main bronchus, and the azygos vein arches over it. The left main bronchus is 5 cm long. It passes under the aortic arch, in front of the esophagus, thoracic duct and descending aorta, and has the left pulmonary artery lying first above and then in front of it. Because the right upper lobe bronchus arises only a short distance below the carina, it is not possible to place a tube in that bronchus without the risk of obstruction of the lower lobe. To overcome this difficulty, right-sided endobronchial tubes have an orifice in the lateral surface of the tube that coincides with the opening of the right upper lobe. No special arrangement has to be made for tubes placed in the left bronchus, as the 5 cm distance between the carina and the left upper lobe bronchus leaves ample room for the cuffed end of an endobronchial tube.

The Lungs (Fig. 13)

Each lung is roughly conical, with an apex, a base, a lateral (or costal) and a medial surface and with three borders—anterior, posterior and inferior. Each lung lies freely within its pleural cavity apart from its attachments at the hilum. The right lung is the larger, weighing on average 620 g compared with 570 g on the left. The lung of the male is larger and heavier than that of the female. Each lung is divided by a deep oblique fissure, and the right lung is further divided by a transverse fissure. Thus, the right lung is trilobed and the left bilobed.

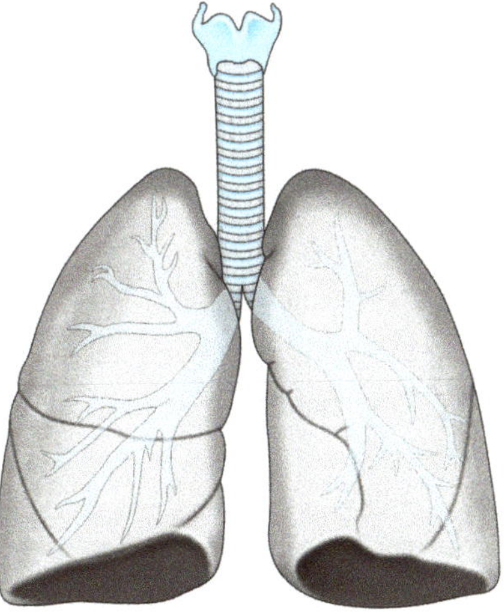

Fig. 13: Lungs.

Bronchopulmonary Segments (Figs. 14A and B)

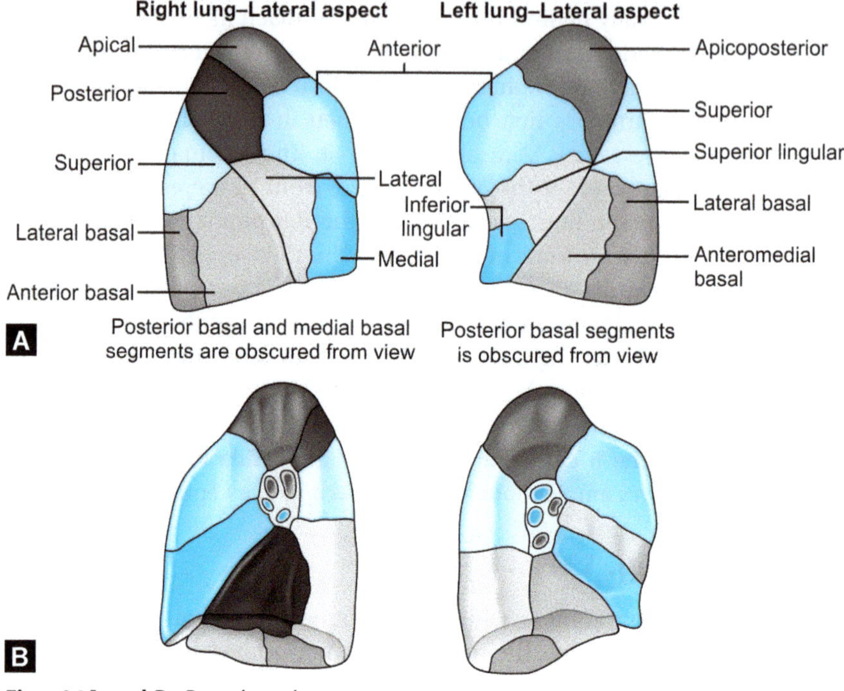

Figs. 14A and B: Bronchopulmonary segments

DIFFERENCES BETWEEN ADULTS AND CHILDREN (AIRWAY) (FIGS. 15A AND B)

Characteristics	*Children (up to 1 year)*	*Adults*
Carina cricoid distance	5–6 cm	10–20 cm
Right bronchus angle	30 (straighter)	20
Left bronchus angle	45	45
Narrowest part of airway	Cricoid	Glottis
Glottic level	C_{3-4} interspace	C_5
Vocal cords	Anteroinferior	Horizontal
Epiglottis	Omega shaped (long, anterior)	Crescent
Corniculate/cuneiform tubercles	Prominent	Minimal
Glottic-epiglottic angle	Small	Large
Prominence of occiput	Large head (compared to body)	Small
Breathing route	Nasal	Mouth or nasal
Laryngoscope preferred	Straight blade	Curved blade

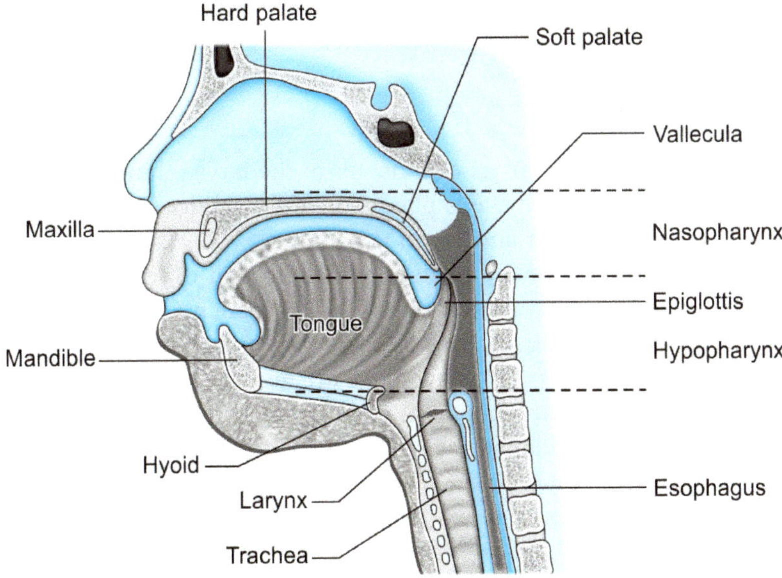

Fig. 15A: Pediatric airway anatomy

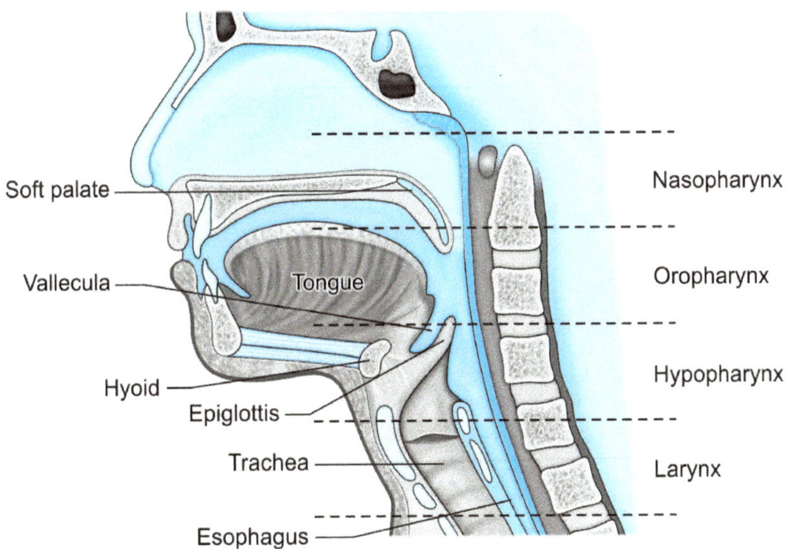

Fig. 15B: Adult airway anatomy.

PHYSIOLOGY

Geetanjali S Verma

FUNCTIONAL ANATOMY

The nose, mouth and pharynx conduct air to the larynx, humidify and filter the air gases. The larynx aids phonation and conducts the gas into the trachea (18 mm diameter and 11 cm length).

It is lined with columnar ciliated epithelium and divides into the left and right major bronchi at the carina (T_4). The bronchi divide 23 times in total (23 generations) (Fig. 16) in order to increase the surface area available for gas exchange. The first 16 generations are termed the conducting zone (no bronchi in his region take part in gas exchange and this forms the anatomical dead space). In an average adult the volume of this space is about 150 mL. From generation 17, small alveoli bud off the bronchi. Generation 17–23 is the respiratory zone where gas exchange occurs. The volume of this zone is about 2–3 liters and there are about 300 million alveoli present within an average lung.

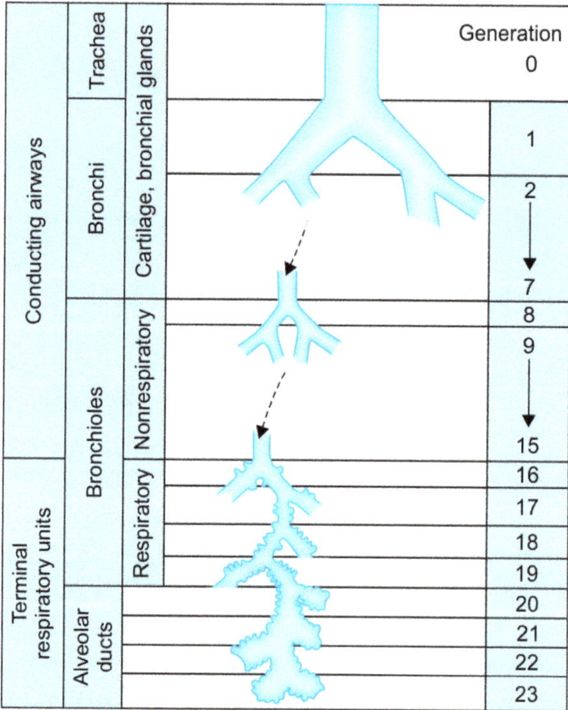

Fig. 16: Division of bronchi into 23 generations.

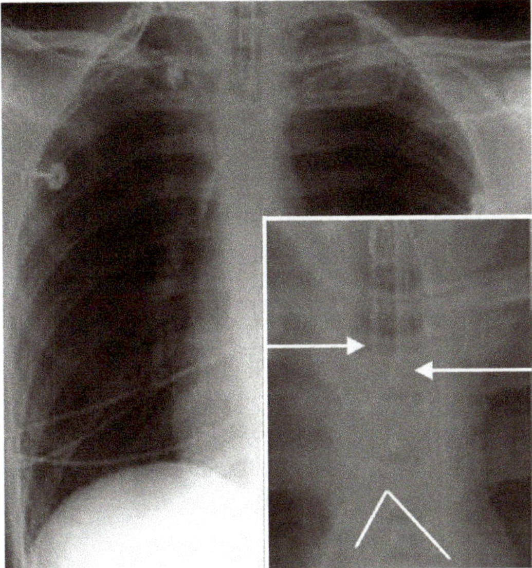

Fig. 17: Chest X-ray depicting ETT in situ.

- The endotracheal tube (ETT) in an adult should lie 1-2 cm superior to the carina (Fig. 17)
- On an X-ray the carina is the point at which the trachea can be seen dividing into the right and left bronchi—around T_4.

STRUCTURE AND FUNCTION OF RESPIRATORY SYSTEM

1. Exchange of O_2 and CO_2
2. Blood reservoir
3. Heat exchange
4. Metabolism—synthesis and catabolism
5. Immunological and mechanical defence blood/gas barrier to diffusion ~50-80 m^2 alveolar walls have two sides
   a. active side ~0.4 mm
   b. service side ~1-2 mm.

Type	*Function*	*Structure*
Conductive	Bulk gas movement	Trachea to terminal bronchioles
Transitional	Bulk gas movement Limited gas exchange	Respiratory bronchioles Alveolar ducts
Respiratory	Gas exchange	Alveoli Alveolar sacs

Cells Types and Functions in the Lung

Type 1 alveolar cells: Derived from type II alveolar cells, provide a thin layer of cytoplasm which covers about 80% of the gas exchange zone. 0.1 mm thick, have 1 nm gap junctions, impermeable to albumin, allow extravasation of mf's—unable to divide—highly sensitive to hyperoxia.

Type II alveolar cells: These cells allow the formation of surfactant and other enzymes. They are rounded cells at septal junctions, resistant to hyperoxia.

Type III alveolar cells: These cells are the main lung defence system—alveolar macrophages.

SURFACE TENSION

A thin film of liquid lines the alveoli and the surface tension of this film is an important factor in the pressure-volume relationship of the lung. The surface tension arises because the attractive forces between adjacent molecules of the liquid are much stronger than those between the liquid and the gas. As a result of that the liquid surface area becomes as small as possible. At the interface between the liquid and the alveolar gas, intermolecular forces in the liquid tend to cause the area of the lining to shrink (the alveoli tend to get smaller). The surface tension contributes to the pressure-volume behavior of the lungs because when the lungs are inflated with saline they have much larger compliance that when they are filled with air (because saline abolishes the surface tension).

This generates a pressure predicted from *Laplace's law*:

$$\text{Pressure} = (4 \times \text{surface tension})/\text{radius}$$

the surface tension contributes a large part of the static recoil force of the lung (expiration).

The surface tension changes with the surface area: The larger the area, the smaller the surface tension.

SURFACTANT

Surfactant is stored in the lamellar bodies of type II alveolar cells and made up of phospholipids, plasma proteins and carbohydrate. It is an amphipathic molecule with a charged hydrophilic head and hydrophobic tail.

Its major constituent is *dipalmitoyl phosphatidylcholine (DPPC)*, which is synthesized in the lung from fatty acids that are either extracted from the blood or are themselves synthesized in the lung.

Functions of surfactant are:

- Reduces surface tension within the alveoli which helps to increase the compliance of the lung
- Improves alveolar stability
- Keeps alveoli dry by opposing water movement from the pulmonary interstitium.

APPLIED PHYSIOLOGY

Lung Volumes and Capacities (Fig. 18)

Primary lung volumes:

i. Residual volume (RV)
ii. Expiratory reserve volume (ERV)
iii. Tidal volume (TV)
iv. Inspiratory reserve volume (IRV)

Secondary derived capacities:

i. Total lung capacity (TLC)
ii. Vital capacity (VC)
iii. Inspiratory capacity (IC)
iv. Functional residual capacity (FRC)

Lung volumes vary with age, sex, height and weight, and are formulated into normograms.

Definitions

Residual volume (RV)	Volume of gas remaining in lungs after a forced expiration	15–20 mL/kg
Expiratory reserve volume (ERV)	Volume of gas forcefully expired after normal tidal expiration	15 mL/kg
Tidal volume (TV)	Volume of gas inspired and expired during normal breathing	6 mL/kg
Inspiratory reserve volume (IRV)	Volume of gas inspired over normal tidal inspiration	45 mL/kg
Total lung capacity	Volume of gas in lungs at the end of maximal inspiration	80 mL/kg
Vital capacity	IRV + TV + ERV	60–70 mL/kg
FRC	ERV + RV	30 mL/kg

(Any 2 or more volumes added together make a capacity)

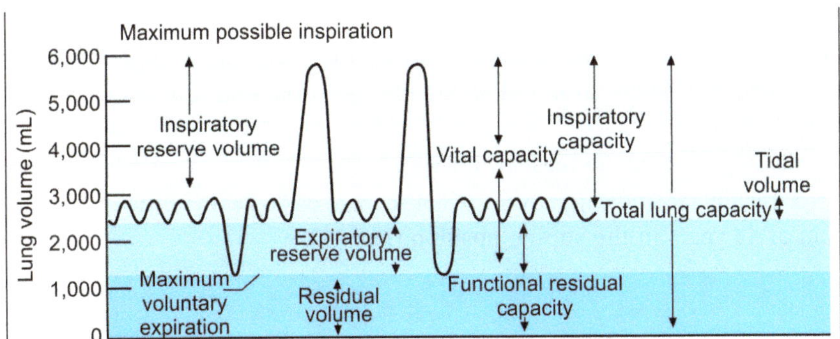

Fig. 18: Lung volumes and capacities.

Functional Residual Capacity

The volume of gas left in the lungs at the end of normal tidal expiration

$$FRC = ERV + RV$$

FRC acts as a buffer:

1. Maintaining relatively constant A and a gas tensions with each breath
2. Preventing rapid changes in alveolar gas with changes in ventilation or inspired gas, e.g. during induction or recovery from anesthesia
3. Increasing the average lung volume during quiet breathing, reducing work of breathing due to shape of compliance curve.

Factors decreasing FRC:

Age, posture—supine position, anesthesia—muscle relaxants, surger—laparoscopic, pulmonary fibrosis/pulmonary edema, obesity, abdominal swelling, pregnancy—increased abdominal pressure.

Factors increasing FRC:

Increasing height of patient, erect position—diaphragm and abdominal organs less able to encroach upon bases of the lungs, emphysema—decreased elastic recoil of lung therefore less tendency of lung to collapse, asthma—air trapping.

Measurement

- Helium dilution
- Body plethysmography
- Nitrogen washout.

Closing Capacity (CC)

This is the volume at which the small airways close during expiration. Under normal circumstances the FRC is always greater than the CC however, if the FRC was to decrease then this would no longer be the case and the small airways may close at the end of normal tidal expiration. This leads to hypoxemia, atelectasis and worsening gas exchange due to increasing V/Q mismatch.

Closing capacity increases with age.

Typically closing capacity = FRC at the age of 66 years in the erect position or 44 years in the supine position (Fig. 19).

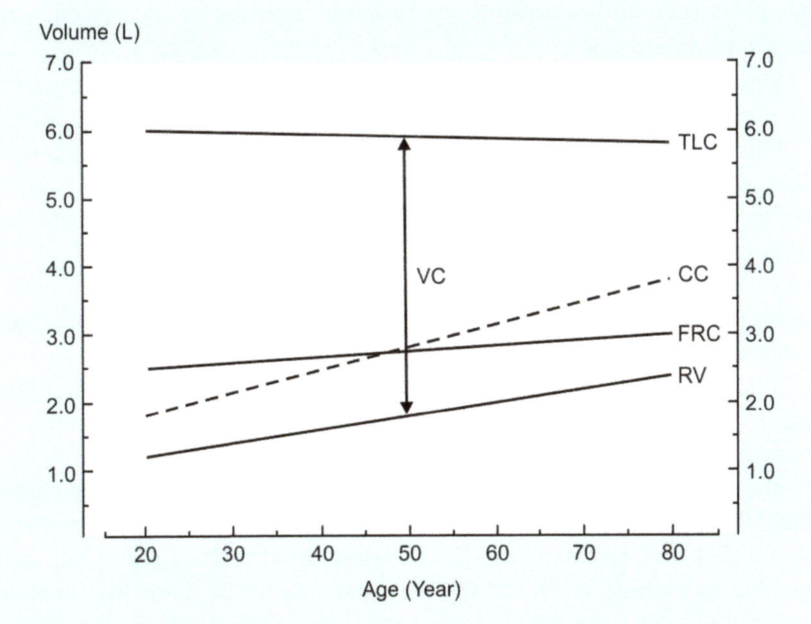

Fig. 19: Relation of FRC & CC.
Source: www.frca.co.uk/Documents/147%20Respiratory%20physiology%20part%201.pdf

Definition of Respiratory Pattern Terminology

Word	*Definition*
Eupnea	"Good breathing": continuous inspiratory and expiratory movement without interruption
Apnea	"No breathing": cessation of ventilatory effort at passive end-expiration (lung volume = FRC)
Apneusis	Cessation of ventilatory effort with lungs filled at TLC
Apneustic ventilation	Apneusis with periodic expiratory spasms
Biot	Ventilatory gasps interposed between periods of ventilation apnea; also "agonal ventilation".

VENTILATION

Airways and Airflow

Inhaled air passes through the conducting airways and eventually reaches the respiratory epithelium of the lungs. The trachea divides into right and left main bronchi, which in turn divide into lobar, then segmental 12 bronchi.

This process continues down to the terminal bronchioles (the smallest airways without alveoli).

Since the conducting airways have no alveoli they do not take part in gas exchange but constitute the anatomical dead space (about 150 mL).

During inspiration, respiratory tubes are lengthened and dilated, especially in deep breathing. Since the airways serve as a barrier as well, harmful foreign material including most microorganisms can not easily enter the lower respiratory passages. The very first barrier starts at the vestibules of the nose, which contain hairs, and healthy, sticky mucus intercepting airborne particles. Caught particles are then ejected by ciliated epithelium, which covers the entire upper respiratory tract.

The larynx and the bifurcation of the trachea are the most sensitive regions and any particles of foreign matter lodged in these regions are removed with a cough reflex.

The alveolated region of the lung includes respiratory bronchioles (divided from terminal bronchioles and have only occasional alveoli on their walls) and alveolar ducts (completely lined with alveoli). This zone is called respiratory zone and the gas exchange occurs here. The distance from the terminal bronchiole to the distal alveolus is only a few mm, but the respiratory zone makes up most of the lung (2.5–3 L).

Blood is brought to the other side of the blood-gas barrier from the right heart by pulmonary arteries, which also form a series of branching tubes leading to the pulmonary capillaries and back to the pulmonary veins. The capillaries lie in the walls of the alveoli and form a dense network that the blood continuously runs in the alveolar wall. At rest, all the capillaries are not open but when the pressure rises (e.g. exercise) recruitment of the closed capillaries occurs. The diameter of a capillary segment is about 10 micrometer (= size of RBC). The pulmonary artery receives the whole output of the right heart, but resistance of pulmonary circuit is very low. This enables the high blood flow to the circuit.

DEAD SPACE

Dead space: volume of gas which does not take part in gas exchange (Figs. 20 and 21).

Types

1. *Anatomical dead space*: This includes any breathing system or airway plus mouth, trachea and the airways up until the start of the respiratory zone—does not take part in air exchange.

   The typical volume in an adult is about 150 mL.
2. *Alveolar dead space*: This occurs when areas of the lung are being ventilated but not being perfused and this leads to what is known as V/Q mismatch.

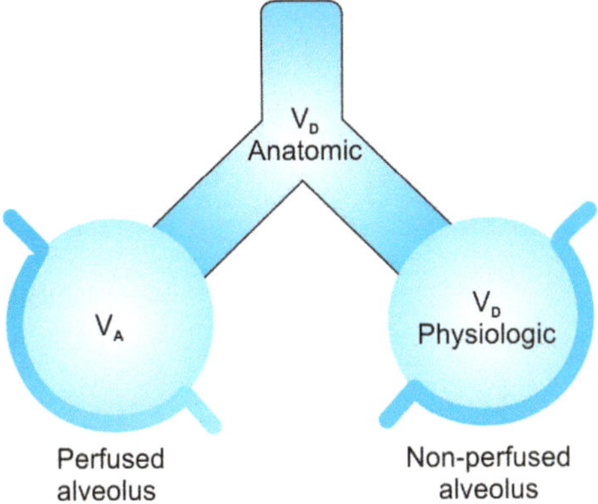

Fig. 20: Dead space

- Ventilated areas which do not participate in gas exchange

Total dead space = Anatomic + Alveolar + Mechanical

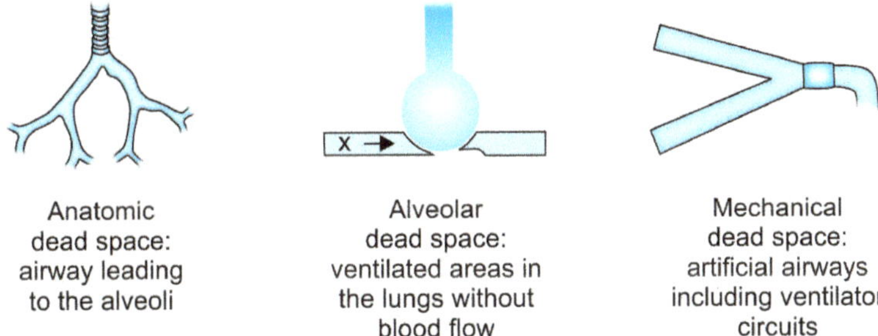

Fig. 21: Dead space.

Large increases in alveolar dead space commonly occur in the following conditions: pneumonia, pulmonary edema, and pulmonary embolism

3. *Physiological dead space* = alveolar + anatomical dead space. Dead space is usually 30% of VT.

Measurement of Dead Space

1. Fowler's method—tracer washout (Fig. 22)
   - Single breath analysis using an indicator gas (N_2, CO_2, O_2, He) to mark the transition between dead space and alveolar gas
   - Following inspiration of 100% O_2, a plot of VEXP vs. %[N_2] gives wash-in phase

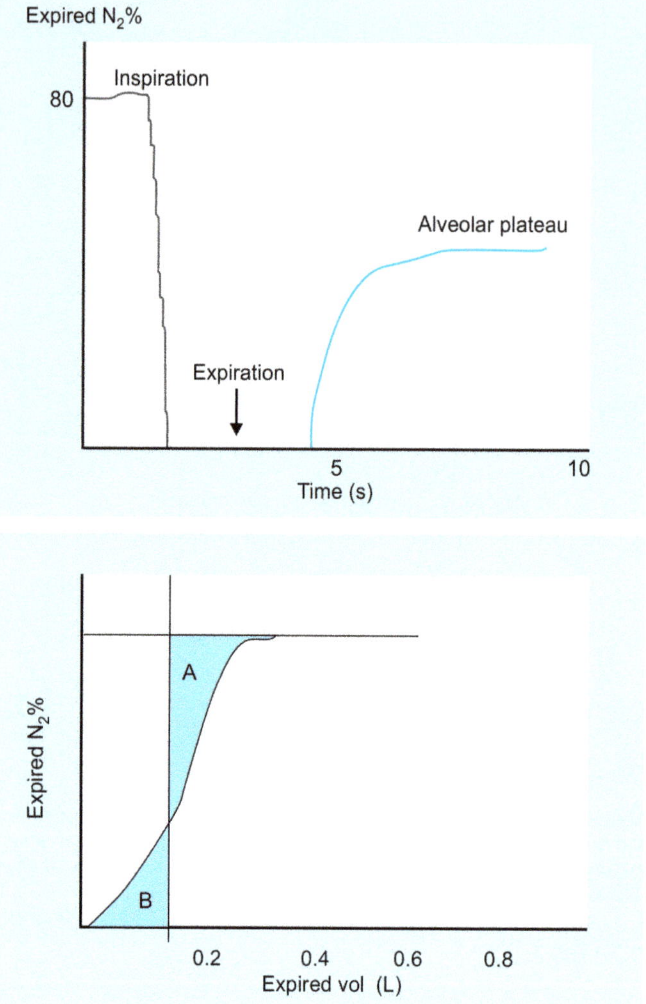

Fig. 22: Fowler's method.

- The mid-point of the wash-in (where area A = area B below) measures the transition from conducting airways to the transition from dead space to alveolar gas
- In patients with nonuniform distribution of ventilation, i.e. regions of the lung with different time constants, a slow "wash-in" is seen and the method is inaccurate.

2. Bohr's method—conservation of mass

   The Bohr equation: It is a complicated equation is based upon the fact that all CO_2 comes from alveolar gas and the exhalation of CO_2 can therefore be used to measure gas exchange or lack of gas exchange, if there is alveolar dead space (no perfusion of these alveoli).

For each tidal volume there will be a proportion of dead space (anatomical) but the amount of gas that is left over should take part in gas exchange.

Abbreviations used in equation:
$FACO_2$- Alveolar CO_2
$FeCO_2$- CO_2 from mixed expired gases
VT- Tidal volume
VD- Dead space volume (physiological)

Bohr's Equation Derivation

$V_T \cdot F_{ECO_2} = V_A \cdot F_{ACO_2}$
But $V_A = V_T - V_D$
Substituting: $V_T \cdot F_{ECO_2} = (V_T - V_D) \cdot F_{ACO_2}$
$V_T \cdot F_{ECO_2} = V_T \cdot F_{ACO_2} - V_D \cdot F_{ACO_2}$
Rearranging: $V_D \cdot F_{ACO_2} = V_T \cdot F_{ACO_2} - V_T \cdot F_{ECO_2}$
$= V_T (F_{ACO_2} - F_{ECO_2})$
Hence, $V_D/V_T = (F_{ACO_2} - F_{ECO_2})/F_{ACO_2}$
Or $V_D/V_T = P_{aCO_2} - P_{ECO_2}/P_{aCO_2}$

RESPIRATORY MECHANICS

Respiratory Muscles

Inspiratory muscles

- Diaphragm—has the ability to contact 10 cm in forced inspiration
- External intercostals—pull the ribs up and forwards
- Accessory inspiratory muscles—scalene muscles (elevate first 2 ribs) and sternomastoids (raise the sternum)
- Muscles of neck and head (seen in small babies in respiratory distress).

Expiratory muscles

Expiration is usually passive and relies on the elastic recoil of the lungs and the chest wall.

Under anesthesia or extreme exercise, expiration may become active due to the activation of abdominal muscles. Muscles have their use in forced expiration.

- Abdominal wall muscles—rectus abdominis, internal and external oblique
- Internal intercostal muscles—pull ribs down and inwards.

Compliance (Figs. 23 and 24)

Elastic recoil is usually measured in terms of compliance.

Compliance is defined as the volume change per unit pressure change. It is expressed in mL/cm H_2O

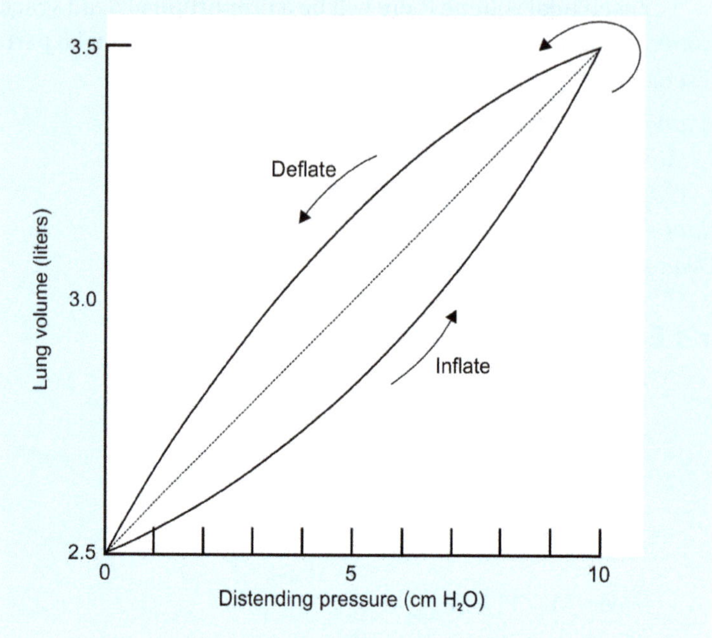

Fig. 23: Lung-chest wall pressure–volume curve.

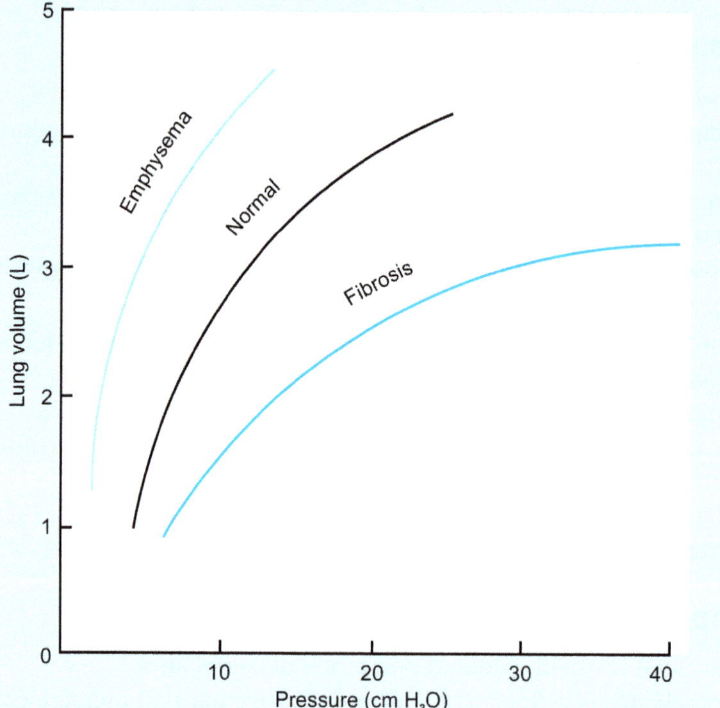

Fig. 24A: Compliance curve.

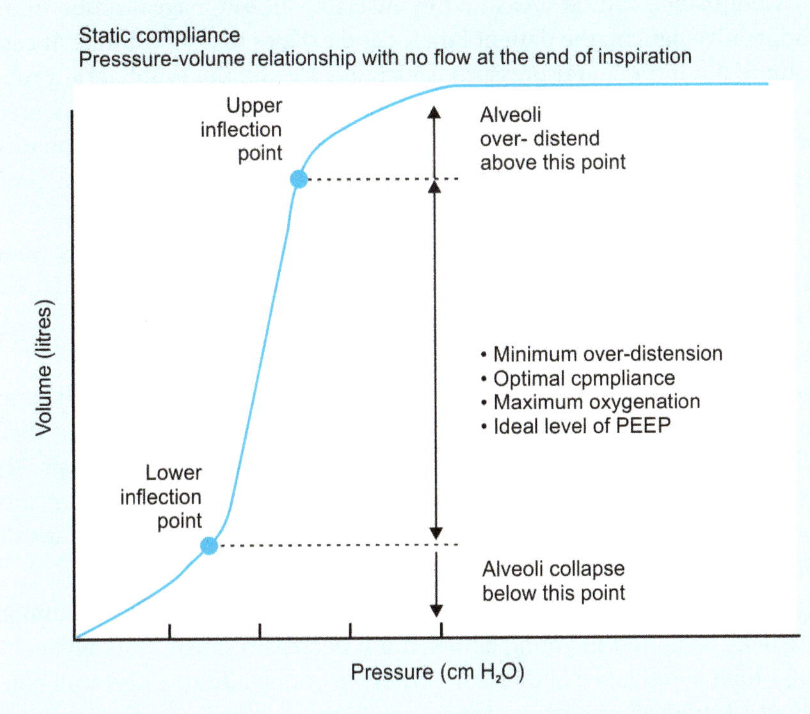

Fig. 24B: Static compliance.
Source: frca.co.uk

$$\text{Compliance} = \Delta V/\Delta P$$

It is classified into chest wall, lung or total lung compliance (distensibility).

Chest wall compliance (CW) = change in chest volume/change in transthoracic pressure.

Normally, it equals 200 mL/cm H_2O

There are 2 types of compliance: static and dynamic

Static compliance is measured during plateau pressure.

Dynamic compliance varies and is calculated with measurement of tidal volume at a given intrathoracic pressure during which there is airflow through the lungs at any point during inspiration or expiration.

Lung compliance (CL) = change in lung volume/change in transpulmonary pressure.

A variety of factors affect this like lung volume, pulmonary blood volume, extravascular lung water and pathological processes (inflammation, fibrosis)

Total compliance (CT) = 1/CT = 1/CL + 1/CW = 100 mL/cm H_2O

Compliance can be measured by inserting an esophageal probe into a cooperative patient, the patient inhales and exhales to a set volume. At each volume the intrapleural pressure is estimated using the esophageal probe. A pressure volume curve can then be plotted. If during the measurement process no gas flow occurs at each set volume then this is static compliance. (Gas flow ceases and equilibration occurs.) If gas flow continues throughout measurement then this is dynamic compliance.

Compliance increases in old age and emphysema as elastic lung tissue is destroyed. It is decreased in pulmonary fibrosis, pulmonary edema, atelectasis and in the extremes of lung volume.

Factors affecting compliance are:

Disease: In atelectasis, when the lung is relatively stiff, the point of balance (resting expiratory volume) will be reached at a lower lung volume, as there will be greater pull inwards; this will predispose to further atelectasis. The excessively compliant emphysematous lung has less elastic recoil; resting expiratory volume will then be greater, since the natural tendency for the chest wall to expand is maintained.

Age: The immature lung in the infant is less elastic than in adulthood. Elasticity is highest in young adults and it decreases slowly with advancing age—lung compliance is therefore lowest in young adults. Chest wall compliance is highest at birth and slowly declines with age.

Posture: Thoracic compliance is lower in the supine position, as the gravitational pull of the abdomen, which existed in the upright position, is reversed and the diaphragm is pushed into the chest by the abdominal contents.

Anesthesia: Several factors (supine position, airway closure, changes in intrathoracic blood volume, accumulation of fluid, direct effect of drugs, altered muscle tone, external pressure) influence compliance under anesthesia; generally compliance is decreased.

Obesity: The effect is compounded by supine or lithotomy position.

Work of Breathing

It is the work required by the respiratory muscles to overcome the mechanical impedance to respiration. It is the sum of work requires to overcome both elastic and airflow resistance.

The energy required for the work of breathing is mainly used in the process of inspiration as energy is required to overcome airway resistance, the elastic recoil of the tissues and the chest wall and tissue resistance. The energy stored within the elastic tissues is used to provide for expiration.

- West describes the total work required to move the lung as OABCGO (Fig. 25)

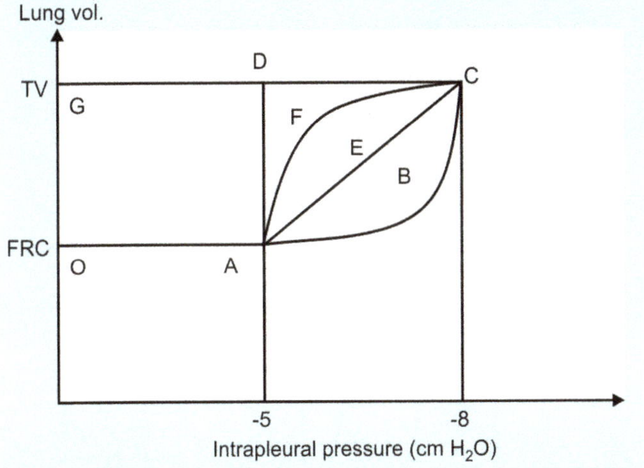

Fig. 25: Work of breathing curve.

- With the work to overcome elastic resistance given by the trapezoid OAECGO the difference between these representing the nonelastic resistance, given by the area ABCEA.
- This is not the work of "breathing", as some work is performed by the stored elastic potential energy of the thoracic cage.
- The true work of inspiration is given by ABCDA, with the elastic component being AECDA.
- As airway resistance, or inspiratory flow rate is increased, so would dPIP, effectively sloping the curve to right, increasing total and viscous work on expiration.
- The work to overcome nonelastic forces (AECFA), falls within work trapezoid and can be accomplished with the stored energy in elastic structures the difference between AECDA-AECFA represents the energy expenditure with which no external work is done is released as heat.

REGULATION AND CONTROL OF BREATHING (FIG. 26)

Central Control

Breathing is mainly controled at the level of brainstem. The normal automatic and periodic nature of breathing is triggered and controled by the respiratory centers located in the pons and medulla.

Medullary Respiratory Center

a. *Dorsal medullary respiratory neurones*: Associated with inspiration. It has been proposed that spontaneous intrinsic periodic firing of these

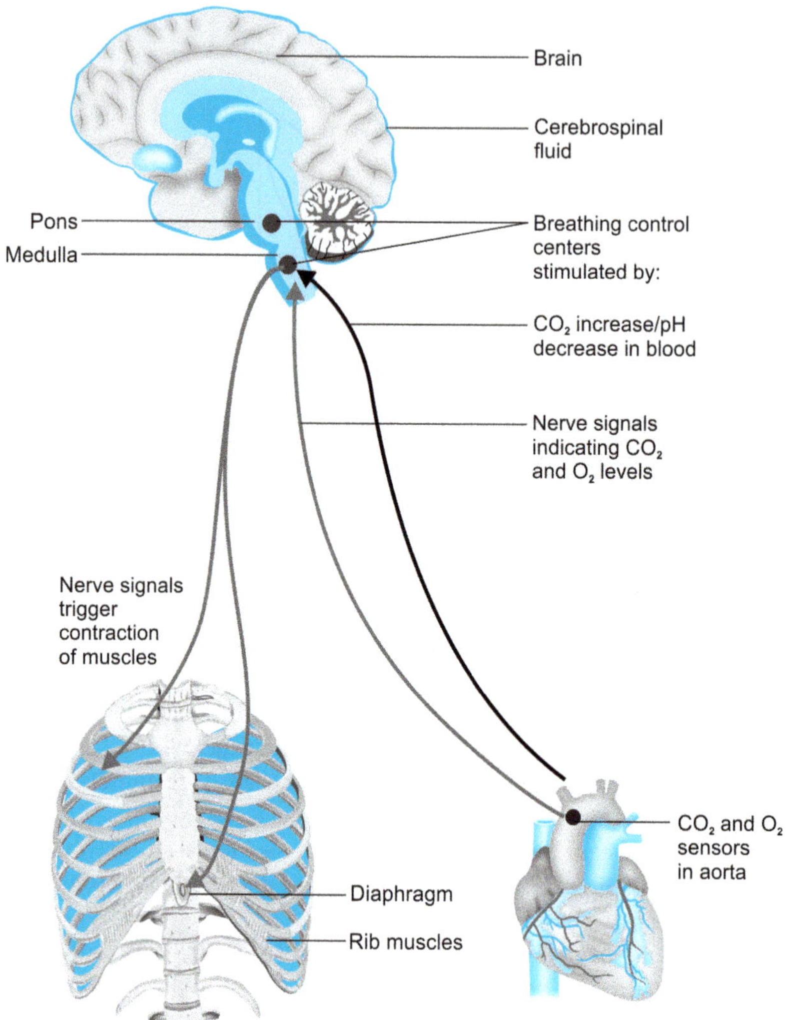

Fig. 26: Centers for regulation of respiration.

neurones responsible for the basic rhythm of breathing. As a result, these neurones exhibit a cycle of activity that arises spontaneously every few seconds and establish the basic rhythm of the respiration. When the neurones are active their action potentials travel through reticulospinal tract in the spinal cord and phrenic and intercostal nerves and finally stimulate the respiratory muscles.

b. *Ventral medullary respiratory neurones*: Associated with control of breathing. These neurones are silent during quite breathing because expiration is a passive event following an active inspiration. However, they are activated during forced expiration when the rate and the depth of the respiration is increased (e.g. exercise). During heavy breathing increased activity of the inspiratory center neurones activates the expiratory system. In turn, the increased activity of the expiratory system inhibits the inspiratory center and stimulates muscles of expiration.

The dorsal and ventral groups are bilaterally paired and there is 8 cross communication between them. As a consequence they behave in synchrony and the respiratory movements are symmetric.

Apneustic Center

It is located in the lower pons.

Exact role is not known. Lesions covering this area in the pons cause a pathologic respiratory rhythm with increased apnea frequency. What is known is nerve impulses from the apneustic center stimulate the inspiratory center and without constant influence of this center respiration becomes shallow and irregular.

Pneumotaxic Center

It is located in the upper pons.

These neurones have an inhibitory effect on the both inspiratory and apneustic centers. It is probably responsible for the termination of inspiration by inhibiting the activity of the dorsal medullar neurones. It primarily regulates the volume and secondarily the rate of the respiration. In the lesions of this area normal respiration is protected, thus it is believed that upper pons is responsible for the fine-tuning of the respiratory rhythm. Hypoactivation of this center causes prolonged deep inspirations and brief, limited expirations by allowing the inspiration center remain active longer than normal. Hyperactivation of this center on the other hand results in shallow inspirations.

The apneustic and pneumotaxic centers function in coordination in order to provide a rhythmic respiratory cycle: Activation of the inspiratory center stimulates the muscles of inspiration and also the pneumotaxic center. Then the pneumotaxic center inhibits both the apneustic and the inspiratory centers resulting in initiation of expiration. Spontaneous activity of the neurones in the inspiratory center starts another similar cycle again. Breathing in some extent is also controled consciously from higher brain centers (e.g. cerebral cortex). This control is required when we talk, cough and vomit. It is also possible voluntarily change the rate of the breathing. Hyperventilation can decrease blood partial carbon dioxide pressure (PCO_2) due to loss of CO_2 resulting in peripheral vasodilatation and decrease in blood pressure. One can also stop breathing voluntarily. That results in an increase in arterial partial oxygen pressure (PO_2), which produces an urge to breathe. When eventually PCO_2 reaches the high enough level it overrides the conscious influences from the cortex and stimulates the inspiratory system. If one holds his breath long enough to decrease PO_2 to a very low level one may loose his consciousness. In an unconscious person, automatic control of the respiration takes over and the normal breathing resumes. Other parts of the brain (limbic system, hypothalamus) can also alter the breathing pattern, e.g. affective states, strong emotions, such as rage and fear. In addition, stimulation of touch, thermal and pain receptors can also stimulate the respiratory system.

SENSORS/OTHER RECEPTORS (FIG. 27)

Mechanoreceptors

These receptors are placed in the walls of bronchi and bronchioles of the lung. The main function of these receptors is to prevent the overinflation of the lungs. Inflation of the lungs activates these receptors and activation of the stretch receptors in turn inhibits the neurones in inspiratory center via vagus nerve. When the expiration starts activation of the stretch receptors gradually ceases allowing neurones in the inspiratory neurones become active again (Hering-Breuer Reflex). It is particularly important for infants.

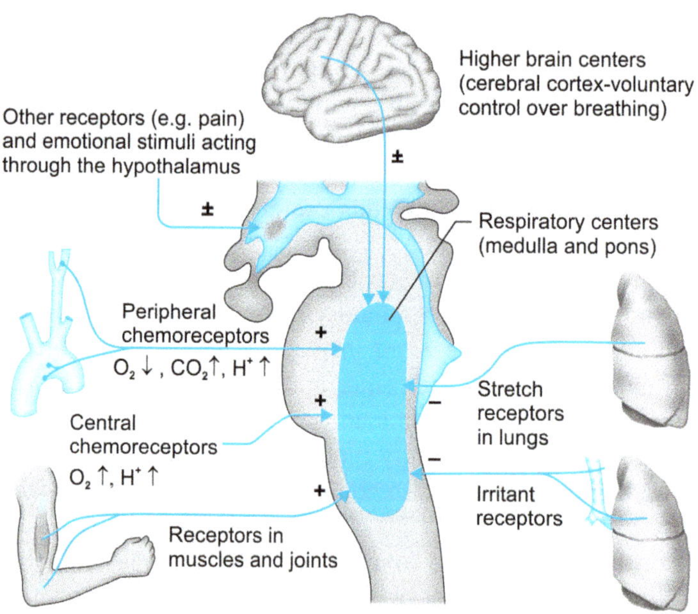

Fig. 27: Receptors for regulation of respiration.

In adults it is functional only during exercise when the tidal volume is larger than normal.

Chemoreceptors

The respiratory system maintains concentrations of O_2, CO_2 and the pH of the body fluids within a normal range. Any deviation from these values has a marked influence on the respiration. Chemoreceptors are specialized neurones activated by changes in O_2 or CO_2 levels in the blood and the brain tissue, respectively. They are involved in the regulation of respiration according to the changes in PO_2 and pH. O_2-sensitive chemoreceptors (Peripheral chemoreceptors) are located at the bifurcation of the carotid artery in the neck and the aortic arch. They are small vascular sensory organs encapsulated with the connective tissue. They are connected to the respiratory center in the medulla by glossopharyngeal nerve (carotid body chemoreceptors) and the vagus nerve (aortic body). Central chemoreceptors are located bilaterally in the chemosensitive area of the medulla oblongata and exposed to the cerebrospinal fluid (CSF), local blood flow and local metabolism. They actually respond to changes in H^+ concentration in these compartments. When the blood partial PCO_2 is increased CO_2 diffuses into the CSF from cerebral vessels and liberates H^+. (When CO_2 combines with water forms carbonic acid and liberates H^+ and HCO_3^-).

$$CO_2 + H_2O \leftrightarrow H_2CO_3 \quad H_2CO_3 \leftrightarrow HCO - 3 + H^+$$

An increase in H^+ stimulates chemo receptors resulting in hyperventilation which in turn reduces PCO_2 in the blood and therefore in the CSF. Cerebral vasodilatation always accompanies an increased PCO_2 and enhances the diffusion of CO_2 into the CSF. Because CSF has less protein than blood it has a much lower buffering capacity. As a result changes in pH for a given change in PCO_2 is always bigger than the change in blood.

CO_2 level is a major regulator of respiration. It is much more important than oxygen to maintain normal respiration. Even very small changes in carbon dioxide levels (5 mm Hg increase in PCO_2, hypercapnia) in the blood cause large increases in the rate and depth of respiration (100% increase in ventilation). Hypocapnia, lower than normal PCO_2 level in the blood causes in periods in which respiratory movements do not occur. Effects of PO_2 (if the changes occur within the normal range) on respiration is very minor. A decrease in PO_2 is called hypoxia and only after 50% decrease in PO_2 can produce significant changes in respiration. This is due to the nature of O_2-Hb saturation that at any PO_2 level above 80 mm Hg Hb is saturated with O_2. Consequently only big changes in PO_2 produce symptoms otherwise it is compensated by O_2, which is bound with Hb. In stroke patients or physiologically at high altitude blood PO_2 level may drop considerably

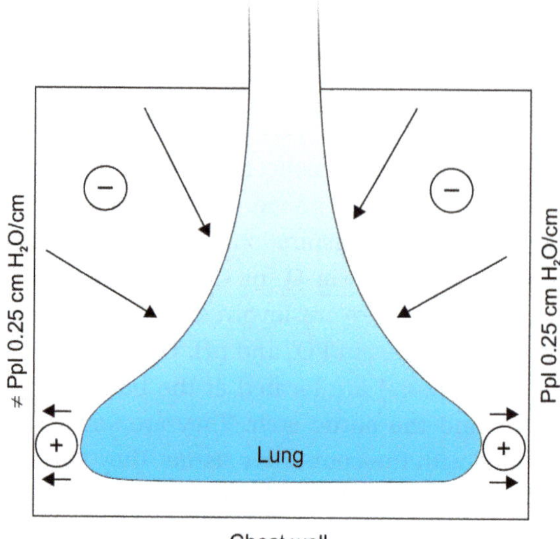

Fig. 28: Distribution of ventilation.

and activate peripheral chemoreceptors and activate stimulation. At high altitude because the ability of the lung to eliminate CO_2 is not affected, in response to increased respiration, blood PCO_2 is decreased. If PO_2 drops under certain level respiratory system does not respond and death will occur.

Distribution of Ventilation

Alveolar pressure is the same throughout the lung; therefore, the more negative intrapleural pressure at the apex (or the least gravity-dependent area) results in larger, more distended apical alveoli than in other areas of the lung (Fig. 28). The transpulmonary pressure (Paw - Ppl), or distending pressure of the lung, is greater at the top and lower at the bottom, where intrapleural pressure is less negative. Despite the smaller alveolar size, more ventilation is delivered to dependent pulmonary areas. The decrease in intrapleural pressure at the base of the lungs during inspiration is greater than at the apex because of diaphragmatic proximity. Thus, because the dependent area of the lung generates the greatest change in transpulmonary pressure, more gas is sucked into dependent areas of the lung.

PERFUSION

Blood flow to and around the lung is similar to any other organ but at much lower pressures than the systemic system (Fig. 29).

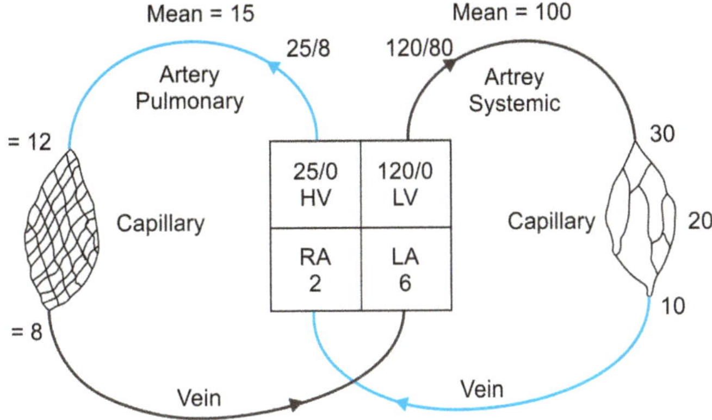

Fig. 29: Pulmonary vs systemic circulation.

The blood vessels in the lungs continually branch and get consistently smaller very like the branching of the airways. The pulmonary arteries whose walls are very thin in comparison to that of the arteries in the main circulation feed the lung up to the level of the terminal bronchioles and then split into the capillary bed. The capillaries have great capability to distend thus enhancing gas exchange and reservoir action. Once the red blood cells have become oxygenated the capillary bed is drained into venules which then join to form the pulmonary veins. It is the ability of the blood vessels to distend and be recruited which allows the pressures in the pulmonary system to stay low despite very high blood flow.

The pulmonary arteries only supply blood flow and oxygen to the lungs and must have the ability to accept huge blood volumes at times. The low pulmonary pressures are important to minimize the work of the right heart.

Pulmonary Vascular Resistance

$$PVR = 80 \times (MPAP - PCWP)/CO$$

The differences between the pulmonary and the systemic circulation:

1. The pressures in the pulmonary circulation are remarkably low.
   Main pulmonary artery pressure: 25 mm Hg (systolic) and 8 mm Hg (diastolic).
   Pressure in aorta: 100 mm Hg.
2. Pulmonary arteries have exceedingly thin walls.
   This anatomical adaptation of the lung is critically important for its function: The lung is required to receive the 24 whole of the cardiac output at all times. Keeping the pulmonary pressure as low as possible allows the right heart answer this demand with a minimum work.
3. Unlike the systemic capillaries, which are organized as tubular network with some interconnections, the pulmonary capillaries mesh together in the alveolar wall, so the blood flows as a thin sheet (capillary bed).

4. Pulmonary circulation can decrease resistance as cardiac output increases by two mechanisms:
    a. *Capillary recruitment*: Opening of initially closed capillaries when cardiac output increases.
    b. *Capillary distension*: The decrease in pulmonary pressure with increased cardiac output (this has several beneficial effects.

    It minimizes the load on the right heart, prevents pulmonary edema, maintains the adequate flow rate of the blood in the capillary and increases the capillary surface area).

Distribution of Blood Flow

Blood flow within the lung is mainly gravity-dependent. Since the alveolar-capillary beds are not composed of rigid vessels, the pressure of the surrounding tissues can influence the resistance to flow through the individual capillaries. Thus, blood flow depends on the relationship between pulmonary artery pressure (Ppa), alveolar pressure (PA), and pulmonary venous pressure. West et al. and West and Dollery created a lung model which divides the lung into three zones (Fig. 30).

Zone 1 conditions occur in the most gravity-independent part of the lung (alveolar pressure is approximately equal to atmospheric pressure; and pulmonary artery pressure).

Zone 2 occurs from the lower limit of zone 1 to the upper limit of zone $3 = P_{pa} > P_a > P_{pv}$. The pressure difference between pulmonary artery and alveolar pressure determines blood flow in zone 2. Pulmonary venous pressure has little influence. Well-matched ventilation and perfusion occur in zone 2, which contains the majority of alveoli (Figs. 30 and 31).

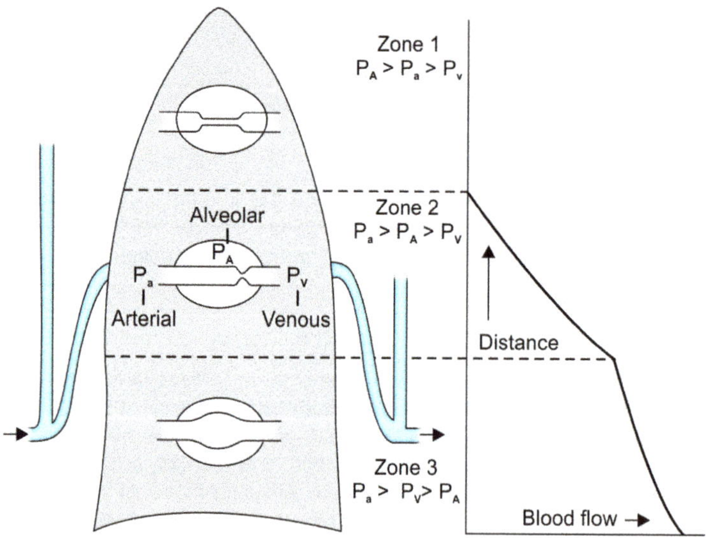

Fig. 30: West zones (upright position)
Source: researchgate.net

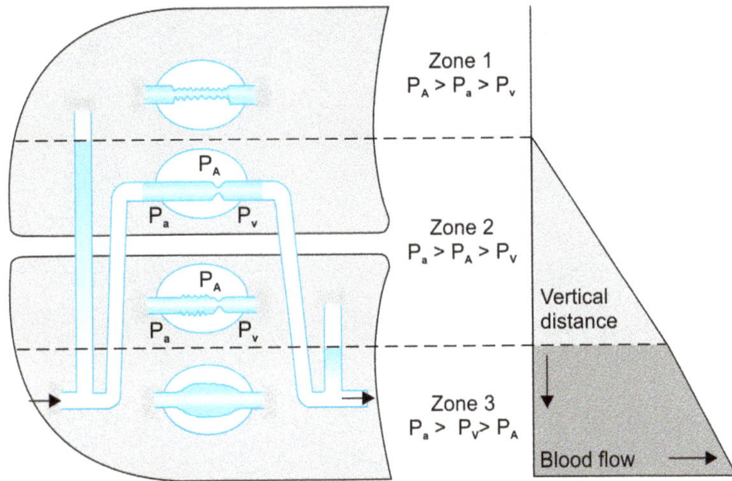

Fig. 31: West zones (lateral decubitus).

Zone 3 occurs in the most gravity-dependent areas of the lung = $P_{pa} > P_{pv} > P_A$. blood flow is primarily governed by the pulmonary arterial to venous pressure difference. Because gravity also increases pulmonary venous pressure, the pulmonary capillaries become distended. Thus, perfusion in zone 3 is lush, resulting in capillary perfusion in excess of ventilation, or physiologic shunt.

Schematic representation of the effects of gravity on the distribution of pulmonary blood flow in the lateral decubitus position. Vertical gradients in the lateral decubitus position are similar to those in the upright position and cause the creation of West zones 1, 2, and 3. Consequently, pulmonary blood flow increases with lung dependency, and is largest in the dependent lung and least in the nondependent lung. Pa, pulmonary artery pressure; PA, alveolar pressure; Pv, pulmonary venous pressure.

Distribution of Ventilation and Perfusion

The efficiency with which oxygen and carbon dioxide exchange at the alveolar-capillary level highly depends on the matching of capillary perfusion and alveolar ventilation. At this level, the combination of lung and the circulatory system must be well-matched.

Ventilation-Perfusion Relationships

The majority of blood flow is distributed to the gravity-dependent part of the lung. During a spontaneous breath, the largest portion of the tidal volume also reaches the gravity-dependent part of the lung. Thus, the nondependent

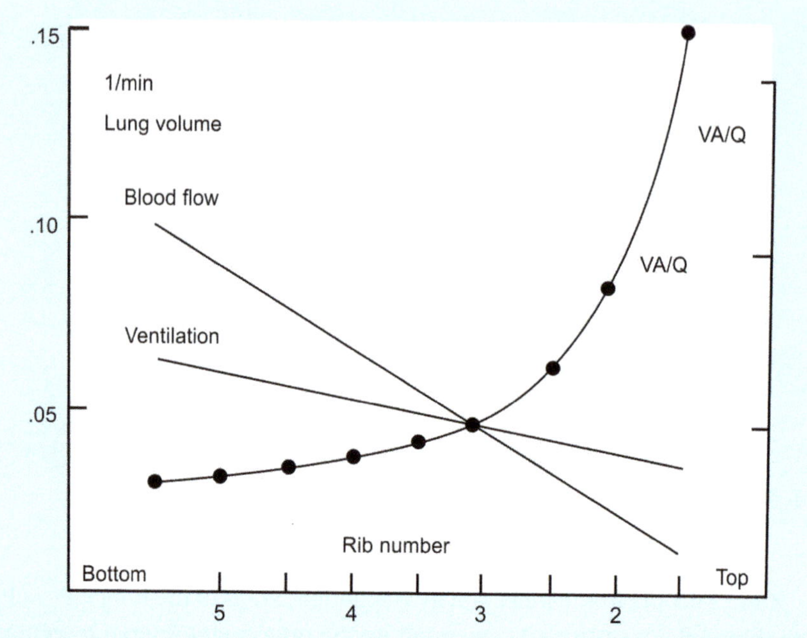

Fig. 32: Ventilation perfusion distribution.

area of the lung receives a lower proportion of both ventilation and perfusion, and dependent lung receives greater proportions of ventilation and perfusion. But, ventilation and perfusion are not matched perfectly, and various V/Q ratios result throughout the lung (Fig. 32).

Any discrepancy between ventilation and blood flow in the lung will result in V/Q mismatch and potentially dangerous irregularities in gas exchange.

If flow of blood to the lung units is to match that of ventilation to the same unit then the ratio of ventilation to perfusion should be in a ratio of 1:1.

If the lung is being underventilated but perfused as normal then we say that the V/Q ratio is <1 (Fig. 33).

If the lung is under perfused then the V/Q is >1 (Fig. 33).

Even in a normal lung the V/Q ratio is not uniformly 1 throughout the lung as perfusion and ventilation both have favored parts of the lung. Differences between the apices and bases of the lungs.

At the apices there is less ventilation than the bases as alveoli are already very stretched however there is proportionally less perfusion therefore the overall V/Q ratio is higher compared to the base of the lung.

Blood flow is directly affected by gravity and naturally has a tendency to flow to the bases of the lungs thus V/Q ratios toward the lower segments of the lung are usually greater than 1. The vertical change in V/Q ratios in the

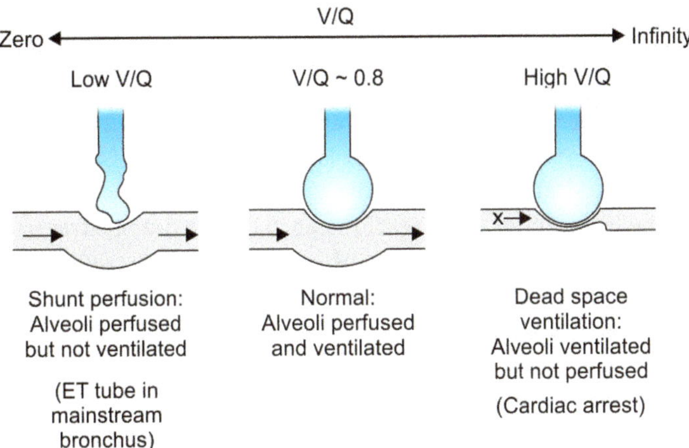

Fig. 33: V/Q in different pathologies.

lung is because although both ventilation and perfusion increase from top to bottom of the lung, perfusion increases much quicker than ventilation.

Thus the V/Q ratio at the top of the lung is 3.3 whereas at the bases it is around 0.6.

Ideal V/Q ratio = 1; believed to occur at approximately the level of the third rib.

Above this level, ventilation occurs slightly in excess of perfusion, whereas below the third rib the V/Q ratio becomes less than 1.

V/Q = 0 in shunt

V/Q = infinity in dead space.

Hypoxic pulmonary vasoconstriction and bronchoconstriction allow the lungs to maintain optimal V/Q matching.

Many pulmonary diseases result in both physiologic shunt and dead space abnormalities. However, most disease processes can be characterized as producing either primarily shunt or dead space in their early stages. Increases in dead space ventilation primarily affect carbon dioxide elimination and have little influence on arterial oxygenation until dead space ventilation exceeds 80 to 90% of minute ventilation. Similarly, physiologic shunt primarily affects arterial oxygenation with little effect on carbon dioxide elimination until the physiologic shunt fraction exceeds 75 to 80% of the cardiac output. Defective to absent gas exchange can be the net effect of either abnormality in the extreme.

GAS EXCHANGE

The partial pressure of oxygen that is inhaled from our natural environment through normal inhalation is not maintained at the same partial pressure by the time it reaches the alveoli and indeed the mitochondria. The process by which this decrease in partial pressure occurs is called the **oxygen cascade**.

- Dry atmospheric air gas - 21% of 100 kPa
  SO: 21 kPa or 160 mm Hg
- However as gas is inspired it is diluted by water vapor which reduces the partial pressure of oxygen water vapor - 6.3 kPa/47 mm Hg
  $PO_2 = 0.21 \times (760 - 47) = 149$ mm Hg or
  $PO_2 = 0.21 \times (100 - 6.3) = 19.8$ kPa
- When the gas reaches the alveoli the partial pressure of oxygen will again decrease as some oxygen is absorbed and CO_2 is excreted. The partial pressure at this point in the oxygen cascade can be determined by using the **alveolar gas equation.**
  $PAO_2 = PIO_2 - PACO_2/RQ$
  The RQ stands for respiratory quotient and is normally 0.8.
  It is determined by the amount of CO_2 produced/oxygen consumed.
  $PAO_2 = 0.21\text{-}5/0.8 = 14$ kPa (106 mm Hg)
- Again when the gas reaches the arterial blood a further small drop in partial pressure will have occurred as blood known as venous admixture with a lower oxygen content mixes with the oxygenated alveolar blood. Venous admixture is made up of blood that has passed through poorly ventilated regions of lung and thus has a lower O_2 partial pressure. Venous admixture is also composed of venous blood which has drained the lungs and left side of the heart. This blood is known as true shunt and drains directly into the left side of the heart. Extraction of oxygen from this blood then causes the end capillary oxygen partial pressure to be 6–7 kPa (40–50 mm Hg)
- In the mitochondria the PO_2 varies hugely from 1–5 kPa (7.5–40 mm Hg). This provides us with an explanation for the following graph, the **oxygen cascade** (Fig. 34).

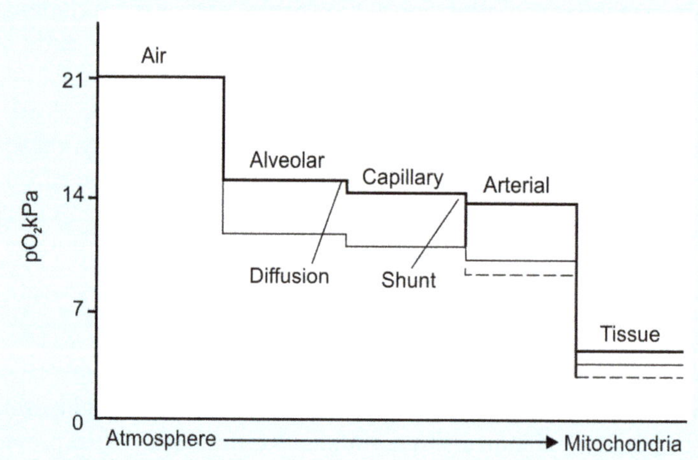

Fig. 34: Oxygen cascade.

The speed and ease of diffusion are controlled by the laws of diffusion. Fick's law of diffusion states that gas transfer across a membrane is directly proportional to the concentration gradient.

Graham's law states that diffusion of a gas is inversely proportional to the square root of the molecular weight of the molecule.

Other factors which increase diffusion:

- Large surface area
- Thin membrane
- High solubility

The following equation incorporates the important factors Diffusion is proportional to A/T D (P_1-P_2):

A = Area T = Thickness D = Diffusion constant P_1-P_2 = Concentration gradient Diffusion in the lungs can be limited in the presence of disease states, e.g. pulmonary edema and thickening of the alveolar membrane in pulmonary fibrosis.

Oxygen Transport

Oxygen is carried in 2 forms in the blood:

- Oxygen combined to hemoglobin (97%). Hemoglobin molecule consists of 2 alpha and 2 beta chains; each chain is formed from an iron-porphyrin molecule—hem. Each hemoglobin molecule can bind 4 oxygen molecules (20 mL oxygen per 100 mL blood) or 15 mL oxygen per 100 mL in venous blood.
- Oxygen dissolved in the blood—this accounts for a minimal amount (0.3 mL per dL).

The amount dissolved obeys Henrys' law—amount is proportional to the partial pressure 0.023 mL per kPa per 100 mL blood oxygen content in the blood. Total content of oxygen in the blood can be calculated from the Oxygen flux equation:

Flux = [CO × Hb × Saturation × Huffners constant (1.39)] + (0.023 × PO_2)

Oxygen dissociation curve (Fig. 35):

- Sigmoid shaped curve relating the fact that binding of oxygen to the hemoglobin molecule is a cooperative process
- Describes the relationship of saturation of hemoglobin with oxygen at varying partial pressures
- Be aware of the P50 -(point at which Hb is 50% saturated)
- Decreasing pH, increasing temperature, 2,3-DPG and CO_2 tension will cause a right shift of the curve
- Increased pH, and reduction in CO_2 tension, temperature and 2,3-DPG produce a left shift of the curve

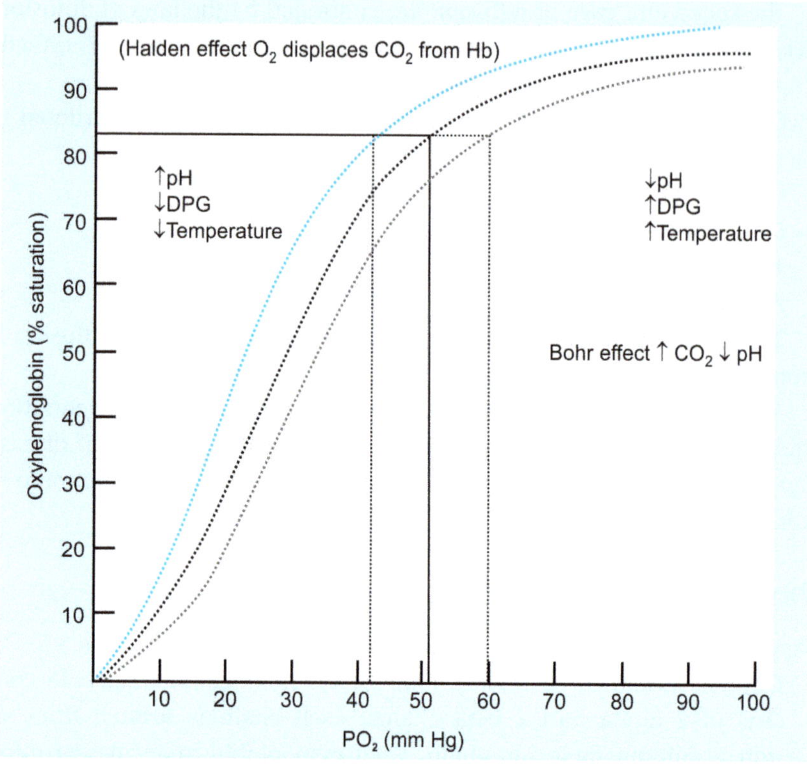

Fig. 35: Oxygen dissociation curve.

- If a right shift occurs the Hb molecule is more likely to offload oxygen to the tissues
- In a left shifted situation the Hb is less likely to release oxygen to the tissues.

2,3-DPG: This molecule binds to deoxygenated Hb - it reduces the affinity of hemoglobin for oxygen and therefore ensures offloading of oxygen to the tissues.

The Bohr effect: This describes the affect that CO_2 has on influencing the release of oxygen to the tissues. On entering red blood cells the following reaction occurs:

$$CO_2 + H_2O \leftrightarrow H_2CO_3 \leftrightarrow H^+ + HCO_3^-$$

An increase in H^+ will cause an acidosis and therefore encourage the release of oxygen from Hb.

In the lungs where the CO_2 is being removed, the alkalosis will encourage the uptake of oxygen.

$$\text{Oxygen Delivery } (DO_2) = \text{Cardiac output} \times \text{arterial } O_2 \text{ content}$$

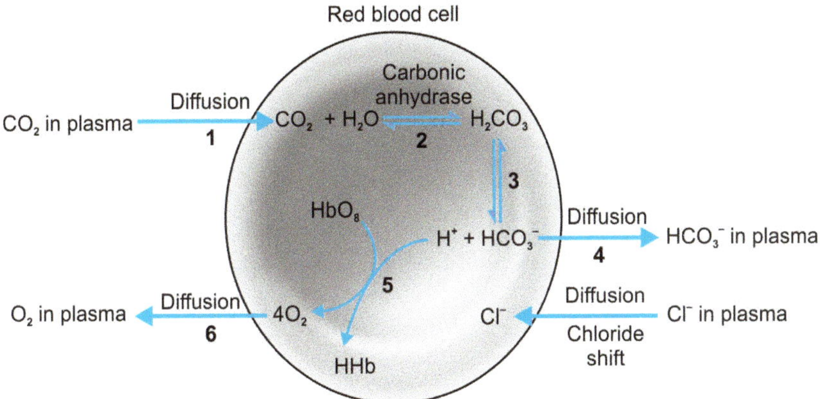

Fig. 36: Chloride shift.

Carbon Dioxide Transport

Carbon dioxide is carried in the blood in 3 ways:

- As bicarbonate - 90%
- As dissolved CO_2 - 5%
- As carbamino compounds - 5%

Carbamino compounds are formed by the reaction of the CO_2 with terminal amino groups of proteins and side chains of arginine and lysine. Hemoglobin is essential for this process to occur since it has 4 amino groups per molecule. Albumin also provides amino groups but only 1 per molecule.

The Hamburger effect (chloride shift) (Fig. 36).

The transport of chloride ions into the cell as a result of outwards diffusion of bicarbonate in order to maintain electrical neutrality.

The Haldane effect:

This phenomenon refers to the increased ability of blood to carry CO_2 when hemoglobin is deoxygenated. Deoxyhemoglobin is 3.5 times more effective than oxyhemoglobin in forming carbamino compounds.

ALVEOLAR-ARTERIAL PO_2 GRADIENT

CO_2 Dissociation Curve (Fig. 37)

The value for the A-a gradient gives the clinician some idea about the amount of VQ mismatch and shunt that is present in the lungs. A typical normal value would be around 0.5-1 kPa (5 mm Hg) though values up to around 15 mm Hg may be accepted.

- It is calculated as PAO_2 - PaO_2.
- The PAO_2 is calculated using the alveolar gas equation.

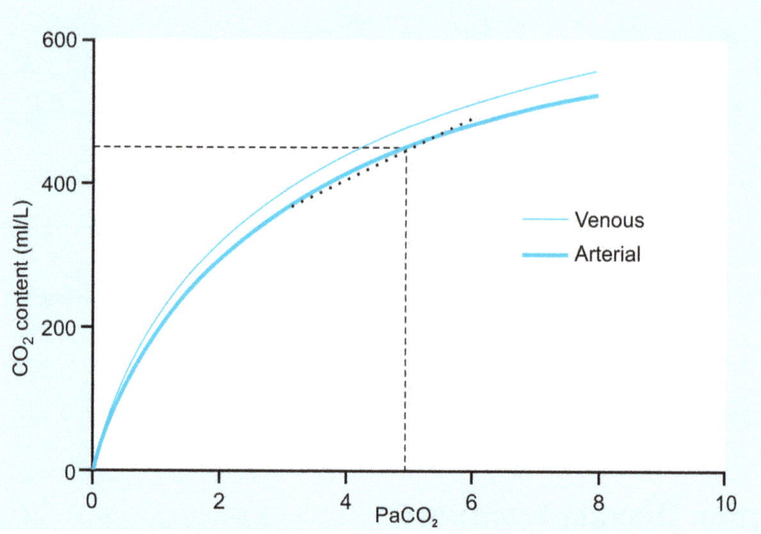

Fig. 37: CO_2 dissociation curve.

Shunt

True shunt refers to a VQ = 0.

That is to say that blood has passed through areas of the lung where no ventilation is occurring. As discussed earlier VQ mismatch is also referred to as shunt. Blood passes through areas of the lung which are poorly ventilated, i.e. VQ < 1.

Physiological shunt refers to the amount of venous admixture which is directly added to main circulatory blood without having passed through the oxygenating mechanism of the lung. Blood from the bronchial veins draining the lung parenchyma and the thebesian veins draining the cardiac muscle represent the physiological shunt (around 5% of cardiac output). The shunt equation allows calculation of the amount of shunt present in an individual subject.

The shunt equation: Qs = Shunted blood flow Qt = Cardiac output Qt-Qs = Blood flow through the lungs minus the shunted blood CcO_2 = Oxygen content of end pulmonary capillary blood CaO_2 = Oxygen content of arterial blood CvO_2 = Oxygen content of mixed venous blood shunt equation (Fig. 38).

The amount of oxygen leaving the lungs is Qt × CaO_2.

This is equal to the shunted blood flow plus the oxygen content from the lung which would be (Qs × CvO_2) + (Qt-Qs) × CcO_2. (shunt flow × mixed venous O_2 content + pulmonary capillary flow × pulmonary capillary O_2 content).

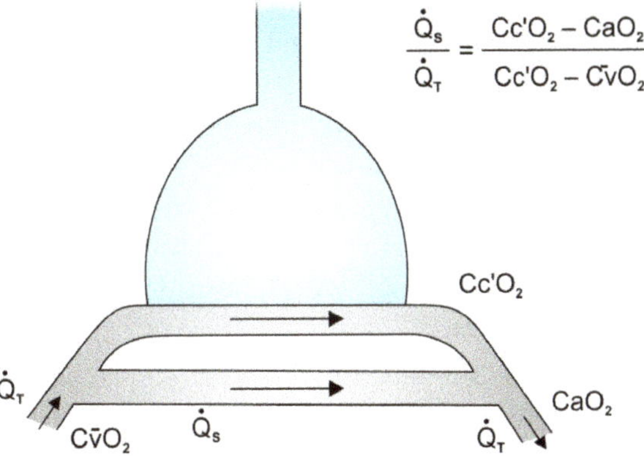

Fig. 38: Shunt equation.

$$Qt \times CaO_2 = (Qs \times CvO_2) + (Qt\text{-}Qs) \times CcO_2$$

When these equations as rearranged it provides the classic shunt equation:

$$Qs/Qt = CcO_2 - CaO_2/\ CcO_2 - CvO_2$$

Carbon Monoxide Diffusing Capacity

Because PO_2 in the pulmonary capillary blood varies with time as it moves through the pulmonary capillary bed, oxygen cannot be used to assess diffusing capacity. A gas mixture containing carbon monoxide is the traditional diagnostic gas used to measure diffusing capacity. Its partial pressure in the blood is nearly zero, and its affinity for hemoglobin is 200 times that of oxygen. Carbon monoxide diffusing capacity (D_{LCO}) collectively measures all the factors that affect the diffusion of gas across the alveolar-capillary membrane. The D_{LCO} is recorded in mL CO/min/mm Hg at standard temperature and pressure, dry.

In persons with normal hemoglobin concentrations and normal V/Q matching, the main factor limiting diffusion is the alveolar-capillary membrane. Small amounts of carbon dioxide and inspired gas can produce measurable changes in the concentration of inspired gas compared with expired gas. There are several methods for determining D_{LCO}, but all methods measure diffusing capacity according to the equation:

$$D_{LCO} = \frac{\text{mL CO transferred/min}}{\text{mean } PaCO_2 - \text{mean capillary } PCO_2}$$

The average value for resting subjects when the single-breath method is used is 25 mL CO/min/mm Hg. D_{LCO} values can increase to 2 or 3 times normal during exercise.

The DLO_2 may be estimated from the D_{LCO} by multiplying D_{LCO} by 1.23, although the D_{LCO} is usually the reported value. D_{LCO} can be divided by the lung volume at which the measurement was made to obtain an expression of diffusing capacity per unit lung volume.

Some of the other factors that can influence D_{LCO} are as follows:

1. *Hemoglobin concentration*: Decreased hemoglobin concentration decreases the D_{LCO}.
2. *Alveolar PCO_2*: An increased $PACO_2$ raises D_{LCO}.
3. *Body position*: The supine position increases D_{LCO}.
4. Pulmonary capillary blood volume.
5. Diffusing capacity is decreased in alveolar fibrosis associated with sarcoidosis, asbestosis, berylliosis, oxygen toxicity, and pulmonary edema. These states are frequently categorized as *diffusion defects,* but low D_{LCO} is probably more closely related to loss of lung volume or capillary bed perfusion.

D_{LCO} is decreased in obstructive disease because of the decreased alveolar surface area, loss of capillary bed, the increased distance from the terminal bronchiole to the alveolar-capillary membrane, and V/Q mismatching. In short, few disease states truly inhibit oxygen diffusion across the alveolar-capillary membrane.

CLINICAL APPLICATIONS

Pulmonary Function Testing

Used in patients with significant pulmonary dysfunction.

Pulmonary Function Tests in Restrictive and Obstructive Lung Disease.

Value	*Restrictive disease*	*Obstructive disease*
Definition	Proportional decreases in all lung volumes	Small airway obstruction to expiratory flow
FVC	↓↓↓	Normal or slightly ↑
FEV_1	↓↓↓	Normal or slightly ↓
FEV_1/FVC	Normal	↓↓↓
FEF_{25} –75%	Normal	↓↓↓
FRC	↓↓↓	Normal or ↑, if gas trapping
TLC	↓↓↓	Normal or ↑, if gas trapping

Flow-Volume Loops (Fig. 39)

The flow-volume loop graphically demonstrates the flow generated during a forced expiratory maneuver followed by a forced inspiratory maneuver,

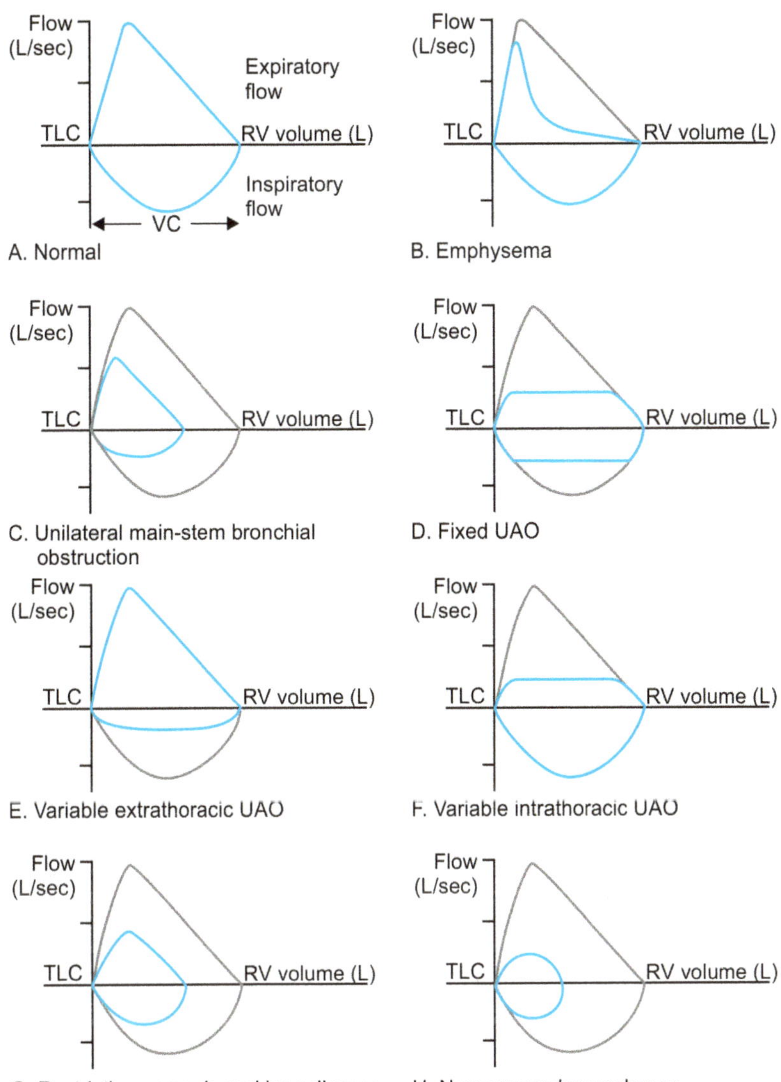

Fig. 39: Flow volume loops.
Source: http://www.warrengoff.com/pft-vim/fvloop/img32.gif

plotted against the volume of gas expired. The subject forcefully exhales completely, then immediately and forcefully inhales to vital capacity. The expired and inspired volumes are plotted on the abscissa and flow is plotted on the ordinate. Although various numbers can be generated from the flow-volume loop, the configuration of the loop itself is probably the most informative part of the test. It helps in distinguishing an extrathoracic from intra thoracic obstruction and guide in its management.

Respiratory Formulas

Formula	*Normal values (70 kg)*
Alveolar oxygen tension	110 mm Hg
$PAO_2 = (PB - 47)\ FIO_2^{-}$; $(PACO_2/R)$	$(FIO_2 = 0.21)$
Alveolar-arterial oxygen gradient	<10 mm Hg
$(A - aO_2) = PAO_2 - PaO_2$	$(FIO_2 = 0.21)$
Arterial-to-alveolar oxygen ratio, PaO_2/PAO_2 ratio	>0.75
Arterial oxygen content	20 mL/100 mL blood
$CaO_2 = (SaO_2)\ (Hb \times 1.34) + PaO_2\ (0.0031)$	
Mixed venous oxygen content	15 mL/100 mL blood
C[v with bar above]O_2 = (S [v with bar above] O_2) (Hb × 1.34) + P[v with bar above]O_2 (0.0031)	
Arterial-venous oxygen content difference	4–6 mL/100 mL blood
C(a-[v with bar above])O_2 = CaO_2 – C[v with bar above]O_2	
Intrapulmonary shunt	<5%
[Q with dot above]sp/[Q with dot above]T = ($Cc'O_2$ – CaO_2)/($Cc'O_2$ – C[v with bar above]O_2) where $Cc'O_2 = (Hb \times 1.34) + (PAO_2 \times 0.0031)$	
Physiologic dead space	0.33
$VD/V_T = (PaCO_2 - P\bar{E}CO_2)/PaCO_2$	
Oxygen consumption	250 mL/min
$VO_2 = CO\ (CaO_2 - CVO_2)$	
Oxygen transport	1,000 mL/min
$DO_2 = CO\ (CaO_2)$	
Respiratory quotient	0.8
[V with dot above]CO_2/[V with dot above]O_2 = R	

(PAO_2: Alveolar oxygen tension; PB: Barometric pressure; FIO_2: Fraction inspired oxygen; $PACO_2$: Alveolar carbon dioxide tension; R: Respiratory quotient; PaO_2: Arterial oxygen tension; CaO_2: Arterial oxygen content; SaO_2: Arterial oxygen saturation; Hb: Hemoglobin concentration; Cv–O_2: Mixed venous oxygen content; Sv–O_2: Mixed venous oxygen saturation; Pv–O_2: Mixed venous oxygen tension; [Q with dot above]SP/[Q with dot above]T: intrapulmonary shunt; $Cc'O_2$: End-pulmonary capillary oxygen content; VD: Dead space gas volume; VT: Tidal volume; $PaCO_2$: Arterial carbon dioxide tension; $P\bar{E}CO_2$: Mixed expired carbon dioxide tension; [V with dot above]O_2, oxygen consumption (mL/min); CO: Cardiac output; [V with dot above] CO_2: Carbon dioxide production (mL/min); DO_2: Oxygen transport).

RESPONSES TO AIRWAY MANIPULATION

Geetanjali S Verma

Direct laryngoscopy and introduction of tracheal tube are noxious stimuli that can provoke a response of cardiovascular, respiratory and other physiological systems.

RESPONSES (FIG. 40)

Cardiovascular System

Hypertension, tachycardia—exaggerated with increased duration an force of laryngoscopy. Increase in arterial pressures starts within 5 seconds of laryngoscopy, peaks in 1-2 minutes and returns to control levels in 5 minutes. Also noted with use of ILMA.

Respiratory System

Laryngospasm—if laryngoscopy attempted during light plane of anesthesia; bronchospasm, coughing, bucking.

Central Nervous System

Elevation of ICT/IOP.

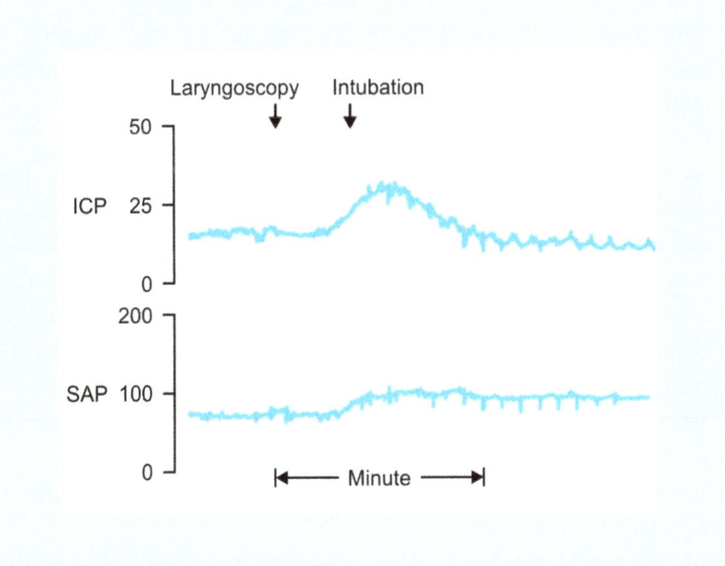

Fig. 40: Response to tracheal intubation.
Source: Bedford RF: Circulatory responses to tracheal intubation. Probl Anesth.

Others

Vomiting, aspiration, latex allergy (Patients with spina bifida, rubber industry workers, atopic patients, and patients with a multiple surgery history are most at risk. Patients with type I hypersensitivity are at risk for developing anaphylaxis with hypotension, rash, and bronchospasm).

PATHWAYS/MECHANISMS

1. Stimulation of proprioceptors (especially mechanoreceptors) located in supraglottic and tracheal region (consist of small-diameter myelinated fibers, slowly-adapting stretch receptors with large-diameter myelinated fibers, and polymodal endings of nonmyelinated nerve fibers) cause laryngospasm, tachycardia and hypertension. Laryngospasm and bradycardia is common in children.
2. Stimulation of glossopharyngeal and vagus nerves—causes widespread autonomic activation of the sympathetic and parasympathetic nervous systems, causing bradycardia and laryngospasm.
3. Stimulation of cardioaccelerator nerves and sympathetic nervous system - causing hypertension and tachycardia (more common in adults) due to release of norepinephrine from adrenergic nerve terminals and secretion of epinephrine from the adrenal medulla.
4. Activation of the renin-angiotensin system (including release of renin from the renal juxtaglomerular apparatus, which is innervated by β-adrenergic nerve terminals) causing hypertension.
5. Stimulation of CNS (especially in patients with pre-existing neuropathology) - elevation of ICT - hypertension and bradycardia (cushing response).
6. Reduced cardiac output - due to PEEP after intubation.
   An increase in mean intrathoracic pressure due to positive-pressure ventilation (PPV) is transmitted to the thin-walled, compressible superior and inferior venae cave, elevating the downstream pressure for venous return and thereby reducing venous blood return to the right atrium. Because the left side of the heart can only pump what the right side delivers, cardiac output and subsequently arterial BP may fall with PPV.
7. Adverse effects of drugs:
   a. Succinylcholine—bradycardia, fasciculations
   b. Atracurium, mivacurium—histamine release—tachycardia
   c. Pancuronium—tachycardia

All the above responses are exaggerated inpatients with pre-existing cardiovascular compromise or intravascular volume depletion.

The neuroendocrine responses to airway manipulation resulting in tachycardia and HTN may result in a variety of complications in patients with cardiac disease, especially myocardial ischemia—seen as ischemic electrocardiographic ST-segment depression and increased pulmonary artery diastolic blood pressure (BP) during intubation in patients with arteriosclerosis.

Increases in systemic arterial pressure (SAP) and intracranial pressure (ICP) in response to endotracheal intubation in a patient with a small brain tumor. Notice the minimal response to rigid laryngoscopy. There is a sustained increase in systemic arterial pressure but only a transient increase in ICP, which returns to normal as cerebrovascular autoregulation becomes operative.

PREVENTION OF RESPONSES

1. Limit laryngoscopy to <15 seconds, minimize attempts.
2. Limit use of cricoid pressure.
3. Use of LMA wherever possible.
4. Use of topical and regional anesthesia.
5. Drugs—fentanyl, propofol, thiopentone, vecuronium (3 minutes pre-oxygenation).
   Use of narcotics—fentanyl 6 μg/kg suppress the response, but can cause respiratory depression.
6. Xylocard—1-1.5 mg/kg IV 90 seconds prior to intubation.
7. *Other drugs*: Pretreatment with phentolamine, 5 mg IV, prevented the hypertensive-tachycardic response to endotracheal intubation during a light barbiturate-succinylcholine anesthetic technique.
   Others: Diltiazem, verapamil, and nicardipine, hydralazine, nitroprusside; nitroglycerin; labetalol esmolol; and clonidine.
8. Inhalational agents - sevoflurane (MAC > 2.5) blunts hemodynamic responses to intubation.
9. Use of N_2O has proved beneficial.
10. Use of awake flexible fiberoptic intubation with effective topical anesthesia eliminates hemodynamic responses to intubation.
11. Use of bronchodilator therapy (in asthmatics) has shown to decrease bronchospasm incidence.

2 Clinical Evaluation of Airway

Geetanjali S Verma

AIRWAY ASSESSMENT

Even though the life-saving scheme has changed from A-B-C to C-A-B, a definitive knowledge of airway assessment and securing the airway remains the priority to help sustain life. An estimated of 28% of all anesthesia related deaths are secondary to inability to mask ventilate or intubate. Thus, prediction of a difficult airway would allow time for selection of equipments, techniques and personnel experienced in difficult airway.

Assessment of the airway would be discussed under 3 subheadings:

1. History
2. Physical examination
3. Radiological indices

HISTORY

Geetanjali S Verma

Patients should be specifically questioned about:

- Previous airway interventions (review old records whenever possible)
- Dental problems (bridges, caps, fillings, appliances, loose teeth)
- Respiratory disease (snoring, sleep apnea syndrome, smoking, coughing, sputum production, and wheezing)
- Arthritis (temporomandibular joint [TMJ] disease, ankylosing spondylitis, osteoarthritis, and rheumatoid arthritis)
- Clotting abnormalities (especially before nasal intubation)
- A history of gastroesophageal reflux disease (GERD)
- Congenital abnormalities and syndromes (especially those involving the head, face, and neck)
- Type I diabetes mellitus—The limited joint mobility syndrome occurs in 30–40% of insulin-dependent diabetics and is thought to be due to glycosylation of tissue proteins that occurs in patients with chronic hyperglycemia.

- History of airway surgery or radiation
- Burns, swelling, tumor, masses
- History of obstructive sleep apnea (OSA) (STOP BANG—Snoring, Tiredness, Obesity, Pressure [HTN], BMI increased, Another person witnessed snoring, Neonates, Gender—more in males).

EXAMINATION

Geetanjali S Verma

GENERAL EXAMINATION

- Level of consciousness
- Look for obvious anomalies: Any masses or swelling around the nose and mouth
- Facies-Pierre-Robin, Treacher Collins, Klippel-Feil, Apert, fetal alcohol syndromes
- Obesity/short neck—BMI is a better predictor of difficult intubation than body mass
- Presence of beard (may interfere with mask ventilation)
- Pregnancy
- Posture
- Cyanosis.

AIRWAY EXAMINATION

Nose (Fig. 1)

- Patency of nostrils

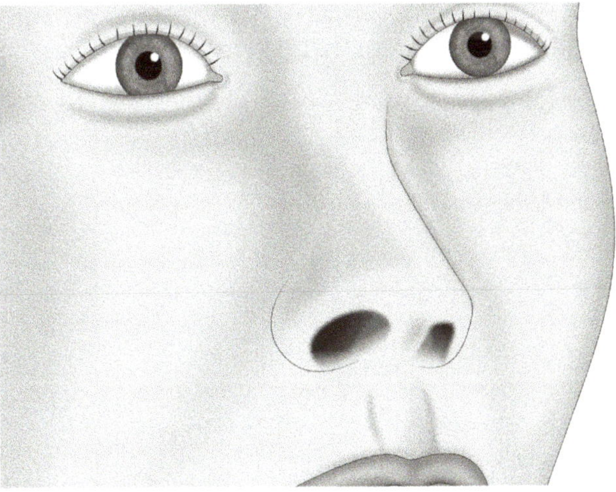

Fig. 1: Look for patency of nostrils.

- Presence of mass or enlarged turbinates
- Malformation of nose (secondary to trauma or burns).

Temporomandibular Joint

- With the middle finger of each hand posterior and inferior to the patient's earlobes, place your index fingers just anterior to the tragus and instruct the patient to open widely. Two distinct movements should be felt: the first is rotational, and the second involves advancement of the condylar head. Listen and palpate for clicks and crepitus, both of which indicate joint dysfunction.
- Insertion of one finger breadth on opening of the joint is also considered adequate.
- TMJ function may also be assessed by asking the patient to insert two or three fingers (of their own hand) held vertically into the oral cavity in the midline. Normal adults are capable of inserting at least three fingers (corresponding to a range of mandibular opening between 40 and 60 mm) (Fig. 2).
    - Patients capable of inserting only two or fewer fingers are considered to have major limitations.

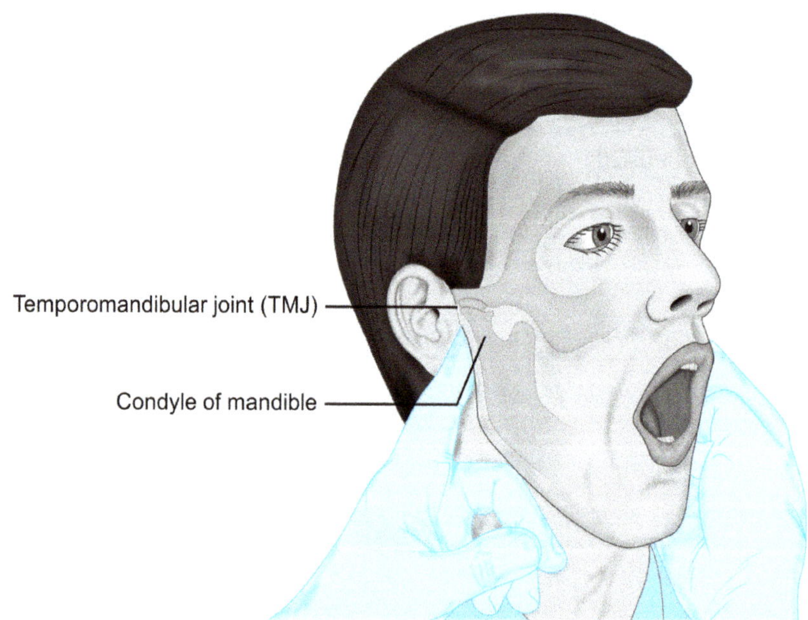

Fig. 2: Temporomandibular joint assessment.

  - If the maximal mandibular opening is less than 30 mm in the adult, oral surgeons suggest that significant TMJ dysfunction is present.
  - If less than 25 mm, it is unlikely that the larynx will be visible using conventional laryngoscopy, since exposure of the larynx depends to a great extent upon the ability to move the mandible and soft tissues forward.
  - If mouth opening is 20 mm or less, a Macintosh 3 or 4 blade will not fit in the mouth and therefore alternative methods of intubation are required.
- It is important to be able to distinguish between limited mouth opening due to muscle spasm and restriction due to joint disease—former responds to muscle relaxation but not the latter.
- *Mandibular protrusion test*: This test is performed by asking the patient to advance the mandible as far as possible and the classification is as follows:
  - *Class A*: The lower incisors can be protruded beyond the upper incisors
  - *Class B*: The lower incisors can be advanced only to the level of the upper incisors
  - *Class C*: The lower incisors cannot reach the level of the upper incisors
- Impaired mandibular protrusion is associated with difficult laryngoscopy and difficult mask ventilation.
- *Upper lip bite test*: This test measures the ability to bite (gently) the upper lip with the lower teeth.

Lips

- Presence of cleft lip
- Absence of the philtrum is a diagnostic feature of fetal alcohol syndrome.

Oral Cavity

- Opening as wide as 2-finger breadths between upper and lower incisors in adults is adequate
- Teeth—presence of loose teeth, missing teeth, dentures (especially removable), and prominent upper incisors
- *Tongue*: Assess size and mobility
- *Palate*: High arched?

Neck and Cervical Spine

- Short?
- Restriction of movement

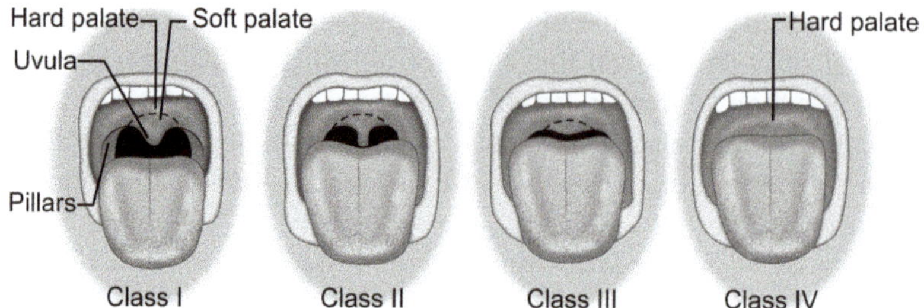

Fig. 3: Mallampati classification.

- *Skin color*: May be indicative of radiotherapy
- *Scars*: Tracheostomy, surgery, burns, etc.
- Masses/swelling (thyroid, tumor, lymph nodes, Ludwig's angina, etc.).

SPECIFIC TESTS FOR ASSESSMENT OF AIRWAY

Mallampati Test (1983) (Fig. 3)

It is performed with the patient in the sitting position, head in a neutral position, the mouth wide open and the tongue protruding to its maximum. Patient should not be actively encouraged to phonate (causes contraction and elevation of the soft palate leading to a spurious picture). Repeat twice to avoid false positives.

Class I: Visualization of the soft palate, fauces; uvula, anterior and the posterior pillars.

Class II: Visualization of the soft palate, fauces and uvula.

Class III: Visualization of soft palate and base of uvula.

In Samsoon and Young's modification (1987) of the Mallampati classification, a IV class was added.

Class IV: Only hard palate is visible. Soft palate is not visible at all.

Class 0 (by Ezri et al.): Epiglottis seen on mouth opening and tongue protrusion.

Atlanto-occipital Joint Extension

It assesses feasibility to make sniffing or Magill position for intubation (i.e. alignment of oral, pharyngeal and laryngeal axes into an arbitrary straight line).

The patient is asked to hold head erect, facing directly to the front. Then he is asked to extend the head maximally and the examiner estimates the angle traversed by the occlusal surface of upper teeth. Measurement can be by simple visual estimate or more accurately with a goniometer (Fig. 4).

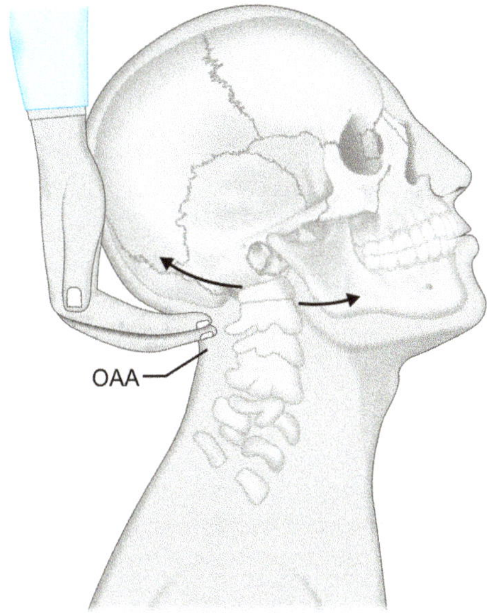

Fig. 4: Atlanto-occipital joint assessment.

Normal angle of extension is 35° or more.

Any reduction in extension is expressed in grades:

Grade I: >35°

Grade II: 22°–34°

Grade III: 12°–21°

Grade IV: <12°

As the grades increase, so does the difficulty of intubation.

Mandibular Space

a. Inter incisor distance

   It is the distance between the upper and lower incisors.

   Normal: 4.6 cm or more

   <3.8 cm predicts difficult airway.

b. Thyromental distance (Patil's test) (distance A in Fig. 5)

   It is the distance from the mentum to the thyroid notch while the patient's neck is fully extended. It assesses how readily the laryngeal axis will fall in line with the pharyngeal axis when the atlanto-occipital joint is extended.

   Normal: >6.5 cm

   Alignment of these two axes is difficult if the thyromental distance is < 3 finger breadths or < 6 cm in adults;

   6–6.5 cm is less difficult.

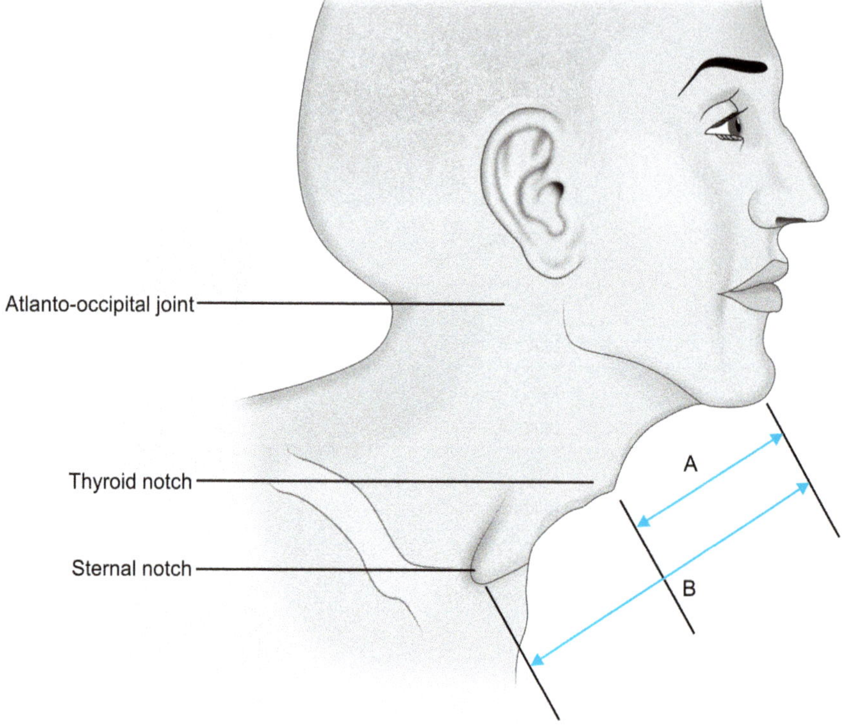

Fig. 5: A: Thyromental distance; B: Sternomental distance.

c. Sternomental distance (distance B in Fig. 5)
   It is measured with the head fully extended on the neck with the mouth closed.
   A value of less than 12 cm is found to predict a difficult intubation.
d. Mandibulohyoid distance
   It is the measurement of mandibular length from chin (mental) to hyoid.
   Normal: >4 cm or three finger breadths.

Direct Laryngoscopy

Cormack and Lehane Grading (Fig. 6)

Grade I: Visualization of entire laryngeal aperture.
Grade II: Visualization of only posterior commissure of laryngeal aperture.
Grade III: Visualization of only epiglottis.
Grade IV: Visualization of just the soft palate.
Grades III and IV predict difficult intubation.

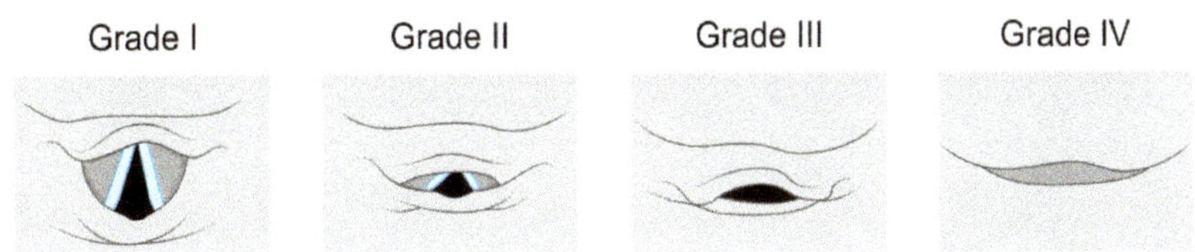

Fig. 6: Cormack and Lehane grading.

Finger Breadth Test (1-2-3-4)

- Temporomandibular mobility—One finger
- Mouth opening—Two fingers
- Measurement of mento-hyoid distance (4 cm) in adult—Three fingers.
- Measurement of distance from chin to thyroid notch (5 to 6 cm)—Four fingers.

Special Tests For Diabetic Patients

a. *Palm print*: The patient is made to sit; palm and fingers of right hand are painted with blue ink, patient then presses the hand firmly against a white paper placed on a hard surface (Figs. 7A to C). It is graded as:
   Grade 0: All the phalangeal areas are visible.
   Grade 1: Deficiency in the interphalangeal areas of the 4th and 5th digits.
   Grade 2: Deficiency in interphalangeal areas of 2nd to 5th digits.
   Grade 3: Only the tips of digits are seen.

b. *Prayer sign* (Fig. 7A): Patient is asked to bring both the palms together as 'Namaste' and sign is categorized as:
   Positive: When there is gap between palms.
   Negative: When there is no gap between palms.

SCORING SYSTEMS

i. *Wilson and colleagues*
   They took 5 variables in consideration—weight, head, neck and jaw movements, mandibular recession, presence or absence of buck teeth.
   Risk score was developed between 0 and 10.
   They found that higher the risk score, greater the accuracy of prediction with a lower proportion of false positives.

ii. *Ame and colleagues*
   Apart from the above indicators by Wilson et al., it also included presence or absence of overt airway pathology. The sensitivity and specificity level of this system was above 90%.

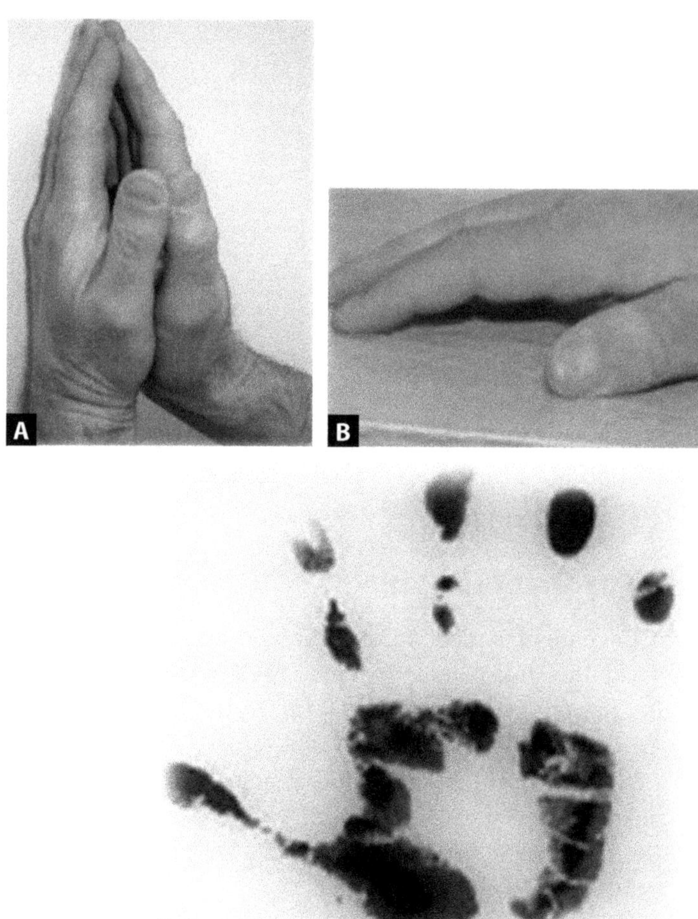

Figs. 7A to C: A: Prayer sign; B, C: Palm print sign.

iii. *Lemon airway assessment*

L = Look externally (facial trauma, large incisors, beard or moustache, large tongue)

E = Evaluate the 3-3-2 rule (incisor distance-3 finger breadths, hyoid-mental distance-3 finger breadths, thyroid-to-mouth distance-2 finger breadths)

M = Mallampati (Mallampati score > 3)

O = Obstruction (presence of any condition like epiglottitis, peritonsillar abscess, trauma)

N = Neck mobility (limited neck mobility).

The score with a maximum of 10 points is calculated by assigning 1 point for each.

Higher scores indicate difficult intubation.

RADIOLOGICAL ASSESSMENT

Geetanjali S Verma

i. Cervical spine X-ray (lateral)
   - *Mandibulohyoid distance*: An increase in the mandibulohyoid distance resulted in an increase in difficult laryngoscopy.
   - *Atlanto-occipital (A-O) gap*: A-O gap is the major factor which limits the extension of head on neck. Longer the A-O gap, more space is available for mobility of head at that joint with good axis for laryngoscopy and intubation. Radiologically there is reduced space between C1 and occiput.
   - *Relation of mandibular angle and hyoid bone with cervical vertebra and laryngoscopy grading*: A definite increase in difficult laryngoscopy was observed when the mandibular angle tended to be more rostral and hyoid bone to be more caudal, position of mandibular angle being more important.
   - *Anterior/posterior depth of the mandible*: White and Kander (1975) have shown that the posterior depth of the mandible, i.e. the distance between the bony alveolus immediately behind the 3rd molar tooth and the lower border of the mandible is an important measure in determining the ease or difficulty of laryngoscopy.
   - *C1-C2 gap*: Calcified stylohyoid ligaments are manifested by crease over hyoid bones on radiological examination. Laryngoscopy is difficult because of inability to lift the epiglottis from posterior pharyngeal wall as it is firmly attached to the hyoidbone by the hyoepiglottic ligament.

ii. Fluoroscopy for dynamic imaging (cord mobility, airway malacia, and emphysema)

iii. Esophagogram (inflammation, foreign body, extensive mass or vascular ring)

iv. Ultrasonography (assessment of anterior mediastinal mass, lymphadenopathy, differentiates cyst from mass and cellulitis from abscess)

v. Computed tomography/MRI (congenital anomalies, vascular airway compression)

vi. Video-optical intubation stylets (combines viewing capability with the familiar handling of intubation devices).

PEDIATRIC AIRWAY ASSESSMENT

Geetanjali S Verma

HISTORY

- Snoring, apnea, and day time somnolence (OSA)
- Stridor and hoarse voice
- Difficulty in feeding/phonation
- Nasal congestion and impaired smelling (adenoiditis)
- Prior surgery or radiation treatment to face or neck
- Review of previous anesthetic records with attention being paid to history of oropharyngeal injury, damage to teeth, awake tracheal intubation or postponement of surgery following an anesthetic.

EXAMINATION

- Evaluate size and shape of head
- Gross features of the face
- Size and symmetry of the mandible
- Presence of submandibular pathology, size of tongue, shape of palate, prominence of upper incisors, range of motion of jaw, head and neck.
- The presence of retractions (suprasternal/sternal/infrasternal/intercostal) should be sought for they usually are signs of airway obstruction
- Breath sounds—Crowing on inspiration (extrathoracic airway obstruction), noise on exhalation (intrathoracic lesions). Noise on inspiration and expiration usually is due to a lesion at thoracic inlet
- Cyanosis
- Mouth breathing or drooling (enlarged adenoids)
- Macroglossia and retrocline of the lower incisors are known to be associated with sleep apnea
- Loose deciduous dentition commonly occurs in children between 6 and 12 years old.

Mallampati and Cormack-Lehane classifications may be used in young adults.

The specific assessment tests mentioned for adults are not suitable for neonates in assessing difficult airway.

COPUR scale for airway evaluation

C: Chin (Side view)

Normal	1
Small/moderately hypoplastic	2
Markedly recessive	3
Extremely hypoplastic	4

O: Opening of Mouth	
>40 mm interdental space	1
20–40 mm	2
10–20 mm	3
<10 mm	4
P: Previous Intubation/OSA	
Previous attempt easy	1
No history of intubation/OSA	2
OSA/previous difficult intubation	3
Extremely difficult intubation/tracheostomy/patient Unable to lie supine	4
U: Uvula	
Whole uvula visible	1
Uvula partially visible	2
Uvula concealed, soft palate seen	3
Soft palate not visible	4
R: Range of Movement (look up and down)	
>120°	1
60–120°	2
30–60°	3
<30°	4

Prediction points:

5-7 points : normal

8–10 : laryngeal pressure may help

12 : increased difficulty, awake fiberoptic intubation (AFOI) preferred

14 : AFOI/advanced methods to prefer

16 : dangerous airway, consider awake intubation, potential tracheostomy

>10 score imply difficult airway.

INVESTIGATIONS

- Obtaining *blood gas and O_2 saturation* is important to determine patient's ability to compensate for airway problems.
- *Transcutaneous CO_2 determinations* are very helpful in infants and young children.
- *Radiological evaluation of the airway* offers noninvasive data on the structure of the pediatric airway. Standard radiographs provide information about the anatomy of the airway, with fluoroscopy being an additional tool.
- *Cephalometric radiography* is used to study the relationships between bony and soft tissue landmarks.

- *Computed tomography and magnetic resonance imaging* have been valuable in providing anatomical details comparable with endoscopy.
- *Endoscopy*: Provides views of the nasal fosse, choanae, pharynx and larynx, even in the neonate. It is also possible to achieve dynamic views of laryngeal and upper airway function.
- *USG studies*: Assist in evaluation of functional and organic airway disorders, assess the dynamic state of certain pathologies.
- *Sleep studies (Polysomnography)*: Best investigation to ascertain the severity of sleep disordered breathing in children. Measurements of the upper airway pressure-flow characteristics may be useful in evaluating upper airway function and sleep nasendoscopy has been used to determine the site of obstruction during sleep.

MNEMONICS

Difficult Bag Mask Ventilation: *MOANS/BONES*

M: Mask seal (beard/blood/mandibular hypoplasia)
O: Obesity and obstruction
A: Age
N: No teeth
S: Stiff lungs

(Bones: > 2 parameters positive = difficulty)

B: Beard
O: Obesity
N: No teeth
E: Elderly > 65 yrs
S: Snorer

Difficult Intubation: *LEMON*

L: Look: a rapid 'gut-feeling' assessment
E: Evaluate the 3-3-2 rule
M: Mallampati score see note below
O: Obesity/obstruction (stridor in particular is worrying)
N: Neck mobility

Difficult bag and mask ventilation (BMV) and Intubation: *HAVNOT*

H: History - including previous airway problems
A: Anatomy - anatomical features that may cause difficulty
V: Visual clues - such as obesity and the presence of a beard
N: Neck mobility and accessibility (including immobilization)
O: Opening of the mouth
T: Trauma

Difficult Placement of SGA (supraglottic airway devices): *RODS*

R: Restricted mouth opening
O: Obstruction of upper airway
D: Disrupted upper airway (trauma/burns)
S: Stiff lung/poor compliance

Difficulty in Surgical Airway Placement: BANG

B: Bleeding tendency
A: Agitated patient
N: Neck scarred/movement restriction
G: Growth in local area

Difficult Airway Assessment:

D: Dentition
D: Distortion
D: Disproportion
D: Dysmobility

3 Anesthetic Pharmacology

Geetanjali S Verma

PREOXYGENATION

Geetanjali S Verma

- Oxygen consumption during apnea is approximately 250 mL/minute (3 mL/kg per minute).
- In a healthy preoxygenated patient the safe apnea time is up to 8 minutes, compared to 1 minute if they were breathing room air.

GOALS

- Achieve SaO_2 = 100%.
- Denitrogenate the lungs (which serve as a large oxygen reservoir during apnea—450 mL of oxygen is present in the lungs when breathing room air; which increases to 3,000 mL when a patient breathes 100% oxygen).
- Oxygenate the blood.

BASICS

Arterial oxygen content (CaO_2): Hb × 1.36 × SaO_2 + PaO_2 × 0.003

(Where 1.36 is estimated mass volume of oxygen that can be bound by 1 g of Hb, SaO_2 is arterial oxyhemoglobin saturation [when fully saturated SaO_2 = 100%], 0.003 is the solubility coefficient of oxygen in human plasma).

The CaO_2 of blood with an hemoglobin (Hb) concentration of 15 g/dL is about 20 mL of oxygen per 100 dL of blood. In addition, about 0.3 mL of oxygen per 100 dL of blood is in physical solution. This amount of dissolved oxygen normally accounts for only 1.5% of the total oxygen, but this contribution increases when PaO_2 is increased (dissolved oxygen is linearly related to PaO_2). The venous oxygen content (CvO_2) of blood with a mixed venous oxygen tension (PvO_2) of 40 mm Hg and mixed venous oxyhemoglobin saturation (SvO_2) of 75% can be calculated accordingly.

Body Oxygen Stores during Room Air and 100% Oxygen Breathing

Store	*Room air*	*100% oxygen*
In the lungs (functional residual capacity	450 mL	3000 mL
In the blood	850 mL	950 mL
Dissolved or bound in tissue	250 mL	300 mL
Total	1550 mL	4250 mL

THE NEED FOR PREOXYGENATION (FIG. 1)

The alveolar gas equation is used to calculate PAO_2:

$$PaO_2 = PiO_2 - [PaCO_2/R]$$

When breathing air (21% O_2):

$$PaO_2 = 0.21 \times (101.3 - 6.7) - 5.3/0.8 = 13.2 \text{ kPa}$$

This is equivalent to 13% (273 mL) of oxygen in an functional residual capacity (FRC) of 2100 mL, the remaining contents being 75% nitrogen, and the 7% water vapor and 5% carbon dioxide used in the alveolar gas equation calculation.

For the purposes of calculation, oxygen consumption at rest is 3.5 mL/kg/min. In a 70 kg adult, approximately 250 mL/min of oxygen is consumed.

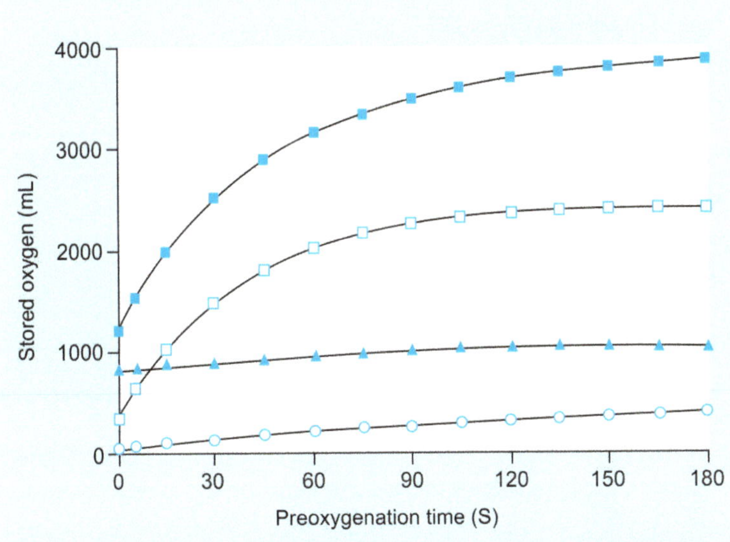

Fig. 1: Variation in volume of oxygen stored in the functional residual capacity (❑), the blood (▲), the tissue (o), and the whole body (▪) with duration of preoxygenation.

Thus, the FRC provides a reservoir of oxygen = 70 seconds worth of oxygen consumption. All of this oxygen cannot be extracted from the alveoli; once the PaO_2 falls below 6kPa, there will be little concentration gradient to maintain flux of oxygen to hemoglobin. The amount of usable oxygen in this reservoir is therefore likely to be only around 150 mL. Actual time to desaturation depends on a complex set of factors (balance between O_2 and CO_2 conc, obesity, pregnancy, pediatrics). Preoxygenation is a highly efficacious way of extending the time to exhaustion of oxygen reserves and desaturation.

When breathing 100% Oxygen:

$PaO_2 = (101.3 - 6.7) - [5.3/0.8] = 88$ kPa

This is equivalent to approximately 88% (1800 mL) of oxygen in the FRC equal to >7 minutes worth of oxygen consumption, or around ten times the amount of usable oxygen compared to breathing room air. This demonstrates that replacing the nitrogen in the FRC with oxygen greatly increases available reserves.

Factors Affecting the Efficacy and Efficiency of Preoxygenation

Factors affecting efficacy
Inspired oxygen concentration
Leak
System used
FGF, type of breathing (TVB or DB)
Duration of breathing
v_A/FRC
Factors affecting efficiency
Capacity of oxygen loading
PaO_2 and FRC
CaO_2 and CO
vO_2

(CaO_2: Arterial oxygen content; CO: Cardiac output; DB: Deep breathing; FGF: Fresh gas flow; PaO_2: Alveolar oxygen concentration; TVB: Tidal volume breathing; V_A/FRC: Alveolar ventilation to function residual capacity ratio; vO_2: Oxygen consumption).

Techniques of Preoxygenation

Tidal volume breathing
Traditional tidal volume breathing (3–5 min)
One vital capacity breath followed by tidal volume breathing
Deep breathing
Single vital capacity breath
4 deep breaths (4 inspiratory capacity breaths)
8 deep breaths (8 inspiratory capacity breaths)
Extended deep breathing (12–16 inspiratory capacity breaths)
One vital capacity breath followed by deep breathing

HOW TO DETERMINE COMPLETE PREOXYGENATION

- End-Tidal Oxygen Concentration > 80% (but the highest achievable ETO_2 should always be aimed)
- *Time*: 3 minutes with normal tidal ventilation and a good seal
- *Number of breaths*: 8 vital capacity breaths in 60 sec or 4 vital capacity breaths in 30 sec.

CALCULATING THE NEED FOR THREE MINUTES

O_2 carried in Hb= Hb conc x O_2 saturation x 1.39
O_2 dissolved in plasma= O_2 partial pressure x 0.022 mL/100 mL plasma

At the end of quiet expiration, FRC = 2500 mL

Given alveolar ventilation of 4L/min, and FRC of 2.5L, time constant = 2.5/4 = 0.625 minutes

Exponential washing of O_2:
After 1 time constant (0.63 minutes), preoxygenation of 37% complete
After 2 time constants (1.25 minutes), preoxygenation of 68% complete
After 3 time constants (1.9 minutes), preoxygenation of 95% would be complete.

APNEIC MASS MOVEMENT OXYGENATION

Preoxygenation followed by oxygen insufflation (using oro or nasopharyngeal cannula) during subsequent apnea maintains SaO_2 by apneic diffusion oxygenation.

In the apneic adult, total-body oxygen consumption is approx. 230 mL/min while the output of CO_2 to the alveoli is about 21 mL/min and the rest (about 90%) of CO_2 production is buffered within the body tissues. The lung volume initially decreases by the net gas exchange ratio of 209 mL/min. Thus, a pressure gradient is created between the upper airway and alveoli, resulting, if the airway is patent, in a subsequent mass movement of oxygen down the trachea into the alveoli. Conversely, CO_2 is not exhaled because of this mass movement of oxygen down the trachea and the alveolar carbon dioxide concentration ($PaCO_2$) shows an initial rise of about 8 to 16 mm Hg in the first minute and a subsequent fairly linear rise of about 3 mm Hg/min.

RAPID SEQUENCE INTUBATION

Geetanjali S Verma

Rapid sequence induction (RSI) is an established method of inducing anesthesia in patients who are at risk of aspiration of gastric contents into the lungs. The aim is to intubate the trachea as quickly and as safely as possible. This technique is employed daily during emergency surgery.

Factors associated with a high risk of aspiration include:

1. Abdominal pathology, especially obstruction or ileus
2. Delayed gastric emptying (e.g. pain, trauma, opioids, alcohol, vagotomy)
3. Incompetent lower esophageal sphincter, hiatus hernia, gastroesophageal reflux disease
4. Altered conscious level resulting in impaired laryngeal reflexes
5. Neurological or neuromuscular disease
6. Pregnancy
7. Difficult airway
8. Metabolic disturbances

SELLICK'S MANEUVER

Introduced by Sellick in 1961 to control regurgitation until intubation with a cuffed endotracheal tube was completed.

The maneuver consisted of "occlusion of the upper esophagus by backward pressure on the cricoid ring against the bodies of cervical vertebrae to prevent gastric contents from reaching the pharynx."

Sellick provided evidence that extension of the neck and application of cricoid pressure obliterated the esophageal lumen at the level of the 5th cervical vertebra (as seen in a previously placed soft latex tube distended with contrast media to a pressure of 100 cm H_2O).

The initial pressure of 10N to be applied in awake subjects and then slowly increased to 30N as the patient loses consciousness. Cricoid pressure should be released once tracheal intubation is confirmed.

Contraindications to the use of cricoid pressure:

i. Suspected cricotracheal injury
ii. Active vomiting
iii. Unstable cervical spine injuries.

Two handed Sellick's maneuver:

One hand kept behind the head for head and neck extension. The other hand's thumb and forefinger used for giving pressure on the cricoid.

BACK MANEUVER

A technique commonly used during laryngoscopy involves posterior displacement of the larynx by putting backward pressure on the thyroid or cricoid cartilage.

BURP MANEUVER: BACKWARD, UPWARD AND RIGHTWARD PRESSURE

Introduced by Knill in 1993 as a modification of Back maneuver.

It involves displacement of larynx as follows:

a. Posterior against the cervical vertebrae
b. As far as superior as possible
c. Slight displacement to the right.

This procedure displaces the thyroid cartilage dorsally in a way that the larynx is pressed against cervical vertebra body, 2 cm in cephalic direction, until resistance appears. Subsequently, it is displaced 0.5–2.0 cm to the right.

When the trachea is located in an anterior anatomic position (especially in small children) using this modification of cricoid pressure greatly facilitates the intubator's viewing of the larynx.

When the Sellick's maneuver was combined with BURP, the view worsened in 30% of patients in comparison to the control.

THE TECHNIQUE OF RAPID SEQUENCE INTUBATION (FIG. 2)

The equipment must be checked—working suction, capnography, and an adequate selection of endotracheal tubes and laryngoscopes. The trolley must tip to a head-down position easily. A wide bore IV cannula is connected to running fluid to ensure speedy circulation of drugs to the brain. The patient should be positioned in the optimal intubating position.

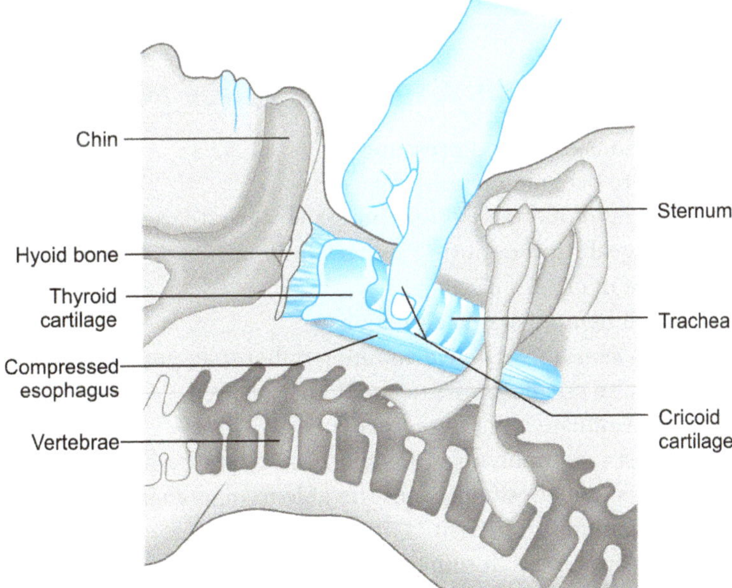

Fig. 2: Cricoid pressure in RSI.

Preoxygenation with oxygen 100% is essential to maximize the oxygen available to the patient from their functional residual capacity during induction. Oxygen is administered for 3–5 min or until the expired oxygen fraction is >85%.

A pre-calculated dose of induction agent is administered, followed immediately by a neuromuscular blocking agent. Cricoid pressure at 20–40 N or 2–4 kg (10N = 1 kg; >40N can cause esophageal rupture) is applied before loss of consciousness. After the jaw has relaxed and succinylcholine-associated fasciculations have ceased, the trachea is intubated. Placement of the endotracheal tube must be confirmed by ventilation, capnography and/or auscultation of the chest. After tube position and adequate seal are confirmed the cricoid pressure may be released.

Drugs for RSI

Induction agents
• Sodium thiopentone 3–7 mg/kg • Propofol 2–4 mg/kg • Etomidate 0.3 mg/kg • Ketamine 1–2 mg/kg
Neuromuscular blocking agents
• Succinylcholine 1 mg/kg • Rocuronium 1.2 mg/kg (reversal with sugammadex 16 mg/kg)

How is 40 N clinically determined?

It is the force that prevents swallowing of liquids in awake patients or the force that causes discomfort while pinching one's nose.

Cricoid yoke is a device that facilitates cricoid pressure of 44N.

COMPLICATIONS OF RAPID SEQUENCE INTUBATION

- Complications of cricoid pressure:
  - Failure to occlude the esophagus
  - Distortion of the larynx disrupting the view at laryngoscopy
  - Esophageal rupture during active vomiting
  - Fracture of cricoid cartilage
  - Minimal hemodynamic alterations
  - *Nausea/vomiting*: If active vomiting rather than passive regurgitation occurs, the cricoid pressure should be released.
- Failure to ventilate a paralyzed patient.
- Drugs most commonly used for RSI have relatively high incidences of anaphylaxis; the anesthetist must be able to treat anaphylaxis and support a compromised patient.
- The risk of awareness during the procedure is unlikely to have a dangerous outcome but is very distressing for patients.

DRUGS FOR INTUBATION

Geetanjali S Verma

6As of Premedication
- Anxiolysis
- Amnesia
- Antiemetic
- Antacid
- Anti-autonomic
- Analgesia

INTRAVENOUS INDUCTION

Most frequently used route where IV line is present.

INDUCTION AGENTS

The patient loses consciousness quickly as the concentration in the brain rises. The drug is then redistributed to other tissues causing fall in plasma concentration, which causes recovery.

Drug	*Induction dosage (mg/kg)*	*Speed of induction (sec)*	*Duration of action (mins)*	*Important effects on systems*	*Adverse effects*
Propofol	1.5–2.5	30–45	4–7	• Hypotension • Respiratory depression • Decreased cerebral blood flow (CBF) and intracranial pressure (ICP)	• Pain on injection • Myoclonic activity • Hiccoughs
Etomi-date	0.2–0.3	30–40	3–6	• Respiration depression • Decreased CBF and ICP • Anticonvulsant	• Pain on injection • Myoclonus • Hiccoughs
Thio-pentone	3–5	20–30	9–10	• Hypotension • Respiratory depression • Decreased CBF and ICP • Anticonvulsant	
Keta-mine	1–2	50–70	10–12	• Increased systemic vascular resistance (SVR) • Bronchodil mini-mum respiratory depression • Increased ICP • Analgesia	Hallucinations
Mida-zolam	0.1–0.3	40–70	10–15	• Hypotension • Respiratory depression • Mild anticonvulsant	

NEUROMUSCULAR BLOCKING AGENTS

	Depolarizing	*Non-depolarizing*		
Mechanism of action	Resemble Ach —act as Ach receptor agonist	Block Ach receptors—act as competitive antagonists		
Drugs	Succinylcholine		Steroid	Benzyl isoquinolinium
		Long acting	Pancuronium, pipecuronium	D-Tubocurarine, Doxacurium
		Inter-mediate	Vecuronium, rocuronium	Atracurium, Cisatra-curium
		Short		Mivacurium

Drug	*Dose of intuba-tion (mg/kg)*	*Main-tenance dose (mg/kg)*	*Time to intuba-tion (sec)*	*Dura-tion of action (mins)*	*Effects*	*Other comments*
Succinyl-choline	1.5	–	40–60	4–6	• Bradycardia (vagal stimu-lation) • Hyperkalemia (arrhythmias) • Malignant hyperpyrexia • Increased intraocular pressure (IOP) • Histamine release	• Used in RSI • Cautious use in – Glaucoma – Myopa-thies – Burns – Pseudo-choline-sterase defi-ciency
Atracu-rium	0.5–0.6	0.15–0.2 (30–50 mg/h)	90–120	20–25	• Histamine release • Hypotension	• Sponta-neous degradation (Hofmann elimination)*
Rocuro-nium	0.6–0.7	0.15–0.2 (30–50 mg/h)	90–100	20–30		• Alternative in RSI
Vecuro-nium	0.1	0.02–0.03 (6–10 mg/h)	90–120	15–20		
Mivacu-rium	0.15–0.2	0.1	100–120	10–15	• Histamine release in large doses	
Pancuro-nium	0.1	0.015	120–150	35–45	• Hypertension • Tachycardia	

ASSESSMENT OF NEUROMUSCULAR BLOCKADE

Clinical

- Head lift 5 sec
- Hand grip 5 sec
- Ability to produce vital capacity breath (>10 mL/kg)
- Tongue suppressor test

Peripheral nerve stimulation

- Train-of-four (TOF)
- Single twitch
- Double burst
- Tetanic stimulation
- Post-tetanic activity

ANALGESICS: OPIOIDS

Act on opioid receptors: most important are Mu and kappa.

Analgesia: mu, κ

Euphoria: mu

Sedation: κ

Depression of ventilation: mu, κ

Physical dependance: mu

Drug	*Dose (IV)*	*Onset of action*	*Duration of action (mins)*
Morphine	0.1–0.15 mg/kg	5–10 mins	40–60
Fentanyl	1–3 µg/kg	2–3 mins	20–30
Alfentanil	10 µg/kg 0.5–2 µg/kg/min	30–60 sec	5–10
Remifentanil	0.1–0.3 µg/kg/min	15–30 sec	Infusion dependent
Pethidine	1–2 mg/kg (IM)	15–20 mins	30–60

Effects on Systems

Cardiovascular system (CVS)	:	Peripheral venodilation, bradycardia (vagal stimulation)
Respiratory system (RS)	:	Bronchospasm, anti tussive
Gastrointestinal (GI)	:	Biliary sphincter spasm, nausea, vomiting, delays GI motility, urinary retention
Central nervous system (CNS)	:	Anlagesia, sedation, euphoria, depression of ventilation/vasomotor centre, nausea/vomiting
Endocrine	:	Release of antidiuretic hormone (ADH) and catecholamines
Others	:	Itching

INHALATIONAL INDUCTION

MAC: Minimal Alveolar Concentration

The concentration of an agent required to prevent movement in 50% subjects when exposed to a noxious stimulus at 1 atm pressure.

- Preferred in children/without IV line
- Slower induction than IV agents
- Sevoflurane is the most preferred agent
- Iso/Des/En - flurane, being pungent cause irritation of the airway, thus increasing chances of bronchospasm.

Agent	MAC in O_2 (%)	Effects	Comments
Sevoflurane	2.2	• Vasodilation • Depresses ventilation	
Isoflurane	1.3	• Hypotension, tachycardia • Depresses ventilation	Pungent
Desflurane	6.0	• Hypotension, tachycardia • Depresses ventilation	Pungent
Halothane	0.75	• Hypotension • Myocardial depression • Arrhythmias • Increased CBF and ICP	Halothane hepatitis*
Enflurane	1.6	• Hypotension • Depresses ventilation	Pungent

Nitrous Oxide

- Colorless
- Sweet smelling
- Non-irritating
- Moderate analgesic property
- Low anesthetic potency (MAC 105%)
- Effects:
  - CVS: Myocardial depression, exacerbated in pre-existing cardiac dis
  - RS: Increases RR, decreases VT
  - CNS: Cerebral vasodilation (increases ICP)
  - Others: Diffuses into air cavities (ear, sinuses, gut, etc.)
    - **Diffusion hypoxia***
    - Bone marrow supression, inhibits DBA synthesis
    - Teratogenic

***Diffusion Hypoxia/Fink Effect/3rd Gas Effect**

When a patient is recovering from N_2O anesthesia, large quantities of N_2O cross from the blood into the alveolus (down its concentration gradient) and thus O_2 and CO_2 in the alveolus are diluted by this gas. This causes the partial pressure of oxygen to decrease and leads to hypoxia. The decrease in CO_2 could also potentiate this effect as ventilation would be suppressed, leading to potential hypoxemia.

Contd...

Contd...

Halothane Hepatitis

Type I

Benign, self-limiting, and relatively common (up to 25–30% of those that receive halothane).

Mild transient increases in serum transaminase and glutathione S-transferase concentrations and by altered postoperative drug metabolism.

Results from reductive (anaerobic) biotransformation of halothane rather than the normal oxidative pathway.

Type II

Associated with massive centrilobular liver necrosis, fulminant liver failure, Fatality rate 50%.

Clinically: Fever, jaundice, and grossly elevated serum transaminase levels. Immune mediated.

Hofmann Elimination

Spontaneous non-enzymatic breakdown at physiological pH and temperature.

ADJUNCTIVE MEDICATIONS

(Discussed in Prevention of Aspiration)

STAGES OF ANESTHESIA

1st: Consciousness lost
Puplls equal and reactive
Muscle tone normal
Breathing by intercostal muscles and diaphragm

2nd: Stage of excitation
Pupils dilated
Eye lash reflex lost
Breath holding/coughing

3rd: Stage of surgical anesthesia
Reduced respiratory activity, intercostal muscles paralyzed
Muscle tone reduced
Layngeal reflex lost
Pupils dilated
Ends with diaphragmatic paralysis

4th: Stage of medullary depression
Loss of all reflexes
Pupils dilated and fixed
Apnea

ANESTHETIZING AIRWAY FOR AWAKE INTUBATION

Supraja Nagaiah

Successful airway management requires a range of knowledge and skill - specifically, the ability to predict difficulty with airway management, to formulate a plan and necessary skill to execute it. Flexible scope intubation of the trachea in an awake, spontaneously ventilating patient is the gold standard for the management of difficult airway. In 1993, the American Society of Anesthesiologists (ASA) published the first Practice Guidelines for Management of the Difficult Airway, which was updated in 2013. It defines the difficult airway as "the clinical situation in which a conventionally trained anesthesiologist experiences difficulty with ventilation of the upper airway via a mask, difficulty with tracheal intubation, or both" and provides guidelines for the evaluation of the airway and preparation for difficult airway management, including a "Difficult Airway Algorithm" intended to guide clinical decision making when an anesthesiologist is faced with a known or potential difficult airway. In this chapter, we will discuss about preparation for awake intubation. Evaluation and management is discussed elsewhere. Preparation of airway enables anesthetist to use any mode of airway intervention, invasive or noninvasive.

Advantages of Awake Intubation

1. Patency of the airway is maintained by intact upper pharyngeal muscle tone.
2. Spontaneous ventilation is maintained.
3. A patient who is awake and well topicalized is easier to intubate, because the larynx moves to a more anterior position after induction of anesthesia compared with the awake state.
4. The patient can still protect his or her airway from aspiration.
5. The ability to monitor for neurologic symptoms (e.g., the patient with potential cervical pathology).

Indications for Awake Intubation

Known or suspected difficulty with mask ventilation or tracheal intubation.

Contraindication

No absolute contraindications other than patient refusal, a patient who is unable to cooperate (such as a child, a mentally retarded patient, or an intoxicated, combative patient), or a patient with a documented true allergy to all local anesthetics.

Preparation

Given below are the six basic elements of preparation for awake intubation.

Element	*Underlying concept action*
Explanation	• Patients understands safety
Preoperative preparation	• Maintain oxygenation and safety
Premedication and sedation	• Maintain patient airway control
Dessication	• Dry the airway
Topicalization	• Anesthetize and obtund reflexes
Procrastination	• Awake intubation (AI) cannot be rushed

Explanation

In this section, the focus is placed on elective patients, for whom there is time for airway evaluation and meaningful communication. Previous anesthesia records should be read carefully. Special attention is given to intubation records. Look for patient position, equipment used and complications encountered.

After the anesthesia practitioner has made the decision that AI is necessary, communication with the patient and psychological preparation is of the utmost importance to maximize the odds for a successful AI. One should in a careful, unhurried manner describe to the patient conventional intu bation contrasted with AI. Focusing on the fact that the former is easier and less time-consuming but that the latter is safer in light of the patient's own anatomy or condition, one must communicate to the patient that the knowledgeable, caring physician is willing to take extra measures to ensure the patient's safety.

Preoperative Preparation

Preparation depends on acuteness of the situation. In emergency situation, as in cervical trauma or stridor, requires immediate intubation in the emergency room. These patients require complete monitoring using pulse oximeter, ECG, noninvasive blood pressure and end-tidal carbon dioxide monitor. These patients are transported to the OR with monitoring and adequate supplemental oxygen.

In the elective scenario, supplemental O_2 should be provided, if appropriate (high-dose O_2 may be detrimental in some patients, such as those who rely on hypoxic respiratory drive), and position should be considered (e.g. the patient who is morbidly obese may experience dramatic physiologic changes when supine and should be transported in a wheelchair or on a gurney in a semi-recumbent position) while transporting the patient to OR.

Administration of supplemental O_2 should be considered throughout the process of AI management. Arterial hypoxemia has been well documented during bronchoscopy, with an average decrease in arterial oxygen tension (PaO_2) of 20 to 30 mm Hg in patients breathing room air, and has been associated with cardiac dysrhythmias. In addition, sedation administered to supplement topicalization of AI may result in respiratory depression. In addition to the standard methods of supplemental O_2 delivery (nasal cannula or face mask), other opportunities include, but are not limited to, delivering O_2 through the suction port of a flexible fiberoptic bronchoscope (FFB), delivering O_2 through an atomizer or nebulizer during topicalization, and elective transtracheal jet ventilation (TTJV) in a patient in extremis.

Proper preparation enhances success. Equipment readiness is of crucial importance. There are many techniques that can be used to secure the airway in the awake patient. Direct laryngoscopy, video laryngoscopy, intubating laryngeal mask airways (iLMAs), FFB, rigid fiberoptic laryngoscopy, retrograde intubation, lighted stylets, and blind nasal intubation have all been used successfully to perform AI. No matter which technique is selected, all of the necessary equipment should be prepared ahead of time and readily available when needed. The practitioner should also have several backup modalities in mind, and the required equipment available, in case the initial technique used is ineffective. A preassembled difficult airway cart saves time. The following box gives the equipment required for difficult airway management suggested by ASA task force on management of difficult airway.

Suggested Contents of the Portable Unit for Difficult Airway Management

Benumof JL (editor). Clinical Procedures in Anesthesia and Intensive Care. Philadelphia, 2002, Lippincott Williams & Wilkins, pp 253–274.

- Rigid laryngoscope blades of alternative designs and sizes from those routinely used; this may include a rigid fiberoptic laryngoscope
- Endotracheal tubes (ETTs) of assorted sizes and styles, such as the Parker FlexTip tube (Parker Medical, Highlands Ranch, CO) or the Endotrol tube (Covidien-Nellcor, Boulder, CO)
- ETT guides, such as semirigid stylets, ventilating tube changer, light wands, and forceps designed to manipulate the distal portion of the ETT
- Laryngeal mask airways of assorted sizes and styles, such as the intubating laryngeal mask airway and the LMA-Proseal (LMA North America, Inc., San Diego, CA)
- Fiberoptic intubation equipment
- Retrograde intubation equipment
- At least one device for emergency nonsurgical airway ventilation, such as a transtracheal jet ventilation stylet or the esophageal-tracheal Combitube (Kendall-Sheridan Catheter Corporation, Argyle, NY)
- Equipment suitable for emergency surgical airway access (e.g. cricothyrotomy)
- An exhaled CO_2 detector
- Pulse oximetry unit.

The items listed in this table represent suggestions. The contents of the portable storage unit should be customized to meet the specific needs, preferences, and skills of the practitioner and health care facility.

Premedication and Sedation

Premedication includes antisialogouges, drugs for antiaspiration prophylaxis and sedative/hypnotics. Antisialogogues will be discussed in next section on dessication which is the most important goal of preparation.

Aspiration Prophylaxis

1. Histamine receptor blockers
2. Proton pump inhibitors
3. Metoclopramide
4. Nonparticulate antacid.

Sedation/Hypnotics

Intravenous sedation may be useful in allowing the patient to tolerate AI by providing anxiolysis, amnesia, and analgesia. Benzodiazepines, opioids, hypnotics, α_2-agonists, and neuroleptics can be used alone or in combination. It is important that these agents be carefully titrated to effect, because oversedation can render a patient uncooperative and make AI more difficult and can also lead to respiratory depression.

Dessication

One of the most important goals of premedication for AI is drying of the airway. Secretions can obscure the view of the glottis, especially when FFB is used. In addition, secretions can prevent local anesthetics from reaching intended areas, resulting in failed sensory blockade, or they can wash away and dilute local anesthetics, diminishing their potency and duration of action. Anticholinergics should be administered at least 30 minutes before topicalization. The anticholinergics used in clinical practice are atropine, glycopyrrolate and scopolamine.

Pharmacologic characteristics of anticholinergic drugs.

Drugs	*Tachycardia*	*Antisialagogue effect*	*Sedation*
Atropine	+++	++	+
Glycopyrrolate	++	+++	0
Scopolamine	+	+++	+++

Doses
Atropine—0.4–0.6 mg IV or IM
Glycopyrrolate—0.2–0.3 mg IV or IM
Scopolamine—0.4 mg IV or IM

Topicalization

Topicalization of the airway with local anesthetics is the primary method of anesthetizing for AI. Many times topical anesthesia alone is adequate for AI. When using local anesthetics, it is important to be familiar with the speed of onset, duration of action, optimal concentration, signs and symptoms of toxicity, and maximum recommended dosage of the drug chosen. The rate and amount of topical local anesthetic absorption vary depending on the site of application, the concentration and total dose of local anesthetic applied, the hemodynamic status of the patient, and individual patient variation. Local anesthetic absorption is more rapid from the alveoli than from the tracheobronchial tree, and more rapid from the tracheobronchial tree than from the pharynx. The most commonly used agents for topical anesthesia of the airway are lidocaine and cocaine.

Lidocaine

Lidocaine, an amide local anesthetic, is the most commonly used agent for airway topicalization. It is available in various concentrations (1–10%) and in preparations including aqueous and viscous solutions, ointments, gels, and creams. For topical anesthesia, the concentration used is 2% to 4%. When nasal AI is planned lidocaine is used with phenylephrine in a 3:1 mixture which provides good vasoconstriction of nasal and nasopharynx mucosa. Lidocaine is an excellent choice for airway anesthesia because of its reasonably rapid onset of 2 to 5 minutes and its high therapeutic index. Its duration of action is 30 to 60 minutes after topical application or infiltration; addition of epinephrine extends the duration to 2 to 3 hours when used for infiltration. It is hepatically metabolized with a half-life of 90 minutes; care should be taken in patients with hepatic failure. The maximum recommended dosage for infiltration of lidocaine without epinephrine is 5 mg/kg of lean body mass. For topicalization of the airway, the maximum dose is less well established. The British Thoracic Society recommends a maximum dose of 8.2 mg/kg. Early symptoms of lidocaine toxicity include euphoria, dizziness, tinnitus, confusion, and a metallic taste in the mouth. Signs of severe lidocaine toxicity include seizures, respiratory failure, loss of consciousness, and circulatory collapse. In asthmatics, lidocaine has been reported to precipitate bronchoconstriction by a nonhistamine-mediated mechanism.

Cocaine

Cocaine, a naturally occurring ester anesthetic, is used primarily for anesthesia of the nasal mucosa when the nasal route is planned for AI. It has a vasoconstrictor property that makes it particularly useful for this application, because the nose is highly vascularized and bleeding can make fiberoptic intubation (FOI) impossible. It is available commercially as a 4% solution (each drop containing 3 mg), and can be applied to the nasal mucosa using cotton pledgets or cotton-tipped swabs. The maximum recommended dosage for intranasal application is 1.5 mg/kg. After topical application of cocaine to the nasal mucosa, peak plasma levels are achieved in 30 to 45 minutes, and the drug persists in the plasma for 5 to 6 hours.Cocaine is primarily metabolized by plasma pseudocholinesterase; it also undergoes slow hepatic metabolism and is excreted unchanged by the kidney. The signs and symptoms of cocaine toxicity include tachycardia, cardiac dysrhythmia, hypertension, and fever. Severe complications include convulsions, respiratory failure, coronary spasm, cardiac arrest, stroke, and death. It must be used with caution in patients with hypertension, coronary artery disease, hyperthyroidism, pseudocholinesterase deficiency, or preeclampsia, and in those patients taking monoamine oxidase inhibitors.

Other Local Anesthetics

Benzocaine is most commonly available as a 20% aerosol spray that is easily applied to the oropharyngeal mucosa. The limiting factor in benzocaine use is the potential development of clinically significant methemoglobinemia. Symptoms of early methemoglobinemia toxicity can be seen with methemoglobin levels of 5% and include cyanosis, tachycardia, and tachypnea. As levels increase to 20% to 30%, patients may develop chest pain, ischemic changes on ECG, hypotension, altered mental status, syncope, or coma. The most severe cases have led to neurologic hypoxic injury, myocardial infarction, and death. Should symptomatic methemoglobin occur, treatment is with methylene blue 1 to 2 mg/kg IV given over 5 minutes.

Tetracaine is an amide local anesthetic agent with a longer duration of action than lidocaine or cocaine. It is available as 0.5% to 1% solutions for local use. It is metabolized through hydrolysis by plasma cholinesterase. Tetracaine is rapidly absorbed from the respiratory and gastrointestinal tract when used to anesthetize the airway, and aerosol doses as small as 20 mg have been shown to precipitate toxicity. Severe toxic reactions after tetracaine overdose include convulsions, respiratory arrest, and circulatory collapse.

Cetacaine is a topical application spray containing 14% benzocaine, 2% tetracaine, and 2% butyl aminobenzoate (a local anesthetic similar to benzocaine). Like 20% benzocaine spray, this combination produces rapid airway anesthesia, but with a prolonged duration of action compared to benzocaine alone. The risk of methemoglobinemia is still a consideration, and cases of severe toxicity have been reported.

Eutectic mixture of local anesthetic (EMLA) cream contains 2.5% lidocaine and 2.5% prilocaine and is considered a topical anesthetic for use on intact skin. Although the manufacturer does not recommend its use on mucosal surfaces because of faster systemic absorption, it has been employed safely as a topical anesthetic for AI. Larijani and colleagues described 20 adult patients who underwent awake FOI using 4 g of EMLA applied over the upper airway. The measured peak plasma concentrations of lidocaine or prilocaine did not reach toxic levels, and methemoglobin levels did not exceed normal values.

Benzonatate, an oral antitussive chemically similar to ester-type local anesthetics, has also been used for airway topicalization. The dose used is 200 mg; the capsules are pierced with a needle, and the patient is instructed to crush the capsules with the teeth or to hold the capsules in the back of the mouth. Oropharyngeal anesthesia is quickly obtained.

Application Techniques

Atomizers (Fig. 3): A common method for applying local anesthetic to the airway is with an atomizer. One system for local anesthetic atomization involves the use of a standard DeVilbiss atomizer with the bulb removed. The atomizer reservoir is filled with 2% to 4% lidocaine. O_2 tubing is connected from the atomizer to an O_2 cylinder with a flow rate of 8 to 10 L/min. A bleed hole is cut in the O_2 tubing; this allows for intermittent application of the local anesthetic when a thumb is placed over the hole in the tubing. The atomizer spray is directed toward the soft palate and posterior pharynx to topicalize the mucosa. Any residual anesthetic agent in the oropharynx should be suctioned out to reduce absorption from the gastrointestinal tract. Disposable plastic atomizers are available for this purpose as well. The device is attached to an O_2 tank, and the phalange is depressed to deliver the local anesthetic solution to the oropharyngeal mucosa. A disadvantage with these methods is the difficulty of controlling the exact amount of local anesthetic administered.

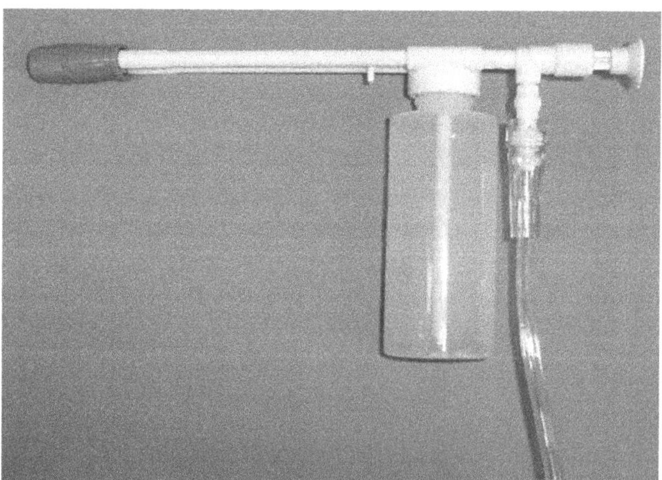

Fig. 3: Typical disposable atomizer.

Nebulizers: Nebulizers may be used to apply local anesthetic to the airway. The advantages of this technique include ease of application and safety. A standard mouthpiece-type nebulizer can topicalize the oropharynx and trachea. If nasal cavity anesthesia is needed, a face mask type nebulizer can be used; the patient is instructed to breathe in through the nose. This approach is especially advantageous for patients with increased intracranial pressure (ICP), open eye injury, or severe coronary artery disease. A typical dose of lidocaine used in a standard nebulizer is 4 mL of 4% lidocaine. This results in a total dose of 160 mg of lidocaine, which is well within the safe dosage range.

"Spray-As-You-Go": In addition to using a nebulizer or an atomizer to anesthetize the vocal cords and trachea, a technique termed "spray-as-you-go" through the FFB can be performed. The technique is noninvasive and involves injecting local anesthetics through the suction port of the fiberoptic bronchoscope (FOB). Two methods have been described. The first requires attaching a triple stopcock to the proximal portion of the suction port to connect O_2 tubing from a regulated O_2 tank set to flow at 2 to 4 L/min. Under direct vision through the bronchoscope, targeted areas are sprayed with aliquots of 0.2 to 1.0 mL of 2% to 4% lidocaine. The physician then waits 30 to 60 seconds before advancing to deeper structures and repeating the maneuver. The flow of O_2 allows higher delivery of a higher fraction of inspired oxygen (FIO_2), keeps the FOB lens clean, disperses mucous secretions away from the lens, and aids in nebulizing the local anesthetic. The second method involves passing a multi-orifice epidural catheter (0.5 - 1.0-mm inner diameter [ID]) through the suction port of an adult FOB. These techniques are especially useful in patients who are at risk for aspirating gastric contents because the topical anesthetic is applied only seconds before the intubation is accomplished, allowing the patient to maintain airway reflexes as long as possible.

Nerve Blocks (Fig. 4)

The following nerve blocks are remarkable for their ease of performance, their minimal risk to the patient, and their speed of onset. Nerve blocks are applied to the nasal cavity and nasopharynx, the oropharynx, the larynx and the trachea and vocal cords.

Clinical Pearls

[Regional and Topical anesthesia for endotracheal intubation. (www.nysora.com)]

- Three major neural pathways supply sensation to airway structures.
- Terminal branches of the ophthalmic and maxillary divisions of the trigeminal nerve supply the nasal cavity and turbinates.
- The oropharynx and posterior third of the tongue are supplied by the glossopharyngeal nerve.
- Branches of the vagus nerve innervate the epiglottis and more distal airway structures.

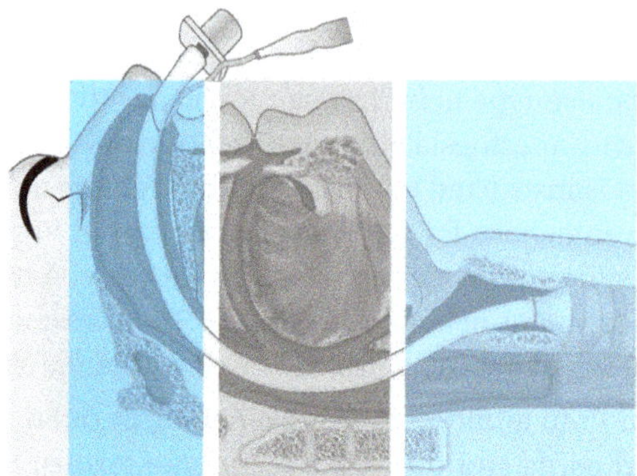

Fig. 4: Innervation of the upper airway.
(*Source*: Brown D [editor]. Atlas of Regional Anesthesia, 2nd edn. Philadelphia, 1999, Saunders).

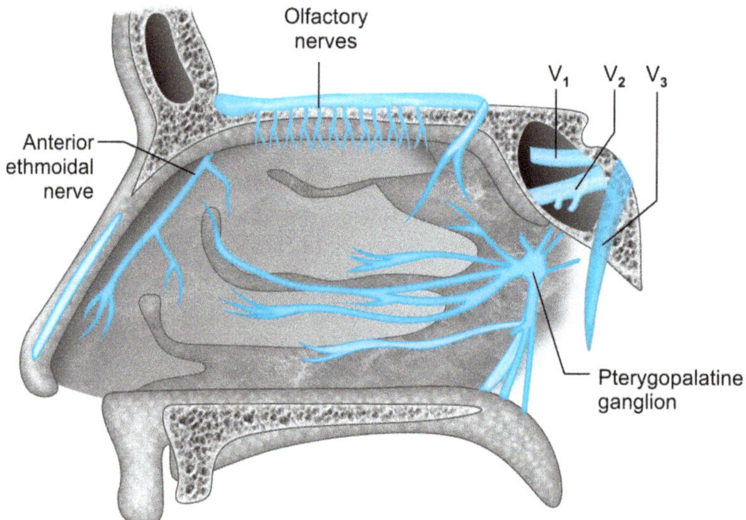

Fig. 5: Innervation of nasal cavity showing anterior ethmoidal, olfactory and trigeminal nerves.
(*Source*: Difficult Airway: Teaching Aids. Irvine, University of California, Department of Anesthesia).

Nasal Cavity and Nasopharynx

The nasal cavity is innervated by the greater and lesser palatine nerves and the anterior ethmoidal nerve (Fig. 5). The palatine nerves arise from the pterygopalatine ganglion which derives sensory nerves from sphenopalatine branches of the maxillary nerve, cranial nerve (CN-v) and innervate the nasal turbinates and most of the nasal septum. The pterygopalatine ganglion is located posterior to the middle turbinate in the pterygopalatine fossa. The anterior ethmoidal nerve arises from the olfactory nerve (CN I) and innervates the nares and the anterior third of the nasal septum.

Nares should first be inspected for a deviated septum by using a nasal speculum and asking the patient to breathe deeply through each individual naris while the opposite naris is occluded.

Nasal cavity can be anesthetized by packing it with cotton pledgets or by performing direct nerve blocks.

Nasal Packing

Place cotton pledgets soaked in either 4% cocaine or 4% lidocaine with epinephrine 1 : 200,000 along the floor of the nasal cavity. The pledgets are advanced posteriorly to the level of the posterior nasopharyngeal wall. The benefits of this technique are that initial topicalization of the nasal cavity is achieved, the angle of endotracheal tube (ETT) insertion can be predicted, and dilation of the nasal cavity is initiated.

Sphenopalatine Nerve Block

Oral approach (Fig. 6): With the patient in the supine position, the physician stands facing the patient on the contralateral side of the nerve to be blocked. Using the nondominant index finger, the physician identifies the greater palatine foramen. It is located on either side of the roof of the mouth between the second and third maxillary molars, approximately 1 cm medial to the palatogingival margin, and can usually be palpated as a small depression near the posterior edge of the hard palate. A 25-G spinal needle, bent 2 to 3 cm proximal to the tip to an angle of 120°, is inserted through the foramen in a superior and slightly posterior direction to a depth of 2 to 3 cm. An aspiration test is performed to ascertain that the sphenopalatine artery has not been cannulated, and 1 to 2 mL of 2% lidocaine with epinephrine 1 : 100,000 is injected. The epinephrine is used as a vasoconstrictor for the sphenopalatine artery, which runs parallel to the nerves, to decrease the incidence of epistaxis. The injection of the local anesthetic should be performed in a slow, continuous fashion (preventing acute increases in pressure within the fossa) to decrease sympathetic stimulation. This block anesthetizes the greater and lesser palatine nerves as well as the nasociliary and nasopalatine nerves, which also contribute to the sensory innervation of the nasal cavity. Complications include bleeding, infection, nerve trauma, intravascular injection of local anesthetic, and hypertension.

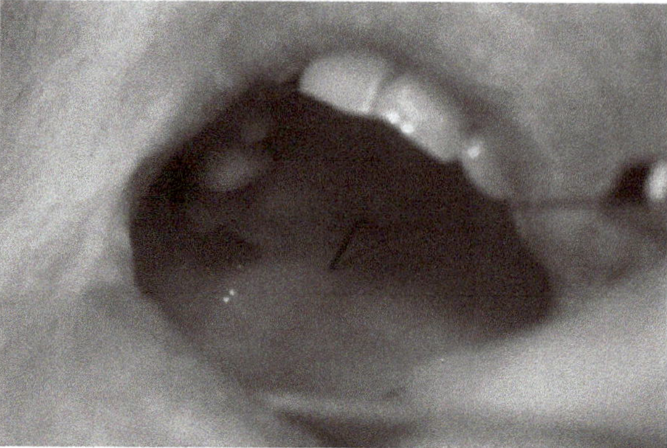

Fig. 6: Right sphenopalatine nerve block, oral approach.

Nasal approach: Noninvasive nasal approaches to the sphenopalatine ganglion block takes advantage of the ganglion's shallow position beneath the nasal mucosa. It involves the application of long cotton tipped applicators soaked in either 4% cocaine or 4% lidocaine with epinephrine 1:200,000 over the mucosal surface overlying the ganglion. The applicator is passed along the upper border of the middle turbinate at an angle of approximately 45° to the hard palate and directed posteriorly until the upper posterior wall of the nasopharynx (sphenoid bone) is reached. The applicator is then left in place for 5 to 10 minutes.

Anterior Ethmoidal Nerve Block

The anterior ethmoidal nerve is blocked by insertion of a long cotton-tipped applicator, soaked in either 4% cocaine or 4% lidocaine with epinephrine 1 : 200,000, parallel to the dorsal surface of the nose until it meets the anterior surface of the cribriform plate (Fig. 7).

OROPHARYNX

The oropharynx, soft palate, posterior portion of the tongue, and the pharyngeal surface of the epiglottis are innervated by the glossopharyngeal nerve. Block of the glossopharyngeal nerve facilitates endotracheal intubation by blocking the gag reflex associated with direct laryngoscopy as well as facilitating passage of a nasotracheal tube through the posterior pharynx. The glossopharyngeal nerve travels anterior along the lateral surface of the pharynx, and its three branches provide sensory innervation to the posterior third of the tongue, the vallecula, the anterior surface of the epiglottis (lingual branch), the walls of the pharynx (pharyngeal branch), and the tonsils (tonsillar branch). Logically, blockade of this nerve bilaterally would result in anesthesia of those structures.

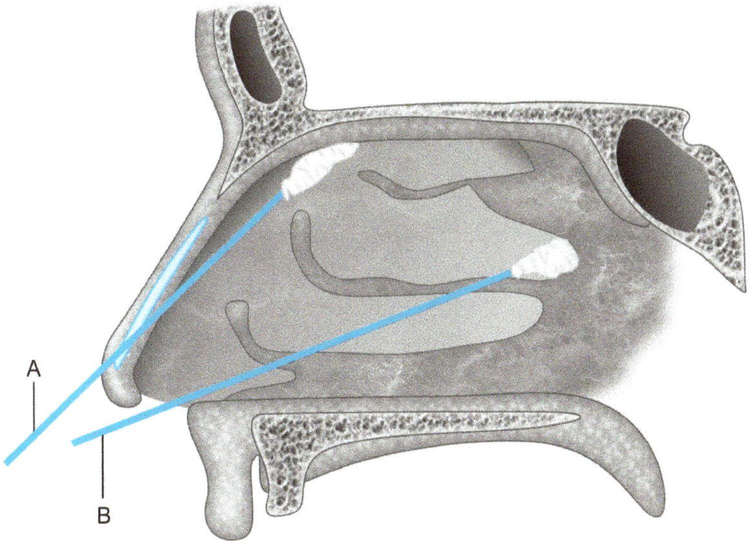

Fig. 7: Left lateral view of the right nasal cavity, showing long cotton-tipped applicators soaked in local anesthetic.
(A) Applicator angled at 45 degrees to the hard palate with cotton swab over mucosal surface overlying the sphenopalatine ganglion. (B) Applicator placed parallel to the dorsal surface of the nose, blocking anterior ethmoidal nerve. (*From Difficult Airway: Teaching Aids. Irvine, University of California, Department of Anesthesia*).

The glossopharyngeal nerve can be anesthetized using either intraoral or extraoral (peristyloid) approaches.

For the intraoral approach, the mouth is opened and the tongue is anesthetized with topical anesthetic. A 3⅓ -in., 22-gaugue needle is used to place 5 mL of local anesthetic solution submucosally at the caudal aspect of the posterior tonsillar pillar (palatopharyngeal fold) (Fig. 8).

To perform the peristyloid approach to the glossopharyngeal block, the patient is placed supine and a line is drawn between the angle of the mandible and the mastoid process. Using deep pressure, the styloid process is palpated just posterior to the angle of the jaw along this line, and a short, small-gauge needle is seated against the styloid process. The needle is then withdrawn slightly and directed posteriorly off the styloid process. As soon as bony contact is lost, 5–7 mL of local anesthetic solution are injected after careful aspiration for blood. Both approaches involve deposition of local anesthetic in close proximity to the carotid artery, and careful aspiration before injection is essential.

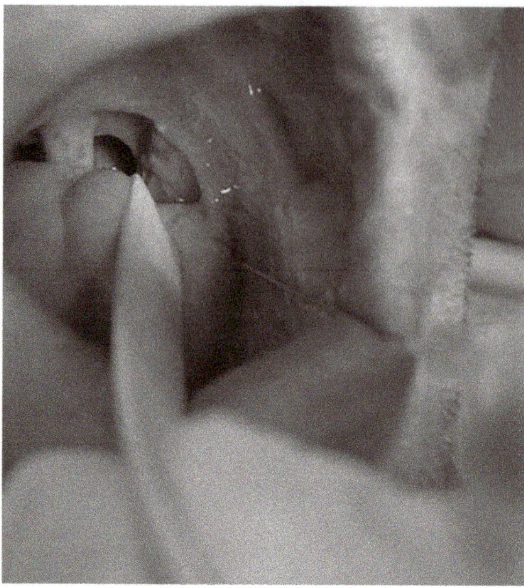

Fig. 8: Intraoral approach to glossopharyngeal nerve block.

Clinical Pearls

[Regional and Topical Anesthesia for Endotracheal Intubation. (www.nysora.com)]

- The glossopharyngeal nerve provides sensory innervation to the posterior third of the tongue, the vallecula, the anterior surface of the epiglottis (lingual branch), the walls of the pharynx (pharyngeal branch), and the tonsils (tonsillar branch).
- It is most easily blocked where it crosses the palatoglossal arch.
- It can be blocked using one of three methods: Topical spray application, direct mucosal contact of soaked pledgets, or direct infiltration by injection (Figs. 8 and 9).
- Glossopharyngeal nerve block is not adequate as a solo technique to facilitate intubation, but in combination with other techniques it is highly effective.

LARYNX

Superior Laryngeal Nerve Block (Fig. 10)

External Approach

The superior laryngeal nerve (SLN), a branch of the vagus nerve, provides sensory input from the lower pharynx and the upper part of the larynx, including the glottic surface of the epiglottis and the aryepiglottic folds.

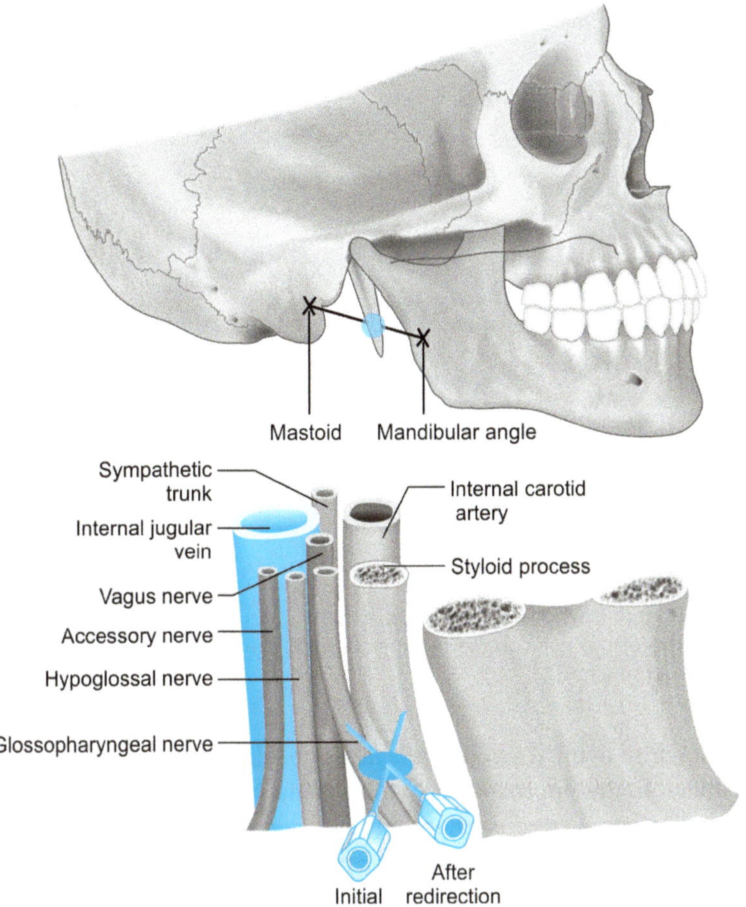

Fig. 9: Glossopharyngeal nerve block, peristyloid approach. A 22-G spinal needle is inserted to contact the styloid process. It is then redirected posteriorly, putting the tip of the needle near the glossopharyngeal nerve.
(*Source:* Brown D, [editor]. Atlas of Regional Anesthesia, 2nd edn. Philadelphia, 1999, Saunders).

Superior laryngeal nerve block is performed bilaterally. A block of this nerve may be achieved using one of three landmarks. Using either the superior cornu of the hyoid or the superior cornu of the thyroid cartilage, a 25-gauge spinal needle is walked off the cornu anteriorly toward the thyrohyoid ligament.

Resistance is felt as the needle is advanced through the ligament, usually at a depth of 1 to 2 cm. After negative aspiration for blood and air, 1.5 to 2 mL of 2% lidocaine is injected and then repeated on the opposite side. The third landmark for the superior laryngeal nerve block is particularly useful in patients who are obese, in whom palpation of the hyoid or the

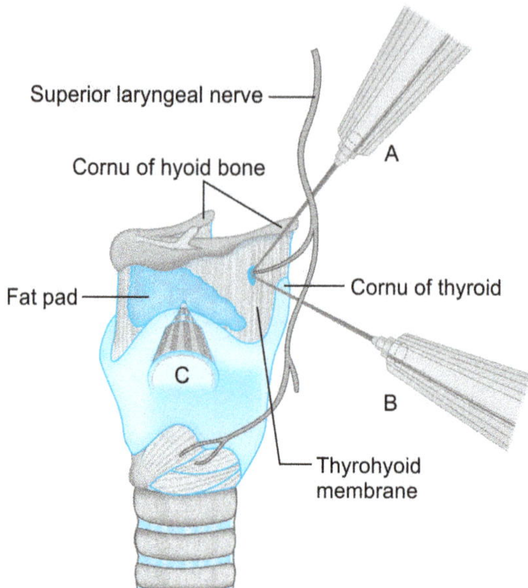

Fig. 10: Superior laryngeal nerve block, external approach using as a landmark the greater cornu of the hyoid bone (A), the superior cornu of the thyroid cartilage (B), or the thyroid notch (C).

superior cornu of the thyroid cartilage may be difficult or uncomfortable for the patient. In this approach, the needle is inserted 2 cm lateral to the superior notch of the thyroid cartilage and directed in a posterior and cephalad direction to 1 to 1.5 cm depth, where 2 mL of 2% lidocaine is infiltrated and, again, repeated on the contralateral side.

Complications include trauma to vocal cords due to deep injections or improper identification of landmarks, injection of LA into carotid artery causing seizures, bradycardia and hypotension. Possible causes of bradycardia and hypotension are (1) vasovagal reaction related to painful stimulation, (2) digital pressure on the carotid sinus, (3) excessive manipulation of the larynx causing vasovagal reaction, (4) large doses of or accidental intravascular administration of local anesthetic drugs, and (5) direct neural stimulation of the branch of the vagus nerve by the needle.

Internal Approach

A noninvasive SLN block can be performed by applying local anesthetic to the pyriform recess. At this anatomic location, the internal branch of the SLN lies submucosally, and blockade is possible by diffusion of concentrated local anesthetic. After adequate topicalization of the oropharynx, the patient is placed in the sitting position with the physician standing on the contralateral side of the nerve to be blocked. The patient's mouth is opened widely with the tongue protruded. The tongue is grasped with the nondominant hand using a gauze pad and gently pulled anteriorly, or it is depressed with a tongue blade. With the dominant hand, a Krause forceps holding a sponge soaked in 4% lidocaine is advanced over the lateral posterior curvature of the tongue along the downward continuation of the tonsillar fossa. The tip of the forceps is advanced until it cannot be advanced any farther; at that point, the handle of the forceps should be in a horizontal position and the tip should be resting in the pyriform recess. The position of the tip of the forceps may be checked by palpating the neck lateral to the posterior-superior aspect of the thyroid cartilage. The forceps are kept in this position for 5 minutes or longer, and then the process is repeated on the opposite side. This approach requires a considerable length of time and is limited to those patients who can open their mouths sufficiently wide.

TRACHEA AND VOCAL CORDS

The sensory innervation of the trachea, inferior larynx, and vocal cords is supplied by the recurrent (inferior) laryngeal nerves, branches of the vagus nerve. The right recurrent laryngeal nerve (RLN) originates at the level of the right subclavian artery; the left originates at the level of the aortic arch, distal to the ligamentum arteriosum. Both ascend along the tracheoesophageal groove to supply sensory innervation to the tracheobronchial tree up to and including the vocal cords, as well as supplying motor nerve fibers to the intrinsic muscles of the larynx (except the cricothyroid muscle). Because the sensory and motor fibers run together, nerve blocks cannot be performed because they would result in bilateral vocal cord paralysis and complete airway obstruction. The alternative is topicalization of the mucosa.

Patient is made to lie in supine position with the neck in extension. In this position, the cervical vertebrae push the trachea and cricoid cartilage anteriorly and displace the strap muscles of the neck laterally so that the cricoid cartilage and the structures above and below it are easier to palpate (Fig. 11). The thyroid cartilage (Adam's apple) is palpated at midline and followed caudally until a depression and a firm ring of tissue are identified. These are the cricothyroid groove and the cricoid cartilage, respectively. Overlying the cricoid groove is the cricothyroid membrane.

The physician should stand at the side of the patient. The patient is asked not to talk, swallow, or cough until instructed. The midline of the cricothyroid membrane is identified as the needle insertion site. The index and middle finger of the nondominant hand can be used to mark this spot and stabilize the trachea (Figs. 12A to D). Using a tuberculin syringe or a 25-G needle,

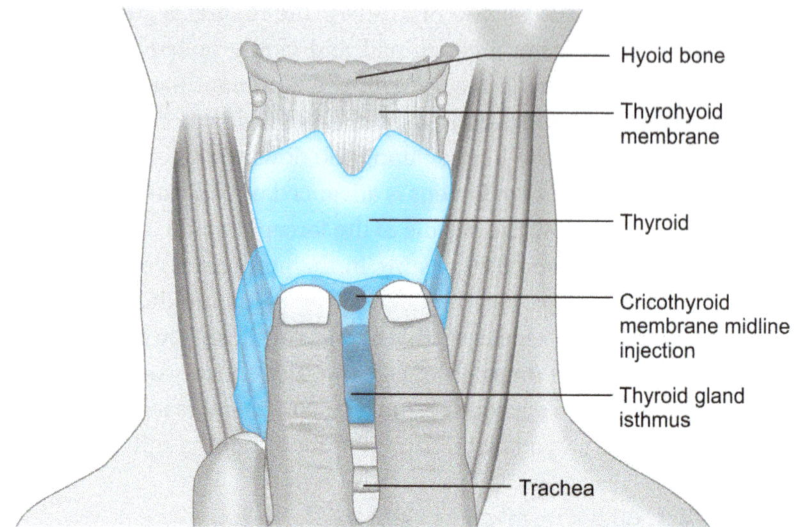

Fig. 11: Translaryngeal anesthesia, anatomic landmarks.
(*Source*: Brown D, [editor]. Atlas of Regional Anesthesia, Philadelphia, Saunders).

the physician raises a small skin wheal. A 20-G angiocatheter attached to a 5-10-mL syringe containing 3-5 mL saline is used. The needle is advanced through the skin perpendicularly or slightly caudally while aspirating. When air is freely aspirated, the sheath of the angiocatheter is advanced slightly, the needle is removed, and a syringe containing 3 to 5 mL of 2-4% lidocaine is carefully attached to the catheter sheath that has been left in place. Aspiration of air is reconfirmed, the patient is warned to expect vigorous coughing, and the local anesthetic is injected rapidly during inspiration (Figs. 12A to D). The sheath of the angiocatheter may be left in place until the intubation is complete in case more local anesthetic is needed and to decrease the likelihood of subcutaneous emphysema. This technique may be performed using a standard 20- or 22-G needle. This may, however, increase the risk of airway injury.

Complications are trauma to vocal cords, avoid directing the needle cephalad. Coughing elicited by this block may result in increased heart rate, mean arterial blood pressure, ICP, and intraocular pressure. As a result, it is contraindicated in patients with elevated ICP or open globe, and care should be taken in patients with significant cardiac disease. It is also relatively contraindicated in patients with cervical instability, although its routine use in these patients has been described without complications. Transtracheal injection should be avoided in patients with local tumor or large goiter. Other complications include subcutaneous and intratracheal bleeding, infection, subcutaneous emphysema, pneumomediastinum, pneumothorax, vocal cord trauma, and esophageal perforation.

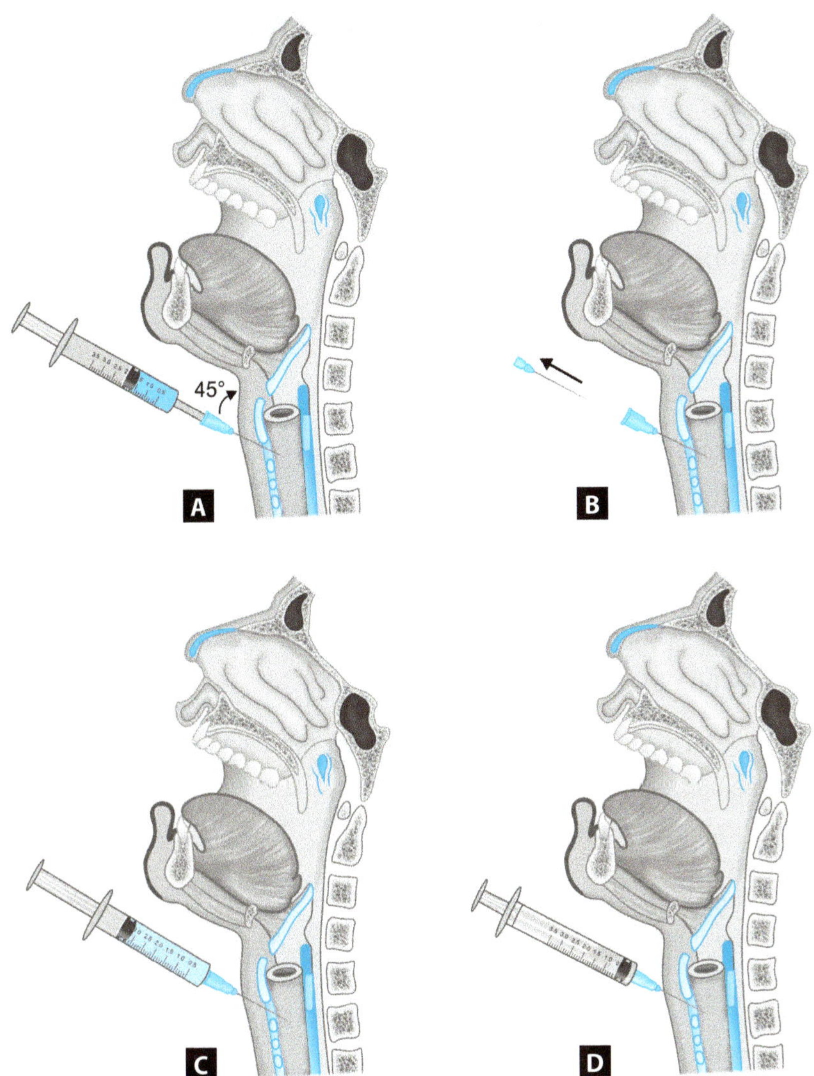

Figs. 12A to D: Translaryngeal anesthesia (midsagittal view of the head and neck). (A) The angiocatheter is inserted at the cricothyroid membrane, aimed caudally. An aspiration test is performed to verify the position of the tip of the needle in the tracheal lumen; (B) The needle is removed from the angiocatheter; (C) The syringe containing local anesthetic attached, the aspiration test is repeated; (D) Local anesthetic is injected, resulting in coughing and nebulization of the local anesthetic (shaded area). (*Source:* The Retrograde Cookbook. Irvine, University of California. Practice guidelines for management of the difficult airway).

PREVENTION OF ASPIRATION

Geetanjali S Verma

IDENTIFY RISK FACTORS

Patient Factors

Full Stomach

- Emergency surgery
- Inadequate fasting time
- Gastrointestinal obstruction.

Delayed Gastric Emptying

- Systemic diseases (diabetes mellitus, chronic kidney disease)
- Recent trauma
- Opioids
- Raised intracranial pressure
- Previous gastrointestinal surgery
- Pregnancy (including active labor).

Incompetent Lower Esophageal Sphincter

- Hiatus hernia
- Recurrent regurgitation
- Dyspepsia
- Previous upper gastrointestinal surgery
- Pregnancy.

Esophageal Diseases

- Previous gastrointestinal surgery
- Morbid obesity.

Surgical Factors

- Upper gastrointestinal surgery
- Lithotomy or head down position
- Laparoscopy
- Cholecystectomy.

Anesthetic Factors

- Light anesthesia
- Supraglottic airways

- Positive pressure ventilation
- Length of surgery > 2 h
- Difficult airway.

Device Factor

- First-generation supraglottic airway devices.

FACTORS THAT INCREASE INTRAGASTRIC VOLUME AND PRESSURE

- *Increased gastric filling*: Air inflation during mask ventilation.
- *Increased gastric acid production*:
  - Gastrin
  - Histamine-2 receptor stimulation
  - Recent ethanol ingestion
  - Recent hypoglycemic episode
- *Decreased gastric emptying*
  - Intestinal obstruction
  - Diabetic gastroparesis
  - Opioids
  - Anticholinergics
  - Sympathetic stimulation (pain and anxiety).

EFFECTS OF ASPIRATION

- Particulate aspiration
  - Airway obstruction
  - Granulomatous inflammation
- Acid aspiration
  - Neutrophilic inflammation
  - Hemorrhagic pulmonary edema
  - Destruction of airway epithelium
  - Loss of type I alveolar cells
  - Loss of surfactant
  - Alveolar instability and collapse
- Disruption of alveolar-capillary membrane
- Plasma leakage from pulmonary capillaries
  - Noncardiogenic pulmonary edema
  - Hypovolemia.

METHODS TO PREVENT ASPIRATION

1. Reducing gastric volume
   - Preoperative fasting
     - Clear liquids - 2 hrs
     - Breast milk - 4 hrs

- Infant formula - 6 hrs
- Non-human milk - 6 hrs
- Light meal - 6 hrs

- Nasogastric aspiration
- Prokinetic premedication
    - Metoclopramide 10 mg IV
    - 30 mins prior

2. Avoidance of general anesthesia
    - Regional anesthesia
3. Anticholinergics
    - Atropine, glycopyrrolate
4. Antiemetics
    - Ondansetron
5. Reducing pH of gastric contents
    - Antacids
        - 0.3 M sodium citrate 30 mL (nonparticulate)
    - H_2 histamine antagonists
        - Ranitidine 50 mg IV or 150 mg PO
    - Proton pump inhibitors
        - Pantoprazole 40 mg IV or PO
6. Airway protection
    - Tracheal intubation (RSI)
    - Second-generation supraglottic airway devices
7. Prevent regurgitation
    - Cricoid pressure <40N
    - Rapid sequence induction
8. Extubation
    - Awake after return of airway reflexes
    - Position (lateral, head down or upright).

DRUGS

Metochlopramide: Gastroprokinetic

Mechanism of action: Central antidopaminergic activity and prolactin stimulation as well as peripheral blockade of dopamine receptors and stimulation of cholinergic function in the upper gastrointestinal tract. It raises lower esophageal sphincter (LES) contractility and barrier pressure and accelerates gastric emptying.

Sodium Citrate

To neutralize the acid pH >7. Larger volumes of sodium citrate can induce nausea, vomiting, or diarrhea.

H_2 Receptor Blockers

H_2-receptor blocker inhibits basal acid secretion as well as that stimulated by the presence of gastrin or food.

Proton Pump Inhibitors

Acetylcholine, histamine, and gastrin stimulate HCl secretion by the gastric parietal cell. Although these agonists stimulate different receptors, their mechanisms of action results in formation of cyclic adenosine monophosphate (cAMP). The cAMP activates the proton pump, H^+,K^+-adenosine triphosphatase (ATPase), which exchanges intraluminal potassium ions for intracellular hydrogen ions. H^+ are thereby secreted from the parietal cell into gastric fluids. Omeprazole (prodrug) is absorbed in the small intestine and is activated in the highly acidic milieu of the gastric parietal cell. Activated omeprazole then remains in the parietal cell for up to 48 hours, inhibiting the proton pump in a prolonged manner. Inhibition of gastric acid secretion can be nearly complete, with no discernible side effects.

Chemical Pneumonitis Criteria

pH < 2.5

Gastric volume > 0.3 mL/kg of body weight (20–25 mL in adults)

4 Instruments

Deva Evu Subhas

AIRWAY EQUIPMENTS

Airway management is one of the essential steps in resuscitation. The need for anesthesiologist to master the skills in airway management cannot be stressed upon more. The knowledge of airway equipment is as important as that of anatomy. We have walked a long way from the days of lifesaving jaw thrust maneuver suggested by Friedrich von Esmarch.

The airway equipments can be categorized as:

1. Equipment used in maintaining patency of airway
2. Equipment used in assisting intubation.

Equipment used in maintaining patency of airway:

These artificial devices were designed to maintain patency of airway. They range from less invasive oropharyngeal airways to tracheostomy tubes. The devices can be further categorized based on anatomy. There are set of devices which are placed above the glottis which are noninvasive in nature and the ones placed below the glottis are generally invasive in nature.

The devices used above the glottis:

1. Oropharyngeal airway
2. Nasopharyngeal airway
3. Supraglottic airway devices (SAD).

OROPHARYNGEAL AIRWAY (FIG. 1)

Deva Evu Subhas

It is a simple device used in maintaining patency of upper airway. Earlier days the airway patency was maintained using maneuvers like jaw thrust. However, with increase in complexity and duration of the procedure, the need for special devices to maintain airway patency arose. Frederick Hewitt started using a metal tube trough the mouth into hypopharynx . The Guedel curved rubber airway was first described in 1935.

The Guedel airway is the most commonly used airway. It is either made of plastic or rubber. The central lumen may be used for suctioning.

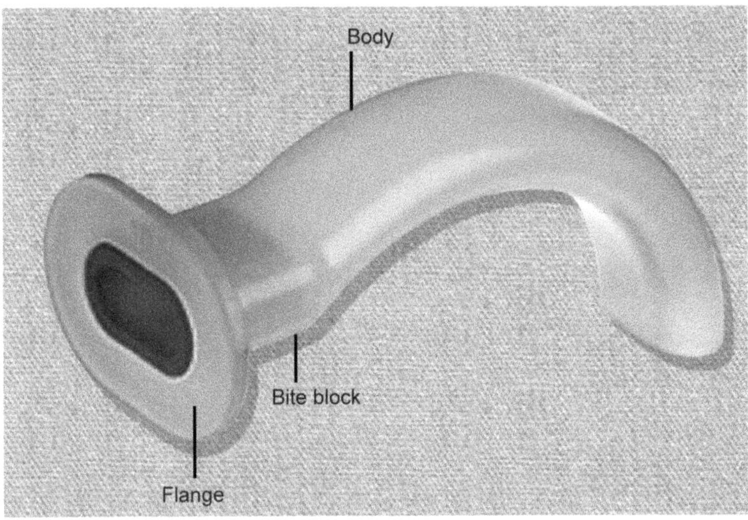

Fig. 1: Oropharyngeal airway (OPA).

The central lumen is reinforced by a harder inner plastic tube at the level of the teeth and by plastic ridges along the pharyngeal section. Oral and pharyngeal mucosae cannot occlude or narrow the lumen from the side. Its oval cross-section allows the four central incisors to make contact with it during masseter spasm. There is a flange at buccal end to prevent swallowing or over insertion.

The Ovassapian airway (Fig. 2) has a large anterior flange to control the tongue. There is a large opening at the level of the teeth to allow a flexible fiberoptic bronchoscope and ETT to be passed through it and later disengaged from the airway. It is often employed during fiberoptic intubations to aid in maintaining upper airway patency.

The oropharyngeal airway (OPA) works by keeping the tongue anterior and thus prevents the tongue from falling back and obstructing the airway. Even though the device is simple to use it has its own problems. The problems include trauma, airway reactivity and obstruction.

The patient's pharyngeal and laryngeal reflexes should be depressed before insertion to avoid worsening obstruction due to airway reactivity. Next step is to measure the appropriate size of OPA, which is determined by measuring the distance between first incisor and angle of mandible. There are two ways of inserting OPA. In the first method, the OPA is inserted using a tongue blade. The mouth is opened, and a tongue blade is placed at the base of the tongue and drawn upward, lifting the tongue off of the posterior pharyngeal wall. The airway is then placed so that the OPA is just off the posterior wall of the oropharynx, with 1 to 2 cm protruding above the incisors. The mouth is inspected to ensure that neither the tongue nor the lips are caught between the teeth and the OPA.

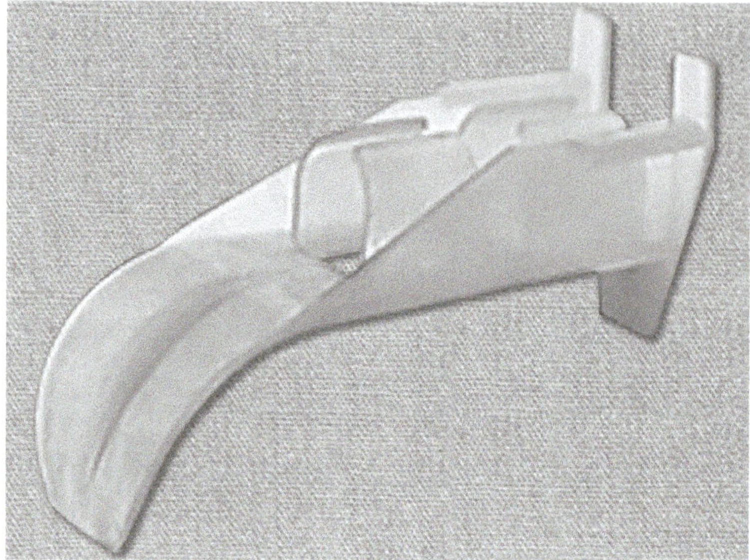

Fig. 2: Ovassapian airway.

An alternative method of placement is to insert the airway backward. Mouth is opened and the OPA is inserted with convex side toward the tongue until the tip is close to the pharyngeal wall of the oropharynx. It is then rotated 180° so that the tip rotates and settles behind the tongue base. There is a chance of dental trauma while insertion.

Airway hyperactivity is a potentially lethal complication of OPA use. Coughing, retching, emesis, laryngospasm, and bronchospasm are common reflex responses. These responses are triggered by stimulating the epiglottis or the vocal cords. Management includes partially withdrawing the OPA, deepening the plane of anesthesia, mild positive airway pressure and a small dose of succinylcholine can be tried.

NASOPHARYNGEAL AIRWAY (NPA) (FIG. 3)

Deva Evu Subhas

It is an alternative airway device for treating soft tissue upper airway obstruction. NPA is less stimulating compared to an OPA and therefore better tolerated in the awake, semicomatose patient or in light plane of anesthesia. They are more preferred in case of oropharyngeal trauma. NPAs are pliable, bent cylinders made of soft plastic or rubber in variable lengths and widths. It has a flange which helps in controlling the depth of insertion by preventing the outer end crossing the nares. NPAs have beveled end which helps in easy insertion and minimizes mucosal trauma.

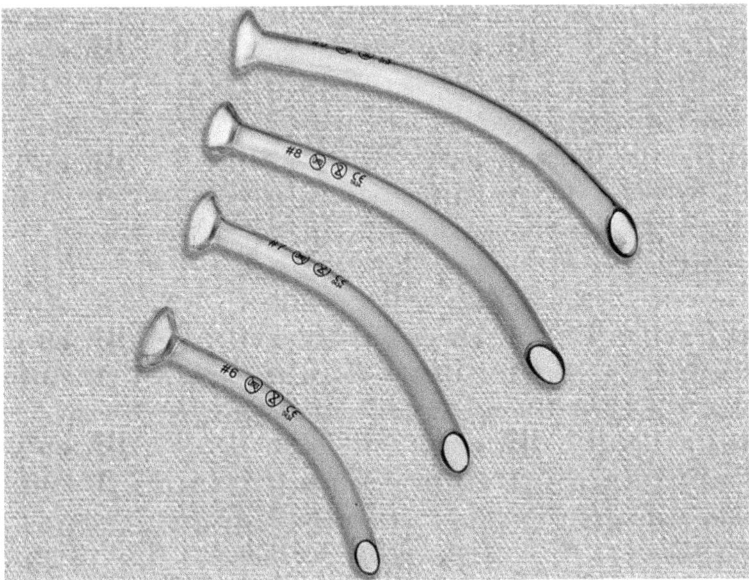

Fig. 3: Nasopharyngeal airway.

Before insertion of an NPA, inspect the nares to determine their size and patency and look for presence of nasal polyps or marked septal deviation. Vasoconstriction of the mucous membranes can be accomplished with cocaine (which has the added benefit of providing topical anesthesia) or phenylephrine drops or spray or cotton swabs soaked in either of these solutions. The NPA should be lubricated using water-soluble lubricant. Then pass the NPA with concave side parallel to the hard palate. Resistance is encountered at the nasopharynx. When there is resistance to passage, try and rotate the NPA 90° counterclockwise, bringing the open part of the bevel against the posterior nasopharyngeal mucosa. As the tube makes the bend (indicated by a relative loss of resistance to advancement), it should be rotated back to its original orientation.

If there is trouble passing NPA with moderate pressure, there are three management options: try a narrower tube, redilate the naris, and try the other naris. If the tube does not pass into the oropharynx, then withdraw the tube 2 cm and then pass a suction catheter through the nasal airway as a guide for advancement of the NPA. Try and avoid stimulating epiglottis or vocal cords. If the patient's upper airway is still obstructed after insertion, then pass a small suction catheter to confirm the patency of the NPA. If patency of the NPA is confirmed, it is possible that the NPA is too short and the base of the tongue is occluding its tip. In this case, a 6.0 ETT can be cut at 18 cm to provide a longer airway.

1. Indications for an NPA include relief of upper airway obstruction in awake, semicomatose, or lightly anesthetized patients; in patients who

are not adequately treated with OPAs; in patients undergoing dental procedures or with oropharyngeal trauma; and in patients requiring oropharyngeal or laryngopharyngeal suctioning.

2. The contraindications (absolute or relative) include known nasal airway occlusion, nasal fractures, marked septal deviation, coagulopathy (risk of epistaxis), prior transsphenoidal hypophysectomy or Caldwell-Luc procedure, cerebrospinal fluid rhinorrhea, known or suspected basilar skull fractures, and adenoid hypertrophy.

The complications of NPAs consist of failure of successful placement, epistaxis due to mucosal tears or avulsion of the turbinates, submucosal tunneling, and pressure sores. Epistaxis is commonly encountered problem. It is usually self-limited. Anterior plexus bleeding can be treated by applying pressure to the nares. If the posterior plexus is bleeding (with blood pooling into the pharynx), leave the NPA in place, suction the pharynx, and consider intubating the trachea if the bleeding does not stop promptly. The patient may be positioned on his or her side to minimize the aspiration of blood.

SUPRAGLOTTIC AIRWAY DEVICES (SADs/SGAs)

Deva Evu Subhas

Ever since laryngeal mask airway (LMA) was introduced by Archie Brain the supraglottic devices have gained popularity over years. It was introduced into clinical practice in 1988. In the first paper on the LMA he described it as "an alternative to either the endotracheal tube (ETT) or the face-mask with either spontaneous or positive-pressure ventilation (PPV)". Even before Brain many people thought supraglottic approach to airway would be less invasive. However LMA was the first device to get into clinical practice. The idea was first conceived way back in 1983. Brain modified Goldman dental nose piece to become cuff and it was glued with diagonally cut endotracheal tube. Over the years of research and experience it was realized that no single LMA can fulfill all requirements. This led to developing various types of LMAs.

First-generation SADs

These are SADs which fit the description 'simple airway device'. They include the cLMA, flexible LMA, and all LMs. In addition, they include the laryngeal tube (LT) and cobra perilaryngeal airway. They may or may not protect against aspiration in the event of regurgitation, but have no specific design features that lessen this risk. They are not considered here further.

Second-generation SADs

The SADs have been designed for safety and have design features to reduce the risk of aspiration. In several cases, the efficacy of that design is unproven. Efficacy for ventilation is often a by-product of design for safety. These include: PLMA, i-gel.

There are certain supraglottic airway devices which are commonly in use. Those devices will be dealt in detail. It makes more sense to deal with second-generation SADs in detail. However it is important to look into certain first generation SADs as they were prototype for the second-generation SADs. It is better to discuss all the LMAs together as they help us understand how the supraglottic airway as such as evolved over time. Then we can discuss certain non-LMA SADs.

CLASSIC LMA (cLMA) (FIG. 4)

It was the simple device first introduced. It was extensively studied. This device was compared with tracheal tubes and mask ventilation. Brimacombe published a meta-analysis in 1995 which highlighted advantages of cLMA over ventilation using tracheal tubes and mask.

Advantages of cLMA

1. There was lesser hemodynamic and intraocular changes with placement and removal of LMA compared to intubation and extubation. There was significant difference in coughing, bucking while awakening the patient.

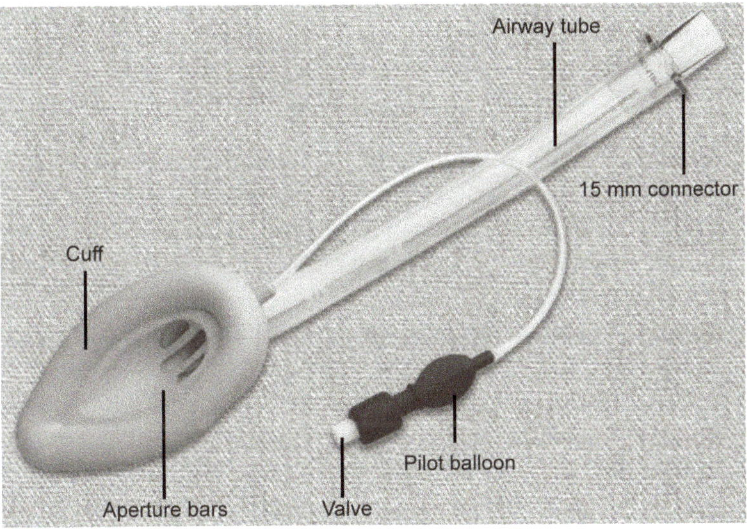

Fig. 4: Classic LMA.

2. cLMA was better in preserving mucociliary function, laryngeal competence and also has the advantage of minimal laryngeal trauma.
3. No need for muscle paralysis or laryngoscopy during placement.
4. Speed and ease of insertion in inexperienced hands is increased.
5. Easy to train. Thus, becomes an important tool during resuscitation in inexperienced hands.
6. Better hemodynamic stability at induction and emergence.
7. Seems to be tolerated well under lighter plane of anesthesia with lesser laryngospasm, bronchospasm and sore throat.

Limitations of cLMA

1. Increased frequency of failed placements.
2. Increased risk of gastric aspiration.
3. Controlled ventilation is not always possible in view of moderate pharyngeal seal. The median seal pressure reached is around 20 cm H_2O. Occasionally it reaches 30 cm H_2O.
4. Does not aid in tracheal intubation.

These limitations led to making of second-generation SADs which were concentrating mainly on improving controlled ventilation and preventing aspiration of gastric contents.

INSERTION TECHNIQUE

There are various insertion techniques described for insertion of cLMA. The LMA insertion originally described was to mimic deglutition. Initially deflate the cuff completely to make it appear like spoon. Lubricate the back of the cuff using water-soluble lubricant like KY jelly. Do not lubricate the front of the cuff as it may block the aperture bar and aspiration of lubricant. Avoid using silicone-based lubricants as they may damage the cuff.

Standard Insertion Technique

1. Make sure that patient is deeply anesthetized.
2. Position the head and neck as for normal intubation.
3. During insertion the LMA to be held like a pen with the index finger placed anteriorly at the junction of the cuff and tube. Press the tip up against the hard palate and verify it lies flat against the palate and that the tip is not folded over.
4. By using the index finger, push the mask backwards while maintaining pressure against the palate. As the mask progresses down, the index finger should keep the mask pressed against the posterior pharyngeal wall as to avoid collision with the epiglottis. Insert the index finger fully into the mouth to complete insertion. Keep moving down until

Table 1: Deciding size of LMA for the patient

Size of the LMA	*Patients weight (kg)*	*Maximum inflation volume (mL)*
1	Up to 5	4
1½	5–10	7
2	10–20	10
2½	20–30	14
3	30–50	20
4	50–70	30
5	70–100	40
6	>100	50

resistance is felt. At this point index finger can be removed while the other hand is stabilizing the LMA. Avoid jerky movements during insertion.

Check that the black line on the tube is in midline. Inflate the cuff without holding the tube, allowing it to position itself correctly. Soon after this the device should be connected to fresh gas flow. Intracuff pressure should not exceed 60 cm H_2O under any circumstance. Overinflation of cuff can weaken the seal.

Thumb Insertion Technique

This technique is favored when the access to the head from behind is difficult or impossible. The steps and principle of insertion are almost same except for the fact that thumb is used instead of index finger. Toward the end the nondominant hand helps in pushing the LMA to its final position.

The information on choosing appropriate size and maximum inflation volumes are highlighted in Table 1.

FLEXIBLE LMA (FIG. 5)

This LMA was introduced in 1994 mainly for head and neck procedures. Spiral coil was incorporated into shaft to make it kink resistant and more flexible. This helps with better surgical access mainly in head and neck procedure.

FASTRACH INTUBATING LMA (FIG. 6)

In 1983, while developing the LMA, Brain conducted a fiberoptic investigation that revealed the LMA's potential as a guide for endotracheal intubation. The same year, he blindly intubated three patients. However the intubating LMA was introduced in 1994 after the cLMA gained popularity. There was demand among clinicians for a device which could serve to ventilate as well as act as a conduit for intubation.

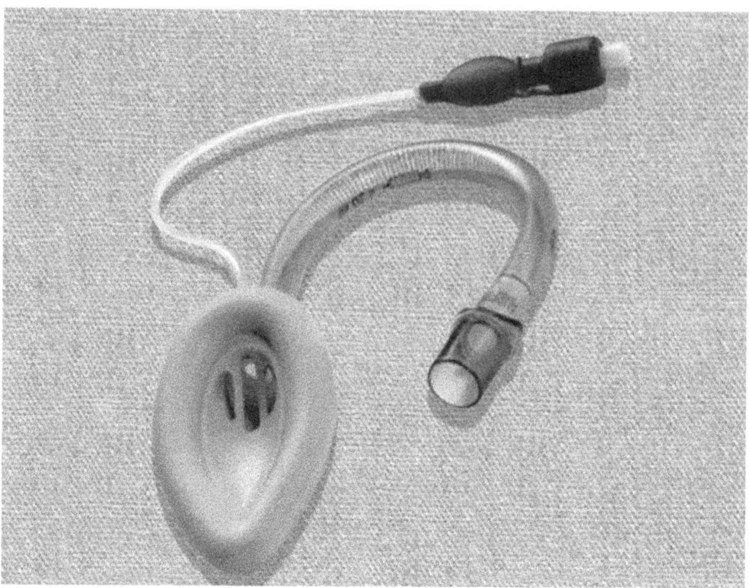

Fig. 5: Flexible LMA.

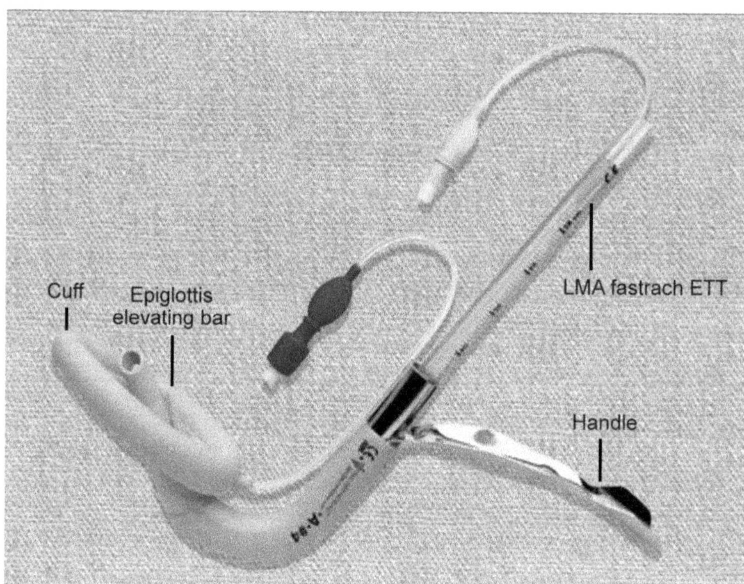

Fig. 6: Fastrach intubating LMA.

The ILMA consists of an anatomically curved, stainless steel tube with a 13-mm internal diameter that is connected firmly at its distal end to the laryngeal mask. The preformed angle was designed based on the data collected from sagittal MRI images with head in neutral position. The two bars at the aperture of the cLMA have been replaced in the ILMA by a single, movable epiglottic elevating bar that pushes the epiglottis out of the way and allows smooth and unobstructed passage of the ETT as it emerges from the distal end of the ILMA's metal shaft. It allows ETT up to 8.5 mm size. The shaft is also kept short so as to avoid need for longer tube.

Many researches were undertaken to improve the rate of blind intubation through the ILMA. However, Chandy's maneuver seems to be the only one which was more consistent. It involves two steps.

i. Rotate the ILMA in sagittal plane till least resistance to ventilation is achieved.
ii. Lift the ILMA slightly (not tilt) from the posterior pharyngeal wall just before blind intubation.

Both maneuvers were done holding the handle. The overall success rates for blind and fiberoptically-guided intubations were 97% and 100%, respectively.

PROSEAL LMA (PLMA) (FIG. 7)

Proseal is a second-generation SAD with a better seal pressure and a drain tube for draining gastric contents. It is a reuse device recommended for about 40 uses. The main advantage over the cLMA is the fact it has double the seal pressure compared to cLMA at intracuff pressure of 60 cm H_2O. Drain tube does not only act as a conduit for draining the gastric contents but also allows passing of gastic tube through it.

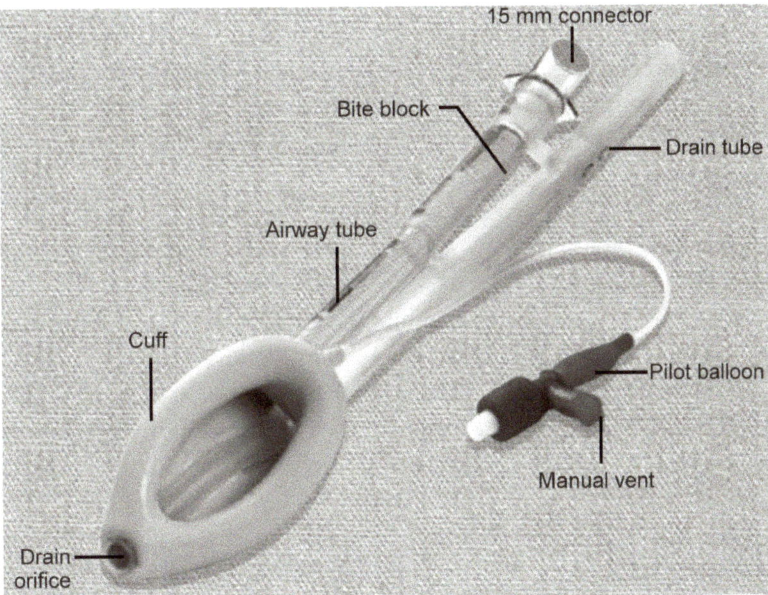

Fig. 7: Proseal LMA.

Insertion Technique

The preinsertion preparation and the principle behind insertion technique is somewhat similar to that of cLMA. The insertion can be successfully made either using the standard technique using index finger or by the thumb insertion technique. In addition to the above-mentioned techniques, a technique using an introducer has been added. The principle of insertion using a dedicated introducer is same as that of the finger techniques. The introducer seem to better while using 1-2½ size LMA. However, at the bigger sizes, there is no significant difference between these three techniques.

Tips to diagnose correct position of the cuff:

i. Observe for the anterior displacement of cricoid while insertion and at inflation.
ii. The correct position will produce perfect seal by the cuff against the glottis with no leak (seal 1). The mask tip should be wedged against the upper esophageal sphincter (seal 2). And the bite block should be at position. The correct mask placement can be checked by placing a small bolus (1-2 mL) of lubricant gel in the proximal end of the drain tube. In a properly placed mask, there should be a slight updown meniscus movement of the lubricant. No movement or the bolus of lubricant is ejected suggests incorrect placement.
iii. In case of incomplete insertion the bite block will be more proximal, there will be leak on ventilation and a leak felt through the proximal end of drain tube (DT). The LMA must be repositioned.
iv. Sometime due to improper deflation of the cuff, the tip of the cuff enters the laryngeal vestibule. This leads to obstruction during ventilation (in spite of deep plane of anesthesia) and leak through the proximal end of DT. The LMA should be removed and reinserted.
v. Next form of malposition is when the tip of the cuff folds back and obstructs the DT. The up-down meniscus movement of lubricating gel is absent. Confirmed by passing a gastric tube through the DT. If the gastric tube does not go past the distal tip, it suggests folding over of the tip. The LMA should be removed and reinserted.

The main advantage of proseal LMA is to prevent aspiration of gastric content. This advantage will be lost in case of malposition. So, it is important to make sure that the cuff is in right position and also that the drain tube is not obstructed.

Table 2 describes the maximum inflation volume, maximum diameter of orogastric tube and introducer sizes for various sizes of proseal LMA.

Table 2: Deciding size of Proseal LMA

Size of the LMA	*Patient weight (kg)*	*Maximum inflation volume (mL)*	*Maximum diameter of orogastric tube (Fr)*	*Introducer size*
1	Up to 5	4	8	1–2½
1½	5–10	7	10	1–2½
2	10–20	10	10	1–2½
2½	20–30	14	14	1–2½
3	30–50	20	16	3–5
4	50–70	30	16	3–5
5	70–100	40	18	3–5

LMA SUPREME (FIG. 8)

This is a single-use LMA made by combining the useful features of ILMA and PLMA together. It is basically a LMA with ease of insertion requiring no finger to be inserted into the oral cavity, head need not be extended with better seal and drain tube for gastric contents.

Salient Features of LMA Supreme

- It is a single-use LMA.
- The LMA supreme has a manifold with an integral bite block, an anatomically shaped airway tube enclosing a drain tube, a redesigned inflatable cuff (through which the drain tube passes), and a cuff inflation line with pilot balloon.

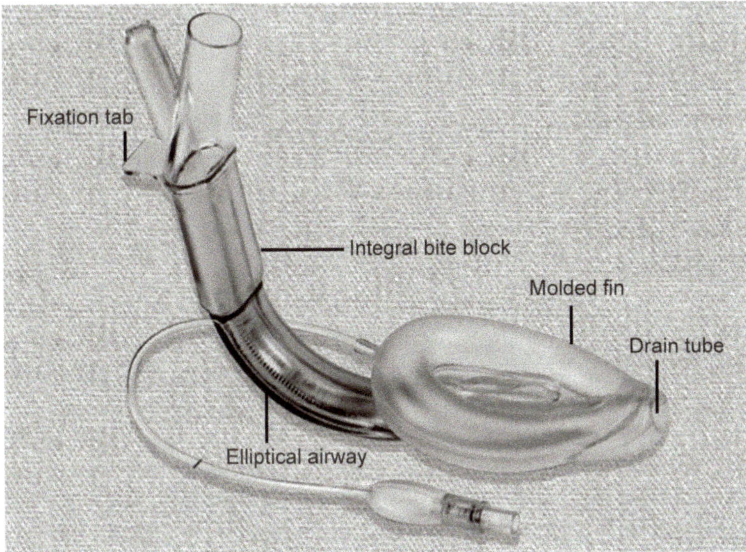

Fig. 8: LMA supreme.

- There is a fixation tab that is molded at right angles to the manifold which helps in easy insertion and fixation after insertion.
- The airway tube is elliptical in shape aiding easy insertion. The airway tube is much stiffer than that of PLMA. However, it is intended to bend with head movement unlike the rigid metal tube of ILMA.
- It has a patented lateral groove on the airway tube which prevents it from kinking.
- The gastric drain tube serves to equalize the UES pressure with atmospheric pressure, drains the gastric contents and acts as a conduit to pass gastric tube.
- The modified shape and enlarged surface area of the inflatable cuff enhances the anatomic fit of the device into the pharynx, permitting higher glottic seal pressures than the LMA classic and LMA unique. The distal cuff is over-molded to strengthen the tip and prevent it from folding over during insertion.
- Two fin-shaped structures extend on either side of the drain tube where it passes through the bowl of the mask, designed to prevent the epiglottis from obstructing the airway.

Insertion Technique

Deflate the cuff completely by pressing between the thumb and index finger while aspirating using a 50 mL syringe. Lubricate the back of the cuff using water-based lubricating gel.

1. Position yourself behind patient's head.
2. Place the head in the neutral or slight "sniffing" position.
3. Press the distal tip against the inner aspect of the upper teeth or gums and slide inwards using a slightly diagonal approach (direct the tip away from the midline. Keep sliding inwards along the hard palate and posterior to the tongue. (a circular motion can be used to negotiate the curvature behind the tongue).
4. Stop progressing further when resistance is felt.
5. Fixation is different compared to other LMAs. First difference is that the fixation is made prior to inflating the cuff. Second is that the fixation is done by applying the tape transversely over the fixation tab. Do not rotate the tape around the proximal end of the LMA.
6. After fixing the LMA the cuff is inflated to cuff pressure of 60 cm H_2O.

Table 3 describes the maximum inflation volume, maximum diameter of orogastric tube and introducer sizes for various size of LMA supreme.

Table 3: Deciding size of LMA supreme

Size of the LMA	*Patient weight (kg)*	*Maximum inflation volume (mL)*	*Maximum diameter of orogastric tube (Fr)*	*Introducer size*
1	Up to 5	5	6	1–2½
1½	5–10	8	6	1–2½
2	10–20	12	10	1–2½
2½	20–30	20	10	1–2½
3	30–50	30	14	3–5
4	50–70	45	14	3–5
5	70–100	45	14	3–5

Disposable Laryngeal Mask Airways

Infection is one of the major problem both for the health care providers and the patients. Even though the LMAs have never been proved to be transmitting infection the uncertainty and fear prevails. LMA unique and flexible single-use are the disposable versions of cLMA and LMA flexible respectively. LMA supreme is also a single-use LMA combining the benefits of ILMA and PLMA. The main difference between the reuse and single-use device is the cuff material. Reuse ones are made of silicone rubber whereas the single-use ones are made of polyvinyl chloride (PVC) plastic.

INDICATIONS/APPLICATIONS OF LMA

There is no clear cut laid down indication as such. The need to use LMA is purely dependent on the skill of the anesthesiologist. So, it is better to start with basic use and move on to doing specialized cases. Any nonemergency case requiring general anesthesia in a patient in the supine position who has an ASA classification of I (ASA I) or II and in whom the surgeon is performing a routine, short procedure that does not involve the alimentary or respiratory tract would constitute an appropriate basic use. Its applications vary from simple diagnostic procedures and short therapeutic procedures such as MRI, lumbar puncture, bone marrow aspiration, central line insertion, minor biopsies, etc. to head and neck surgeries and procedure of respiratory tract. Now LMAs are being used in all specialties including cardiology, neurosurgery, radiotherapy, etc. Cases requiring positive pressure ventilation also are done using LMAs (preferably PLMA or LMA supreme). LMA supreme was used successfully in prone position. So, technically any surgery requiring general anesthesia can be done using LMA depending on the skill and experience of the anesthesiologist. LMA is an important tool in resuscitation and also during difficult airway scenarios. Second generation LMAs are rescue devices in cannot intubate scenario.

COMPLICATIONS

- Sore throat
- Vascular compression or nerve damage—blood supply to tongue, lingual nerve and hypoglossal nerve are more vulnerable
- Risk of aspiration
- There are controversies in using them for surgeries requiring positive pressure ventilation, prone position and prolonged surgeries.

CONTRAINDICATIONS

- Restricted mouth opening
- Anticipated pharyngeal and laryngeal pathology
- Poor compliance requiring peak inspiratory pressure >20 cm H_2O for cLMA and >30 cm H_2O for proseal LMA
- Increased airway resistance
- Patient with increased risk of aspiration such as full stomach, morbid obesity, conditions causing delayed gastric emptying, etc.
- Should not be used in resuscitation of patients who are not profoundly unconscious.

NON-LMA SUPRAGLOTTIC AIRWAY DEVICES

Ambu Laryngeal Masks (Fig. 9)

Ambu designed and started producing Ambu AuraOnce between 2002 and 2004. Ambu AuraOnce is a single-use laryngeal mask with preformed shaft.

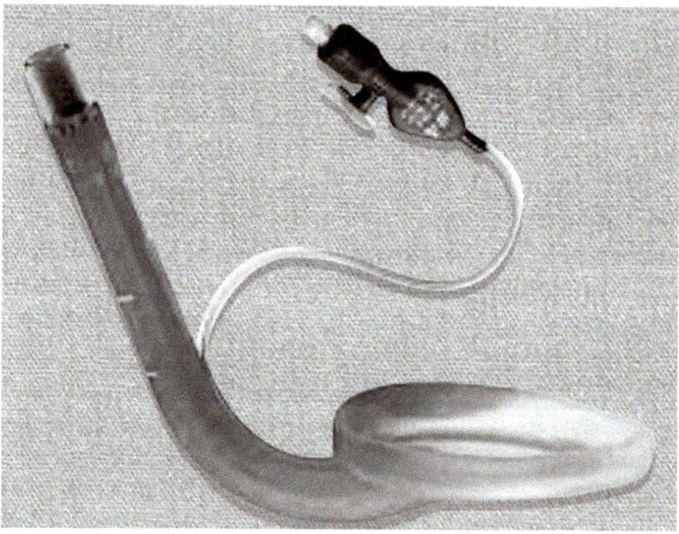

Fig. 9: Ambu LMA.

Ambu Aura40 is a reuse LM. Ambu AuraStraight is a single-use LM with conventional curved shaft. The Ambu AuraFlex is a single-use, reinforced, flexible LM, and the Ambu Aura-i is a modification of the AuraOnce that is designed to facilitate intubation.

Advantages

Its cuff is soft and flexible but has a reinforced tip. These features along with the preformed curve of the stem facilitates insertion. It is molded in a single unit, hence free from ridges that may injure the airway during insertion, and component parts cannot separate during use.

Disadvantages

Its disadvantages are those of all LMs. It is not good for controlled ventilation and the manufacturers recommend limiting peak airway pressure to 20 cm H_2O and the tidal volume to 8 mL/kg. There are no second-generation SADs from Ambu.

The insertion technique, indication, contraindication and complications are all similar to first-generation LMAs.

SOFT SEAL LARYNGEAL MASK (SSLM)

This is a single-use laryngeal mask manufactured by Smiths Medical. It acts as a conduit for intubation. The failure rates are high with blind intubation. Hence use of fiberoptic scope is recommended. The SSLM has a wider ventilation orifice than the LMA classic; larger SSLM sizes can accommodate up to a 7.5 mm ETT. This feature along with absence of aperture bars facilitate intubation. The application, advantages, disadvantages and insertion technique are all same as that of LMA. Some studies showed SSLM to be more difficult to insert among the other LMs. And also associated with increased incidence of blood on the LM and sore throat.

INTUBATING LARYNGEAL AIRWAY (ILA) (FIG. 10)

This is a single-use hypercurved laryngeal airway for intubation. It was invented by Daniel Cook. It took more than 8 years to invent and it was introduced into clinical practice in 2004. Made of medical grade silicon and it is latex-free. There are ridges distal to the connector which helps in achieving better seal. The larger ILA can accommodate up to 8.5 mm ET tube. After intubation the ILA can be removed using Cookgas ILA removal stylet.

The main advantage of ILA over other SADs is that it is designed specifically for intubation. The large bowl and curved tube enhances easy entry through oropharynx. The insertion technique, indication, contraindication and complications are all similar to first-generation LMAs.

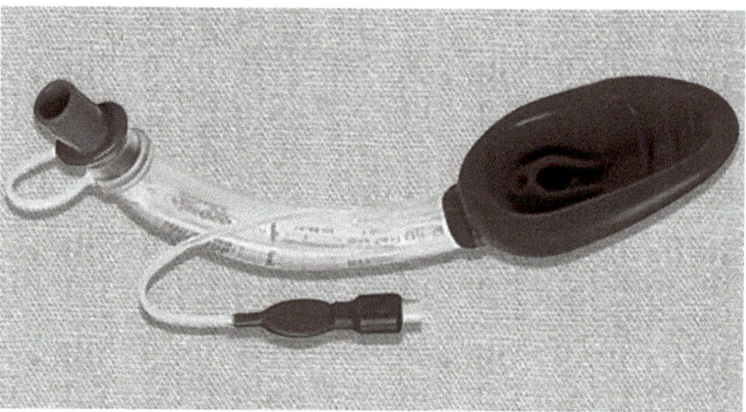

Fig. 10: Intubating laryngeal airway.

LARYNGEAL TUBES

The VBM Laryngeal Tube (VBM Medizintechnik, Sulz, Germany) and King Laryngeal Tube (King Systems, Noblesville, IN) are SAD devices that were introduced in 1999. Between 1999 and 2002, they were put through several modifications like a softer tip, a change from cuff inflation by separate pilot tubes to a single pilot tube, and alterations to the ventilation orifices and proximal cuff. Among the several distinct LTs, some are first-generation and others second-generation SADs.

There are five versions of the LT:

i. Reusable LT
ii. Disposable LT (LT-D)
iii. Reusable Laryngeal Tube Suction II (LTS-II)
iv. Disposable version of the LTS-II (LTS-D)
v. Gastro-Laryngeal Tube (Gastro-LT).

The LTS-II, LTS-D, and LT-G belong to second-generation SADs.

Laryngeal Tubes (LT)

The LT consists of an airway tube with two inflatable balloons or cuffs, one seals the esophageal inlet and the other in the oropharynx. This technically forms a seal above and below the laryngeal inlet allowing the air to flow through orifices between these cuffs. Both these cuffs are inflated using a single pilot balloon. LT is made for silicon rubber and can be reused for 50 times. It contains two main ventilation orifice and also two eyelets (one on either side). LT-D has three eyelets on either side. LT-D is also 1cm longer than the LT.

The LT is inserted along the length of the tongue until the tip lies in the proximal esophagus. Proximal and distal cuffs sit in the oropharynx and esophageal inlet, respectively. Inflate the cuffs. Three black lines seen proximally suggests correct depth of insertion. If the ventilation is not adequate then advance or withdraw the LT until optimal ventilation is achieved.

The main advantage of LT is the ease of insertion. It does not require any extensive training or experience to learn LT insertion. Can be used in spontaneous or controlled ventilation and also a rescue device. Another major advantage is to insert from any position. The fiberoptic bronchoscope and ETT can be advanced through the nose into the oral cavity without deflating the cuffs of the LT. After tracheal intubation has been accomplished, the cuffs of the LT can be deflated and the device removed. The LT is associated with a low incidence of minor traumatic sequelae, such as sore throat, hoarseness, or blood on the device after use. Rare incidence of tracheal insertion reported.

LTS and LTS-II

These are second-generation SADs. LTS was introduced in 2002 with a gastric drainage tube running posteriorly. Even though it was designed to improve the safety of the device, it made the device bulky. Thus, making it difficult to insert and causes trauma. These were the main advantages of LT which is not there in LTS anymore. In 2005, LTS-II (Fig. 11) was introduced which eventually replaced LTS. It was a modified version of LTS to make it less bulky and easy to insert.

The LTS-II has a smaller, considerably longer, and markedly modified tip and a redesigned distal balloon that is ovoid to mimic the shape of the upper esophagus and to provide axial stability for the SAD.

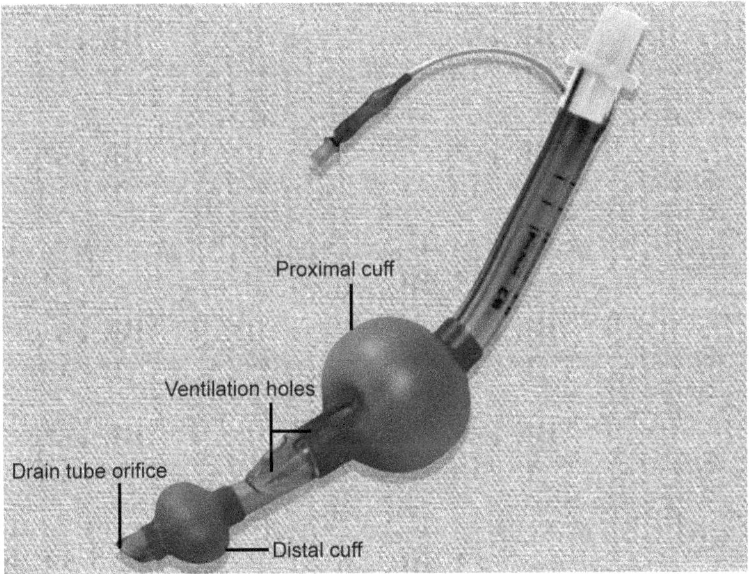

Fig. 11: LTS-II.

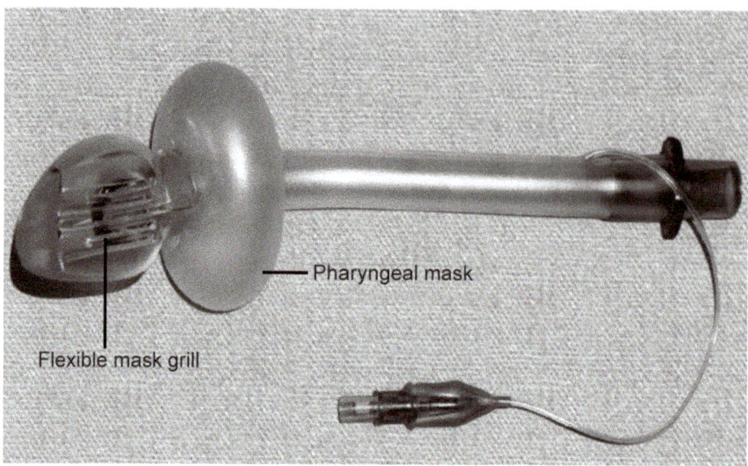

Fig. 12: CobraPLA.

COBRA PERILARYNGEAL AIRWAY (COBRA PLA) (FIG. 12)

The Cobra perilaryngeal airway (CobraPLA, Engineered Medical Systems, Indianapolis, IN) was designed by David Alfery. It was based on a modification of the Guedel oral airway and was marketed in 1997.

The CobraPLA is made of PVC and polycarbonate. It consists of a breathing tube, a circumferential, inflatable cuff proximal to the ventilation orifice; and a distal, widened cobra-like head that surrounds the ventilation orifice. The anterior surface of the head consists of a grill of soft bars which allow gas exchange and also instrumentation of the larynx and upper airway if required. When in the proper position, the head lies in front of the laryngeal inlet and is designed to seal the hypopharynx. The distal tip lies proximal to the esophageal inlet, this feature differentiates it from the SADs. Internal to the head, there is a ramp to direct the breathing gas (or ETT) into the trachea. The head and anterior grill prevents the epiglottis from obstructing the ventilation orifice. The cuff is circumferential and is designed to lie in the hypopharynx at the base of the tongue. When inflated, it raises the base of the tongue, exposing the laryngeal inlet, and it effects an airway seal, allowing positive-pressure ventilation to be carried out.

It is important to choose appropriate size device. The following guidelines helps in choosing correct size: no. 3 for less than 60 kg, no. 4 for 60 to 80 kg, and no. 5 for more than 80 kg. Cobra PLUS PLA comes with a core temperature monitoring device in its adult version and a distal gas sampling port in its pediatric version.

Insertion Technique

Cobra insertion technique is simple. Deflate the cuff completely and check the integrity. Lubricate the device adequately. Fold the distal tip back on to the stem. With the patient in sniffing position the device is inserted through the mouth between tongue and hard palate. The device is correctly seated when modest resistance to further distal passage is encountered. The cuff is inflated after insertion. The cuff inflation should be just about enough to produce adequate seal. Do not over inflate the cuff.

Advantages and Disadvantages

Advantages and disadvantages are similar to that of other first-generation SADs.

TULIP AIRWAY DEVICE (FIG. 13)

The Tulip airway device (Marshall Medical, Bath, United Kingdom) is a first-generation single-use SAD, designed by a British anesthetist Amer Shaikh and brought to market in 2010. Its novel feature is that one size is intended to fit all adults. Its tulip shaped, hence the name. It is made of PVC. The polyhedral cuff inflates below the soft palate and behind the tongue. It has a distal orifice. The stem of the Tulip is curved, and proximally, it has depth

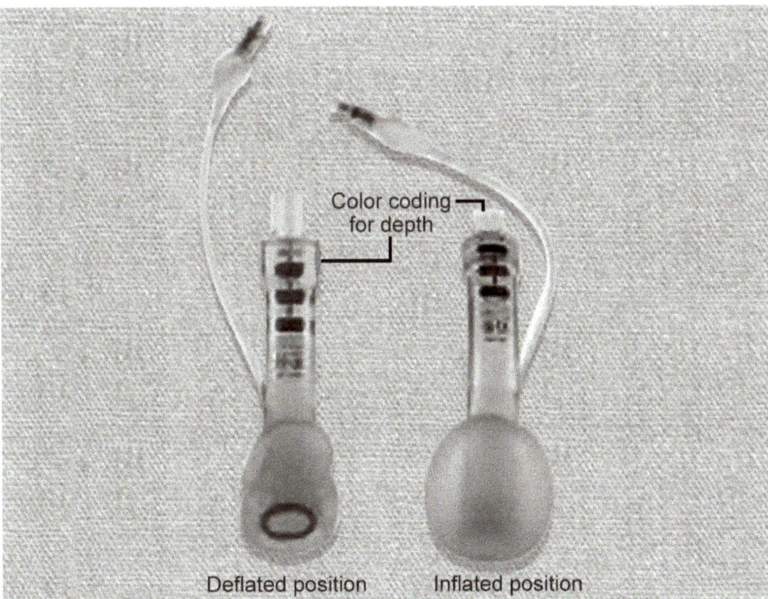

Fig. 13: Tulip airway.

markings in three colors to indicate the correct depth of insertion for small (green), medium (orange), and large (red) adults.

Insertion technique is similar to that of LMA. Hold it like a pen and insert it along the hard palate and soft palate until appropriate marking is reached. Inflate the cuff to 30 mL and add more if needed, but do not exceed 80 mL.

Advantages

- One size fits all adults
- Low cost
- Simplicity of insertion.

Disadvantages

- Lack of airway protection against aspiration as the esophageal orifice is not sealed.
- Controlled ventilation is possible only at a very low pressure.

I-GEL (FIG. 14)

The i-gel (Intersurgical, Wokingham, United Kingdom) is a CE-marked, single-use device. Muhammed Nasir, a British anesthetist designed numerous prototypes of the i-gel. It was marketed in 2007 and has not been modified since its introduction. In 2009, a full range of pediatric sizes was introduced.

This is a single-use, cuffless second-generation SAD. It is made up of a medical-grade thermoplastic elastomer gel (i.e. styrene ethylene butadiene

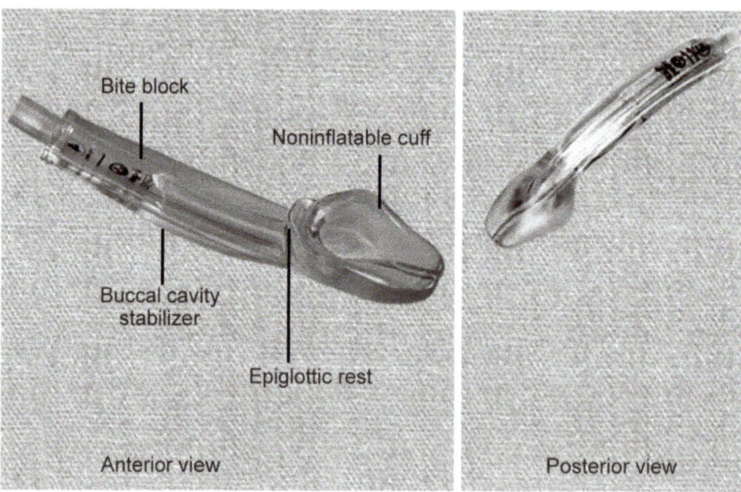

Fig. 14: I-gel.

styrene). It contains a stem and mask portion. The mask creates an anatomic seal with pharyngeal, laryngeal and perilaryngeal structures. The mask is cuffless, so it requires no inflation. There is a ridge at the proximal end of the bowl which prevents it from slipping out of position from base of tongue. The stem is elliptical and curved in cross-section. Its large caliber decreases the chance of displacement or axial rotation after insertion. The stem is firm and noncompressible, acting as an integral bite block. It contains a gastric drainage tube (smaller compared to rest of the second-generation SADs). The biggest i-gel which is size 5 allows maximum 14-Fr gastric tube. A black line at the distal end of the stem helps in determining appropriate depth of i-gel.

Insertion Technique

Choose appropriate sized i-gel. Lubricate the mask along the back and sides using a water-soluble lubricant. After achieving adequate depth of anesthesia insert the i-gel in sniffing position. Insert the device along the roof of the mouth until resistance is met. The tip of the device sitting at esophageal opening suggests correct position. Care should be taken to avoid tongue from getting caught while inserting the device. The device is fixed from "maxilla-to-maxilla" after insertion. The device provides a pharyngeal seal of 20–30 cm H_2O.

Uses

- Maintain airway during anesthesia. Can be used in spontaneous and controlled ventilation
- Used as a rescue airway device
- Conduit for endotracheal intubation.

Advantages

- Insertion is easier and quicker as it is cuffless.
- Broader and elliptical stem provides good stability and reduces risk of displacement.
- Theoretically has benefit of preventing aspiration. (However, this advantage is not proven.)
- The incidence of sore throat, dysphagia, dysphonia, etc. is low.
- Thermoplastic property of the mask allows the mask to undergo some alteration with increase in pharyngeal seal over time.

Disadvantages

- Less suited for head and neck procedure.
- Increase incidence of trauma to dentition, frenulum of tongue, etc.

Table 4: Deciding size of I-gel

i-gel size	*Weight (kg)*	*Maximum ETT size*
1	2–5	3.0
1½	5–12	4.0
2	10–25	5.0
2½	25–35	5.0
3	30–60	6.0
4	60–90	7.0
5	> 90	8.0

- Congestion of tongue due to incomplete insertion.
- Pharyngeal seal is better than that of cLMA, however less compared to PLMA.

  Table 4 gives info on size guideline and ETT size that could be used.

SLIPA: STREAMLINED LINER OF THE PHARYNX AIRWAY (FIG. 15)

The SLIPA (Curveair, London, United Kingdom), was developed by Donald Miller, a UK-based anesthetist. It is a single-use SAD which has no cuff. It is made of plastic with a preformed shape to match the shape of the pharynx.

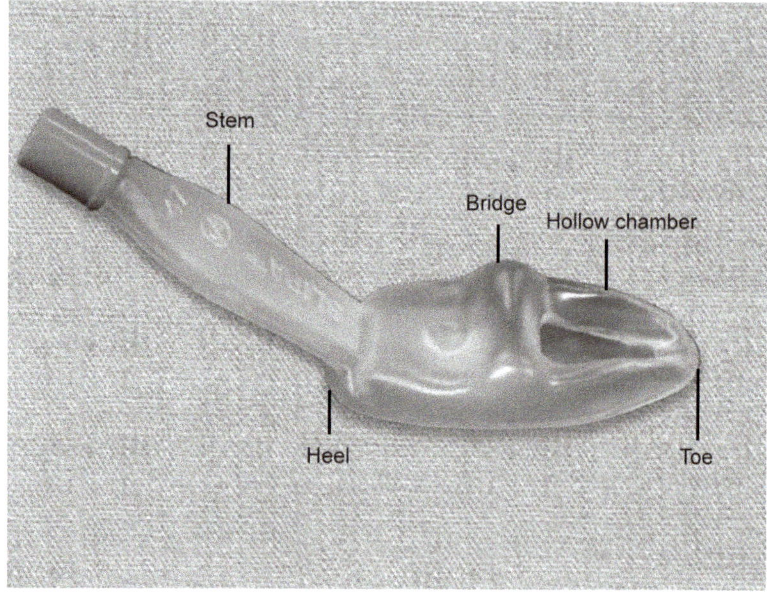

Fig. 15: SLIPA.

Its hollow, blow-molded chamber is shaped like a pressurized pharynx and somewhat like a boot with a toe, a bridge that seals at the base of the tongue, and a heel that anchors the device in a stable position between the esophagus and nasopharynx. The bulges and indentations on the anterior surface were intented to mimic the anatomy of the pharynx. It is designed in such a way to release pressure at vulnerable sites and thereby decreases damage to hypoglossal and recurrent laryngeal nerves.

The hollow design of the anterior surface retains some amount of regurgitated fluid or pharyngeal secretions thus providing some protection against aspiration, making it a second generation SAD. There is no cuff to inflate which makes it important to choose the correct size.

Insertion Technique

The insertion technique is different from that of the classic LMA. The patient is deeply anesthetized and positioned in sniffing position. Lubricate the device adequately. The device is advanced toward the esophagus until the heel of the device spontaneously locates itself in the nasopharynx. It usually passes the oropharyngeal curve with ease. The toe of the SLIPA may be used to lift the base of the tongue in a manner similar to a laryngoscope. Jaw thrust helps in placing the device in correct position. The angle between stem and shoe portion increases as the device moves into position. This angle can get almost perpendicular. When it is in position, further pressure on the stem leads to clear resistance, indicating it is fully inserted. Heel enters the nasopharynx and anchors the device's position and because of this, the manufacturers indicate it is unnecessary to tie the device in place.

The SLIPA can be removed while the patient is still anesthetized. The heel needs to be dislodged from the nasopharynx. The device should be gently pulled anterior and caudal at the same time as opening the mouth. In case of suspected regurgitation the contents can be emptied by passing a suction catheter into the chamber. Alternately remove the device and suction the pharynx.

Advantages

- Inexpensive
- Ease of insertion
- Can be compressed and inserted in case of restricted mouth opening
- Protects against aspiration to some extent
- Decreased incidence of hypoglossal and recurrent laryngeal nerve injury.

Table 5: Deciding size of SLIPA

SLIPA size	*Patient*	*Height range*
47	Very small female	145–160
49	Small female	152–168
51	Medium female	160–175
53	Large female to small male	163–182
55	Medium male	173–193
57	Large male	180–200

Disadvantages

- Cannot be used in prone position or for head and neck procedures.
- Perfect size fit is important leading to need for multiple size to be kept available. The complexity of size selection involving factors like height, width of thyroid cartilage, etc.
- The pharyngeal seal will be lost if the head position is turned to sides.
- The capacity of the chamber to capture regurgitant fluids comes down with change in position to lateral or prone.

  Table 5 shows guidelines in choosing appropriate size SLIPA.

BASKA MASK (FIG. 16)

It has been designed and developed over 11 years by Kanag Baska, an Australian anesthetist. The device came to market in Europe in 2011. It is a

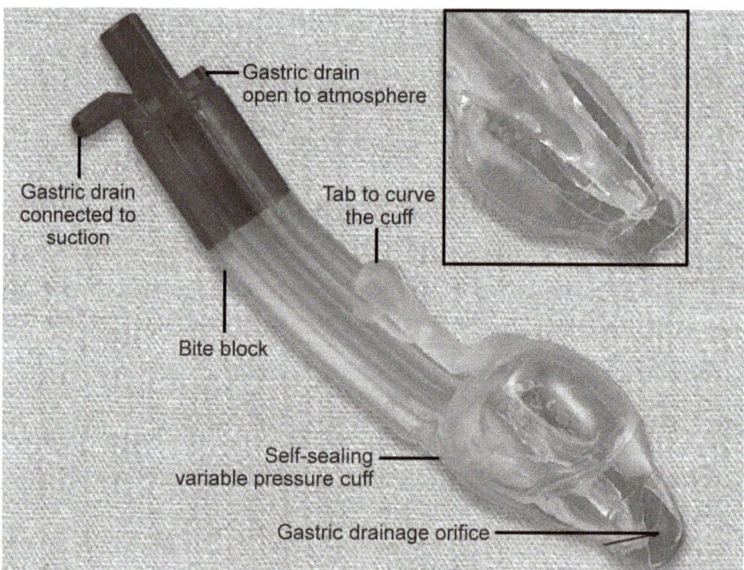

Fig. 16: Baska mask.

single-use, cuffless device made of silicon. The stem is oval in cross-section providing good axial stability. The proximal portion has an integrated bite block and the distal portion is soft and attaches to a soft malleable mask portion. Two drainage tube runs on either side of the stem. The drainage tube runs along both sides and posterior aspect of the mask which ends and extends into mask tip. The soft structure of the mask is compliant enough to change shape when pressure is applied. When positive pressure is applied, the mask distends, increasing the pharyngeal seal, and as that pressure is released, the mask partially deflates, limiting any pressures applied to the pharyngeal tissues. Four sizes are available for small to large adults.

Insertion Technique

The Baska mask is first sealed at both ends with fingers and compressed to assess its integrity. Lubricate the posterior and sides of the mask using a water-soluble lubricant. The device may be inserted with the patient in any head and neck positions, however the neutral position is favored. The device is held in the dominant hand with the thumb, forefinger, and middle finger grasping the base of the mask and compressing it. The device is inserted into the mouth and along the hard palate. The pressure on the device maintained posteriorly using index and middle finger. On reaching the soft palate, the device is advanced into place by advancing the stem of the device. If difficulty is encountered in negotiating the pharyngeal corner, the anterior strap is pulled to flex the device tip and ease it around the corner. There is no cuff to deflate. Confirm the correct position of the device by gentle ventilation. Adjust the device by either withdrawing or pushing the device further. When insertion is not successful we can try using another size. Fix the device after successful insertion.

Advantages

- Easy insertion.
- Increased pharyngeal seal with controlled ventilation because of expandable membranous cuff.
- Continuous suctioning of the pharynx possible.

The device is relatively new with very less studies suggesting advantages and disadvantages.

Combitubes (Fig. 17)

The Esophageal Tracheal Combitube (Combitube; Tyco Healthcare, Mansfield, MA) is a device for emergency intubation. It combines the functions of an esophageal obturator airway and a conventional ETT. It has

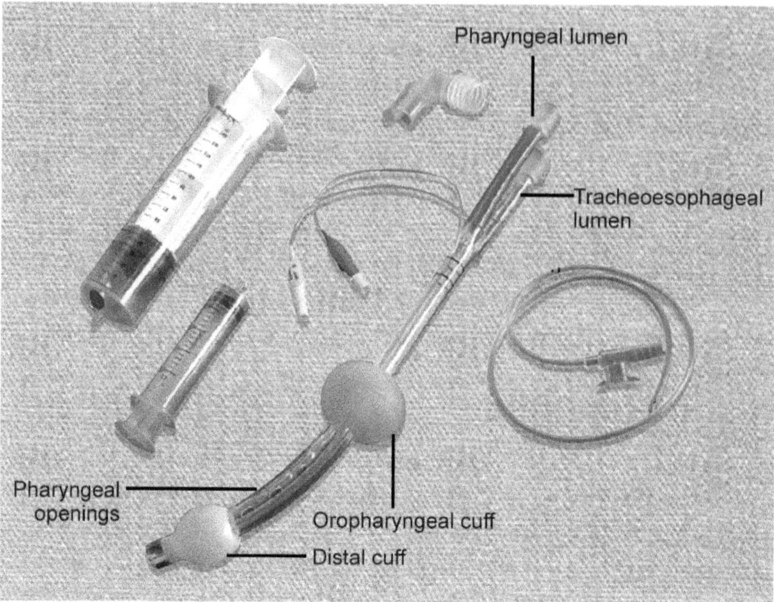

Fig. 17: Combitube.

double cuff; oropharyngeal balloon and a tracheoesophageal cuff. There are two lumen—(i) pharyngeal and (ii) tracheoesophageal lumen. Both the lumens are separated by a partition distally and are present as two separate tubes with standard connector distally. The pharyngeal lumen opens out distally as 8 perforations between both the cuffs. Tracheoesophageal lumen opens as a single opening distally.

Insertion Technique

Conventional Technique

- The lower jaw and tongue lifted using thumb and index finger.
- While pushing the tongue down the Combitube is inserted along the tongue in a curved movement. This helps in avoiding posterior pharyngeal injury.
- The oropharyngeal cuff is inflated first to about 85 mL for a 37-Fr tube. The cuff should not be visible in the mouth.
- Later the distal cuff is inflated to 10 mL with the other pilot balloon.
- First ventilate through the long tube which is pharyngeal lumen. Auscultation showing bilateral equal air entry to the lungs and no air entry to the stomach suggests perfect positioning.
- It can either be located in esophagus (more common) or trachea.

- In case of tracheal position the ventilation is proceeded via the tracheo-esophageal lumen.
- In case of kinking of the tube, it has to be removed and reinserted.

Alternate Technique

- Described by Urtubia and colleagues.
- The upper incisor or alveolar ridge is pulled up using index finger and thumb. Then middle finger is used to push down the chin.
- Recommended to keep the combitube curved until the time of insertion.
- Rest of the technique is similar to that of conventional technique.
- Alternately laryngoscope can also be used in aiding insertion.

Indications

1. Emergency situation requiring intubation, both in and out of hospital
2. Difficult airway situations
3. Decreased interincisor distance. (as small as 15 mm is adequate for combitube insertion
4. Difficult positions and poor illumination are other situations where Combitube comes handy.

Contraindications

- If gag reflex present
- Upper esophageal pathologies like Zenker's diverticulum, caustic substance ingestion, etc.

Advantages

- Blind insertion technique
- Can be used in both esophageal or tracheal position
- Noninvasive compared to cricothyrotomy
- Neck extension is unnecessary
- Useful in difficult airway situation
- Can be inserted from any position
- Allows frequent suctioning of gastric content
- Allows controlled ventilation up to 50 cm H_2O
- Can be used in awake intubation
- Not dependent on the laryngoscope or any other gadgets for insertion.

Disadvantages

- Suctioning of tracheal secretion is not possible
- Hence, prolonged period of ventilation should be avoided.

Complications

- Tongue engorgement
- Esophageal rupture
- Pyriform sinus rupture.

The Devices used below the Glottis

1. Endotracheal tubes
2. Tracheostomy tubes
3. Cricothyrotomy tubes.

ENDOTRACHEAL TUBES (ETT)

Deva Evu Subhas

Endotracheal tube is the best way of establishing a definitive airway, both in elective and emergency situations. Over the years the ET tube has evolved over time from a reusable red rubber tube to a PVC tube, addition of cuff to developing alternate forms of ETT as the need arose.

STANDARD ENDOTRACHEAL TUBE (FIG. 18)

The standard endotracheal tube is a conduit made of PVCs these days. They are all single-use devices. The ETT might have a cuff or without one. The cuff of initial days were high pressure low volume cuffs which was later replaced by low pressure high volume cuffs. The normal cuff pressures to be maintained between 20 and 30 cm H_2O. The cuff is inflated using a pilot balloon.

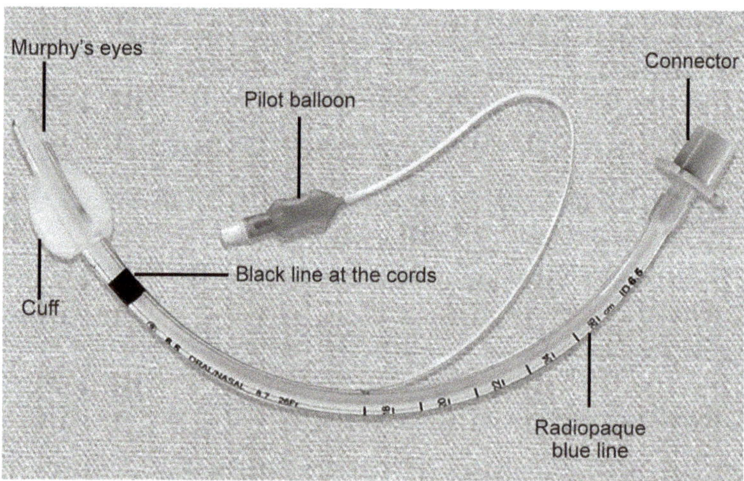

Fig. 18: Endotracheal tube.

The Murphy's eye, so named for Peter Murphy, an English anesthetist, is designed to provide an extra (secondary) portal for ventilation in case the distal lumen is obstructed. Over years the certain additional features have been added like subglottic suction, taper guard endotracheal cuff, etc. There modification to the ETT surface to decrease bacterial adhesion. There are ETT with fiberoptic camera distally which help in easy placement and in tracheal surveillance. Another example is the addition of multiple sensors, for so-called bioimpedance cardiography, that are capable of monitoring stroke volume variation, cardiac output, systemic vascular resistance, and arterial pressures (due to the close proximity of the ETT and the aorta) and thereby, at least theoretically, preventing the need for further invasive technologies.

Complications of Endotracheal Tube Placement

The problems associated with placement:

- Dental and oral problems
- Maxillofacial damage
- Displacement of the arytenoid cartilages
- Vocal cord ulceration or dysfunction
- Airway perforation
- Autonomic hyperactivity
- Failed intubation.

Problem associated with ETT in situ:

- Aspiration
- Vocal cord paralysis, or transient nerve palsy
- Ulceration and granuloma formation in the trachea and on the cords
- Tracheal synechiae
- Subglottic stenosis
- Laryngeal webbing
- Tracheomalacia
- Tracheoesophageal, tracheoinnominate, or tracheocarotid fistula
- Recurrent and superior laryngeal nerve damage.

ALTERNATIVES FOR STANDARD ETT

Reinforced Tubes (Fig. 19)

The reinforced tubes were introduced to overcome the issues related to kinking of the standard endotracheal tubes because of odd positioning. An anode or armored tube with an embedded wire coil is designed to minimize kinking even with quite severe position-induced angulation.

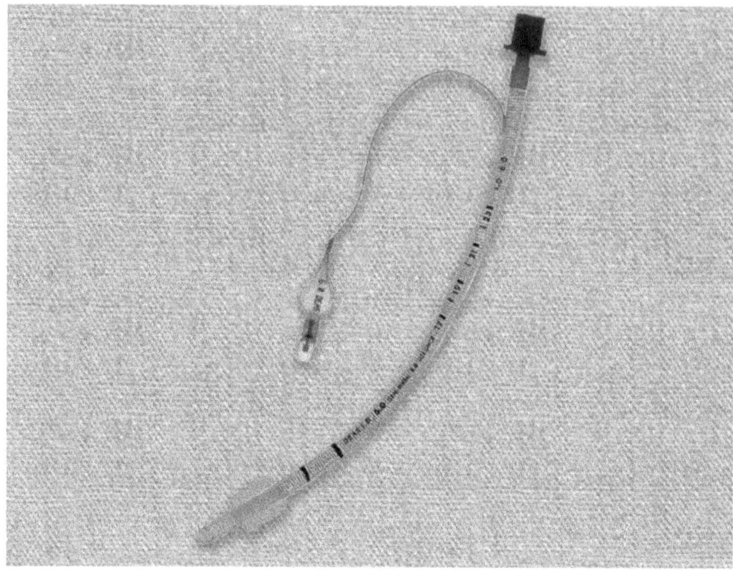

Fig. 19: Reinforced tubes.

Applications

- Used predominantly in head and neck surgeries
- Can be used through tracheostomy lumen
- Can be used during surgery like laryngectomy where tube needs to be moved around the surgical field
- Can used in situations where tracheomalacia is anticipated
- Can be used through ILMA.

Limitations

- Factors like patient biting on the tube might cause kinking beyond a certain threshold
- Accidental extubation frequent. Might require suturing to fix these tubes
- Usually changed to a standard ETT if postoperative ventilation is required.

Preformed Tubes (Fig. 20)

Preformed tubes were designed for better access during certain procedure, predominantly head and neck surgeries. Ring-Adair-Elwyn (RAE) tubes are the ones commonly in use. They are available as oral or nasal RAE tubes. The length of the intra-airway portion and the bend is proportional to the ETT size, i.e. internal diameter.

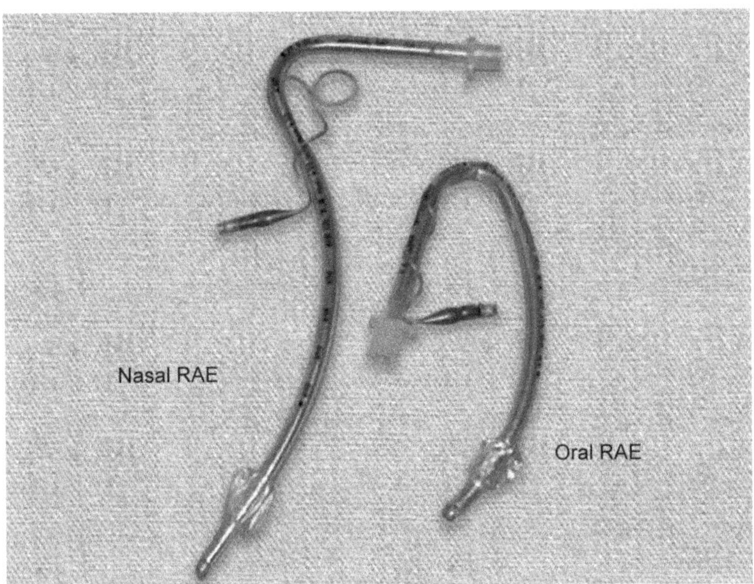

Fig. 20: Preformed tubes. (RAE: Ring-Adair-Elwyn tube)

Applications

- Predominantly in head and neck procedures.
- Improves access during surgery. For example, the access to oral cavity gets better with use of nasal RAE.

Limitations

- High incidence of malpositioning, such as endobronchial migration or accidental extubation is common
- Negotiating a suction catheter through the bent portion is often difficult or impossible.

Laser Tubes

There is a significant risk of airway fire following laser use. All the commonly used materials such as PVC, silicon, etc. are inflammable. Hence require protective wrapping. Commonly used materials for wrapping are aluminium foil, copper foil, metallic tapes, etc. However, none of these are FDA approved. Merocel Laser Guard protective wrap is the only FDA approved wrap which disappeared from market due to poor demand. FDA approved Laser Resistant Tracheal Tubes (LRTT) are available in market. Various manufactures are available with little variations in their features. They are of two types discussed further.

i. Metal shaft

This LRTT is made up of metal shaft. Laser flex by covidien is an example of LRTT with metallic shaft. It contains stainless steel reinforced shaft with double cuff.

ii. Nonmetallic core with metallic overlay

These are the tubes made of PVC or silicon with a metallic overlay. Will give example this category of tubes.

Types of laser tubes

Name	*Manufacturer*	*Material*	*Cuff*	*Comments*
Laser Shield II	Meditronics	Silicon core with aluminium overlay	Single cuff	Used for CO_2 and KTP lasers
Sheridan Laser-Trach	Teleflex Medical	Red rubber with copper foil	Single cuff	Used for CO_2 and KTP lasers
Rusch Laser tubus	Teleflex Medical	Red rubber with copper foil	Dual cuff inside a cuff	All types of laser

Cuff Management

Cuff is vulnerable part of LRTT. It can get punctured or inflamed by the laser. With cuff puncture there is increase in leak of ventilating gas which has high oxygen concentration leading to combustion. Salient points in managing cuff:

- Fill the cuff with saline instead of air, which will help in extinguishing minor fire. First inflate distal cuff and listen to exclude any leak, followed by inflation of proximal cuff.
- Tint the saline with methylene blue for early detection of cuff puncture.
- Sometimes the endotracheal tube needs to be changed in case of severe damage to the cuff.

Double Lumen Tubes

Double lumen tubes—discussed in Chapter 9 on One lung ventilation.

Tracheostomy/Cricothyroidotomy

Discussed in Chapter 7 on Surgical airway.

EQUIPMENTS USED IN ASSISTING INTUBATION

As it has been already discussed the endotracheal tube placement is the most definitive form of airway maintenance. It is important to have knowledge about all equipments that assist in this task.

LARYNGOSCOPE

It is a device used to visualize glottis. The main role it plays is with endotracheal intubation. The laryngoscope has undergone various modifications. And the trend now is to move toward single-use laryngoscope blades.

Historic Aspect

Before the days of laryngoscopes, tactile or blind intubation in awake patients was practiced. Alfred Kristen was first one to suggest that larynx could be directly visualized and came up with an instrument similar to esophagoscope. However, he abandoned this procedure in a years' time. Gustav Killian reviewed work of Alfred Kristen 13 years later and came up with a portable laryngoscope. But his model did not have a light attached. Chevalier Jackson later introduced hand-held laryngoscope with a light at the end. Later other anesthesiologist like Robert Miller, Robert Macintosh designed their own laryngoscopes.

Laryngoscope—Parts (Fig. 21)

Laryngoscopes are made of two main parts—(i) the handle and (ii) the blade.

The handle mainly contains battery power source. In certain type of laryngoscopes with fiberoptic tip, the handle carries the light source.

The blade has the following parts:

- Base to attach to the handle.

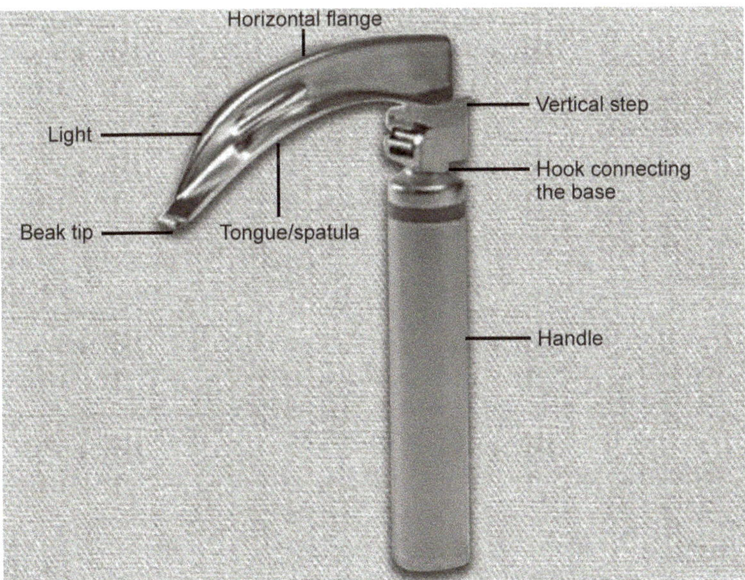

Fig. 21: Parts of laryngoscope.

- Tongue or spatula is that part of the blade which comes in contact with the tongue. It is either curved or straight.
- Left part of the blade is called flanges. It has a vertical and a horizontal component. The vertical part of flange is called vertical step.
- Web contains electric connection and the bulb.

There are also certain set of blades which were designed by decreasing the vertical step. This makes it possible to be used in patients with restricted mouth opening, buck tooth, receding jaw, bull neck, etc. Bizzarri-Giuffrida blade, Callander-Thomas blade, Bucx blade are some to name. Ronald Bowen and Ian Jackson tried creating a blade by combining the advantages of both straight and curved blade. It is called Bowen-Jackson blade. The final design had an almost straight blade with a marked distal curve. Other features such as decreased vertical step and increased angle (100°) between blade and stem were also added. Thus, could be used in patient with decreased mouth opening and also helps in avoiding pressing.

There is loads of blades in the market with slight difference in the design. Hence, lot of which are not in use often. So, those are not described in detail in this chapter. The laryngoscope has evolved over time with multiple variation as below.

- **Left-handed laryngoscopes** for left-handed personnel. This is a mirror image of conventional laryngoscope.
- **Variations with the light bulb**
  - Conventional scopes have light bulb on the blade.
  - Fiber tip operated laryngoscope contains light bulb on the handle. This allows the blade to be autoclaved.
  - LED bulbs are being used instead of the regular bulbs. LED lights are brighter, gives longer life to the batteries.
- **Variations regarding power source**
  - Battery is used as power sources
  - Rechargeable handle units are available these days.
- **Variation in terms of reusability**
  - Most of the laryngoscopes are reusable
  - Single-use versions of laryngoscope blades and laryngoscopes are being used these days in order to prevent spread of infection.
- **Laryngoscope blades with accessory device**
  - Blades with integrated oxygen delivery (oxyscope laryngoscope). Allow supplemental oxygen delivery during laryngoscopy through a separate port.
  - Blades with integrated suction port (Khan's blade, Tull blade). The oxygen supplement port can be used for suctioning or it has a dedicated suction channel. Useful in scenarios where there is bleeding or secretion that needs suctioning.

- Blade with secondary UV light source (IntuBrite). The secondary UV light helps in decreasing the scattering of the white light. This helps in better visualization of the structures.
- Ultralight weight tactile scope (Trulite). It is made of plastic handle with metal blade (Table 6).

Table 6: Different types of blades available

Types of blade	*Curved/straight*	*Comments*
Curved blades		
Macintosh (1943) (Robert Reynold Macintosh)	Curved	• Most popular curved blade • Attaches to handle at 90° • It has different forms: Standard (Fig. 22), English type and German type • English Macintosh (Fig. 23) blade is longer, its curve is more continuous across the entire length of the blade, and the height of the blade flange is shorter • German Macintosh (Fig. 24) version is similar to that of English blade with a glass fiberoptic bundle, LED bulb and a rechargeable batteries. Cleaning is much easier as it does not have much irregularities • Blade tip is placed anterior to the epiglottis in the vallecula
Straight blades		
Magill (1921) (Ivan Magill)	Straight	• Invented by Ivan Magill (1921) • Early laryngoscopes used these blades • Still a standard in veterinary laryngoscopes • Straight blade with 'U' shaped cross-session • Pressure on vagus nerve causes arrhythmias
Miller (1941) (Fig. 25) (Robert A Miller)	Straight	• Most popular straight blade • Straight blade with 'C' shaped cross section • Blade tip is placed posterior to the epiglottis. • Visualization is better than that of curved blade, however ease of placement is better with curved blade
Wisconsin	Straight	• Large straight blade with circular flange

Contd...

Contd...

Types of blade	*Curved/straight*	*Comments*
Soper (1947) (Robert Soper)	Straight	• It was designed as a modification of Macintosh blade • However its predominantly a straight blade with a slightly curved distal tip • Reverse 'Z' vertical step
Gould (1954)	Straight	• Modification of Soper blade • Rubberized flange, decreased vertical step, lengthened and blunted distal tip
Blades with exaggerated angulation		
Belscope		• Straight blade bent 45° at midpoint • No horizontal flanges • If visualization is suboptimal then a prism can be added proximal to the angulation to get an indirect view • Decreased chance of undue pressure to the upper lip • Might require styleted tracheal tube for placement
Choi double angle laryngoscope	Double-angled blade	• Double-angled blade with a spatula incorporating two incremental angles; proximal (20°) and distal (30°) • Light source pointing toward center of the glottis
Orr laryngoscope	Two right angle bends	• Two right angle bends shifts the fulcrum from the upper teeth • Rarely used now
McCoy (Fig. 26)	Lever tip, curved	• Modification of Macintosh blade • It has a hinged tip operated by a lever • Useful in elevating distal structures like epiglottis • Useful in case of difficult intubation like patient on cervical collar • Trauma to epiglottis is a known complication
Pediatric blades		
Oxford (Bryce Smith) blade	Straight	• 'U' shaped flanges and vertical step • Distal end tapers from proximal to distal • Broad horizontal flange prevents the upper lip from obscuring the view • This gives an added advantage in cases like cleft palate
Robertshaw (Fig. 27)	Straight	• Straight blade with 'C' shaped cross section • Blade tip is positioned posterior to epiglottis • Good for neonatal intubation

Contd...

Types of blade	*Curved/straight*	*Comments*
Seward	Straight	• Straight blade with reverse 'Z' shaped vertical step and flange • Straight blade with mid-distal angulation and a tapering width
Laryngoscopes with optically assisted views		
Siker laryngoscopes	Angulated at 135°	• Stainless steel mirror attached by means of copper jacket • Copper improves heat conduction and thus minimizes fogging of mirror • Need practice and expertise for successful intubation • Need styleted ETT
McMorrow-Mirakhur mirrored laryngoscope		• Modification of McCoy blade • The levering tip has a mirror attached to it which will be deployed on activating the levering tip • Mirror and blade should be heated every time before use to minimize fogging
Huffman prism		• Huffman attached a plexiglas prism to a Macintosh 3 blade by means of a steel clip • Thought to decrease pressure on the tongue and hypopharynx • He added another prism distally
Rusch ViewMax (Fig. 28) laryngoscope		(a) ViewMax • Similar to that of a Macintosh blade with a removable lens system ending proximally on an eyepiece • Produces about 20° refraction • Decreased vertical step, hence lesser effectiveness in pushing tongue to one side. Its introduced in the midline (b) True view EVO_2 • The optical system is similar to that of ViewMax but its more angulated • Produces a refraction of 42° • Distinguishing feature of EVO_2 is presence of the oxygen port • Rechargeable fiber lit handle • This could be converted to a video laryngoscope by adding on a camera to the eyepiece

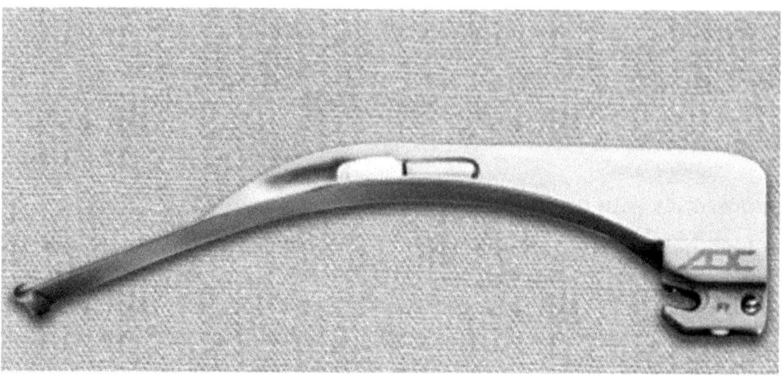

Fig. 22: Standard Macintosh.

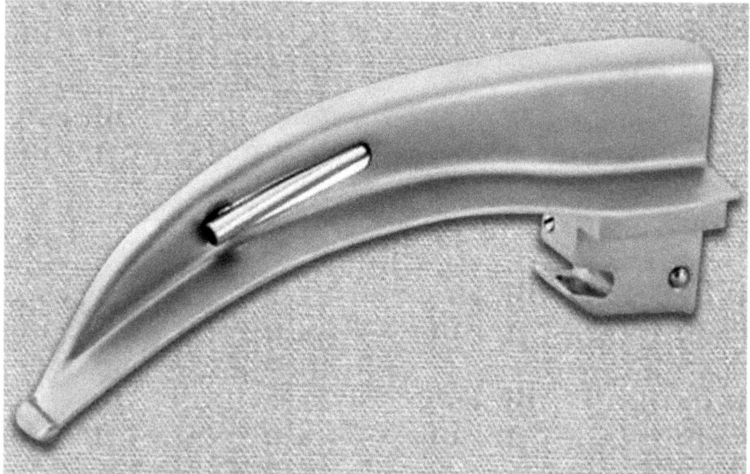

Fig. 23: English Macintosh.

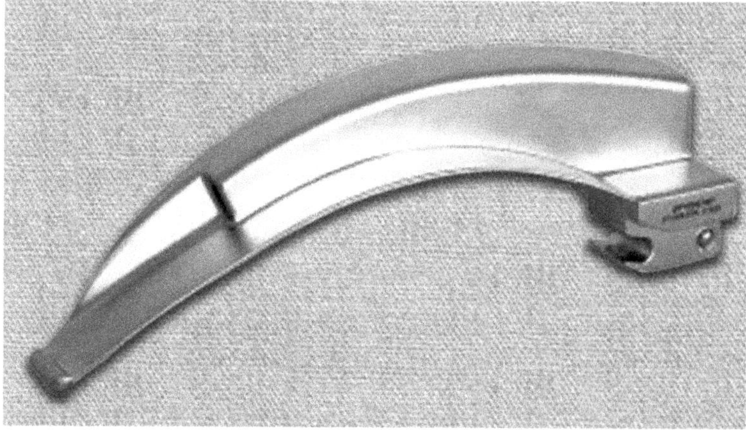

Fig. 24: German Macintosh.

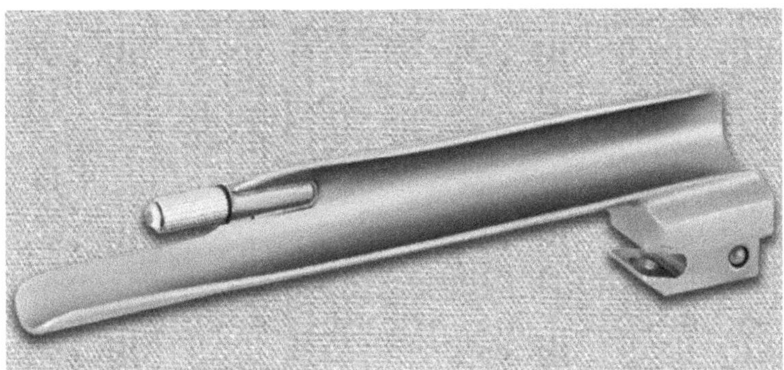

Fig. 25: Miller blade.

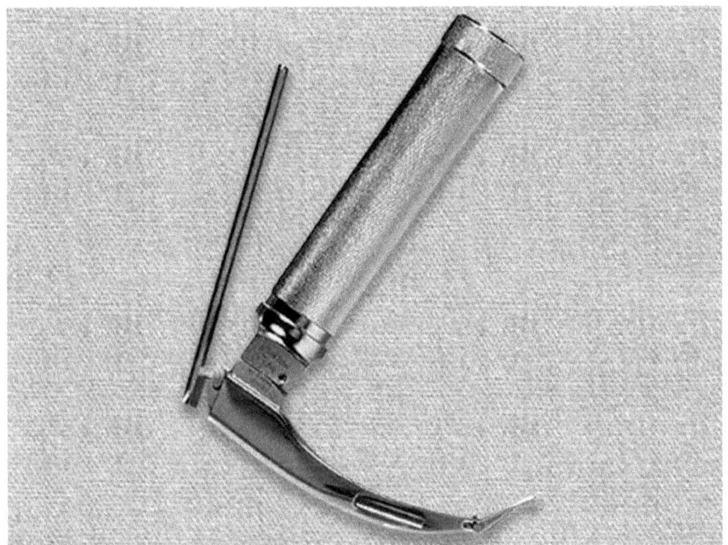

Fig. 26: McCoy blade.

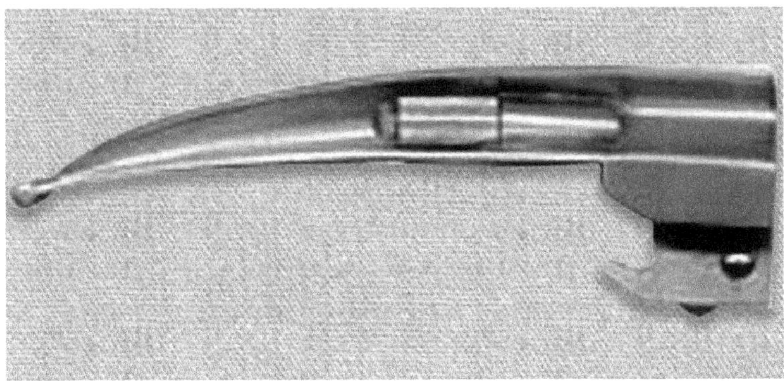

Fig. 27: Robertshaw blade.

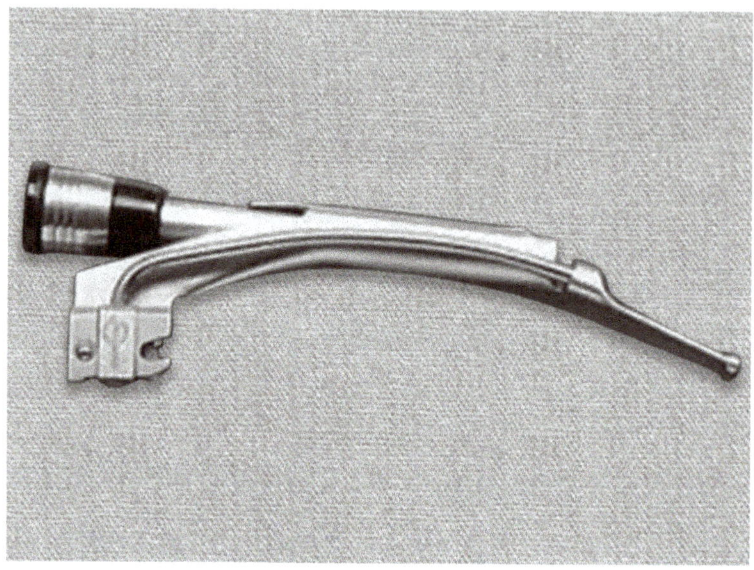

Fig. 28: ViewMax blade.

VIDEO LARYNGOSCOPE (VL)

It seems to have its own advantage in difficult airway cases and also has a role to play in training. Miniaturization of camera chip technology; improved, rechargeable battery power and light output; and affordable, small liquid crystal display (LCD) monitors, all this put together made video laryngoscopy a popular technology, and further led to the introduction of different types of VLs.

The VLs has variations based mainly on the blades. Video system could be added on to the conventional blade like Macintosh. Everybody would be familiar in handling these blades, plus direct laryngoscopy is possible. Next set of system where the blade is highly curved or angulated leading on to better visualization. However direct laryngoscopy is not possible with this system and a styleted ETT curved anteriorly is a must. There is another system where tube guiding channel is incorporated into the system. The use of styleted tube can be avoided.

All the VL systems are available in disposable form. The monitor set up could be external or integrated. External monitor provides better orientation for both laryngoscopist and assistant. Thus, allows the assistant to help. Documentation is possible with external monitor. The integrated system has decreased orientation, difficulty for others to visualize. Advantages of integrated system is its unrestricted movement, less light and space requirement (Table 7).

Table 7: Different types of VL

VL name	*Monitor*	*Features*
Macintosh based VL		
AP advance (Venner Medical, Kiel, Germany)	Integrated, attached to handle via magnet	• Battery powered handle, blade core and monitor • Can be used as direct laryngoscope without attaching the monitor • Comes with two disposable blades similar to Macintosh and one difficult airway blade (DAB) • DAB has a distal angulation and a tube guiding channel
Direct coupled interface (DCI) Video laryngo-scope system (Karl Storz, Tuttlingen, Germany)	External	• Attached to 1943 version of Macintosh blade • DCI system has been displaced by a mobile C – MAC system
C – MAC System (Karl Storz, Tuttlingen, Germany) (Fig. 30)	It has an 7″ external monitor which allows recording on an SD card and also a pocket monitor (2.4″) which attaches wirelessly	• Uses modified Macintosh blade with curvature same as that of 1943 Macintosh version. However, it differs in two aspects; thinner profile and beveled shoulder • C – MAC system has various blades, Macintosh 2, 3 and 4, Miller 0 and 1 and D – Blade • D – blade has exaggerated curvature which comes handy if visualization with regular blades fail • An electronic module (E module) attaches to the blade handle and this allows rapid change of blades • Optical system of the C-MAC consists of a complementary metal-oxide semi-conductor (CMOS) chip set, an optical lens with an aperture angle of 80°, and a high-power, light-emitting diode (LED) at the distal third of the blade with effective antifogging properties • The 7″ external monitor allows capturing of image or video recording • The pocket monitor is a 2.4″ LCD monitor along with a lithium ion battery and E – module. This rechargeable battery supplies both the monitor and the LED light source for about an hour • C–MAC VL generally does not require a sylet along with ETT unless D – Blade is used

Contd...

Contd...

VL name	*Monitor*	*Features*
		• Failed to intubate because of bright environmental light and intubation with the device used as a direct laryngoscope was faster. These were the issues reported. Otherwise overall clinical experience shows better results in difficult airway cases • They also have a C–MAC S system which is similar to the C–MAC system (Fig. 29) except that the blades are single-use, made of plastic
McGrath MAC (Aircraft Medical, Edinburgh, United Kingdom)	Integrated monitor (2.5″ LCD monitor)	• Battery power source is on the handle • Macintosh blades are used. Disposable blades also available (3 and 4) • Direct laryngoscopy is possible • Shown to have improved ease of double lumen tube placement
GlideScope Direct (Verathon Medical, Bothell, WA)	External 7″ monitor	• A Macintosh blade added to the standard glide scope system is called Glidescope direct • Designed mainly for teaching purpose as it allows both direct and indirect laryngoscope • Single-use version is also available
Trueview Picture Capture Device (Fig. 30)	Integrated	• Conventional Trueview EVO_2 is converted to a video laryngoscope by adding a camera and monitor • The camera of the Trueview PCD screen is attached to the eye piece via a magnet
VL with highly curved blade		
Glidescope (Verathon Medical, Bothell, WA) (Fig. 31)	External with 7″ monitor	• Prototype for indirect video laryngoscope • Made up of medical grade plastic • Sizes fitting small children to adult are available • Single-use version (Glidescope cobalt AVL) which comes with a disposable plastic sheath covering the blade • Insertion is little different from that of a regular Macintosh blade. It does not require reaching up to valeculla and no need for the kind of force needed for the regular Macintosh blade • The ETT should be styleted and a distal curve of 60° to 90° to be maintained ("Hockey Stick" formation)

Contd...

Contd...

VL name	*Monitor*	*Features*
		• Achieve a good glottic view prior to inserting the ETT • The tube advanced posterior and alongside the blade • Care to be taken not to injure the pharynx while advancing the ETT • The ETT should be placed at the glottic opening, then the ETT alone should be advanced, holding back the stylet • The ETT should be placed at the glottic opening, then the ETT alone should be advanced, holding back the stylet • Indirect laryngoscopy is an alternate technique for direct laryngoscopy. Hence requires practice and mastering the skill • A study by Aziz and colleagues reported overall success rate of 97% and 3% could not be intubated • Even though the visualization of glottis improves with Glidescope there is still difficulty in passing the ETT
McGrath series 5 (Aircraft Medical, Edinburgh, United Kingdom)	Integrated	• Fully portable system • The blade is highly angulated and the length is adjustable • Comes with a single-use plastic sheath • Scopy and insertion technique are similar to that of Glidescope
Video Laryngoscope with Tube guiding channel		
The King Vision (King Systems, Noblesville, IN) (Fig. 32)	Integrated (can be connected to external monitor too)	• Highly angulated blade which is single-use (has a CMOS camera) and a reusable monitor with battery power source • The blades come with or without a tube guiding channel • Preload the ETT through tube guiding channel • Advance the blade toward glottis. Placing the tip of the blade in valleculla and gentle lifting increases the chance of intubation • When the glottis opening comes to view, make sure it is in the center of the screen and then advance the ETT

Contd...

Contd...

VL name	*Monitor*	*Features*
Pentax Airway Scope AWS-S100 (Pentax medicals)	Integrated	• Handle with power source, LED light and charge coupled device camera • Has a single size blade with a port for catheter • Prototype for VLs with tube guiding port • Needs an antifogging solution to be applied every time used
The Airtraq (Prodol Meditec, Guecho, Spain) (Fig. 33)	External	• Single-use device • Two ports available; one to transfer image through the system of lenses and prism on to eyepiece and another one for ETT • Available in various sizes with an added version for nasal and DLT use • Insertion technique is similar to kings VL with an ETT preloaded • Studies have shown it to be better than conventional Macintosh blade. However, there was no benefit in case of prehospital use

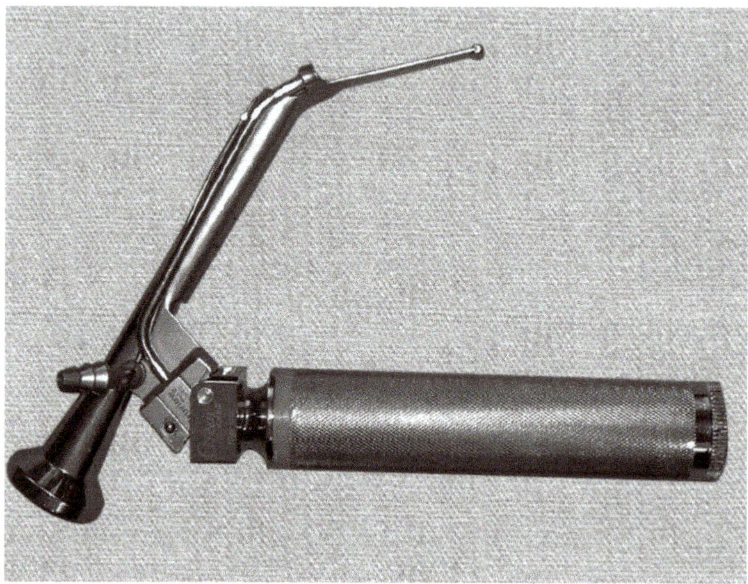

Fig. 29: Trueview.

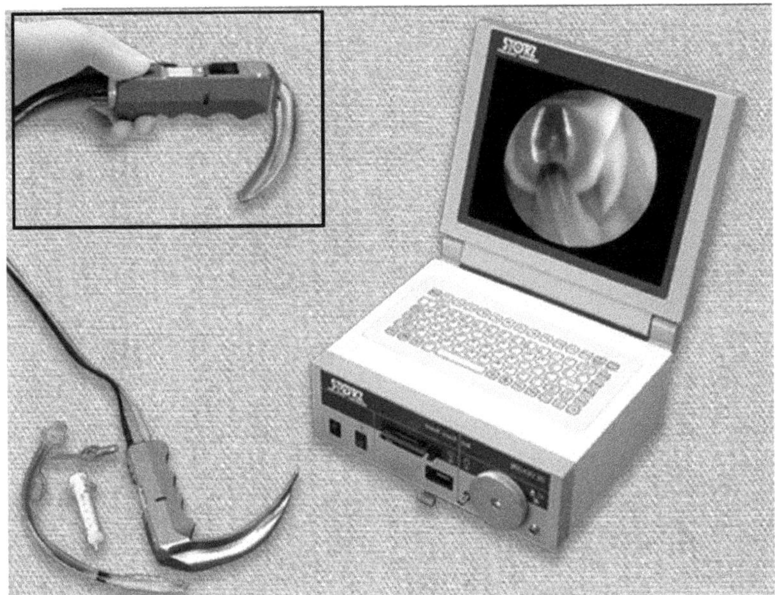

Fig. 30: C-Mac system.

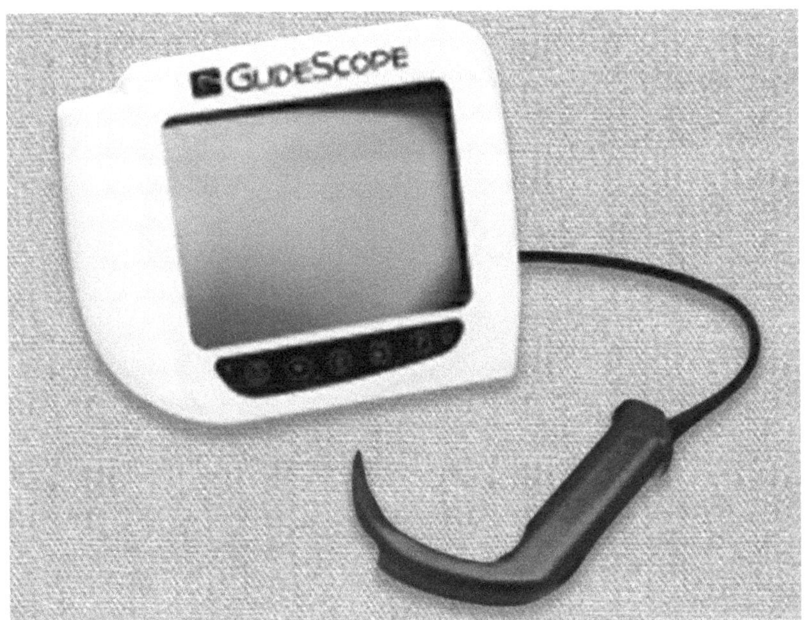

Fig. 31: Glidescope.

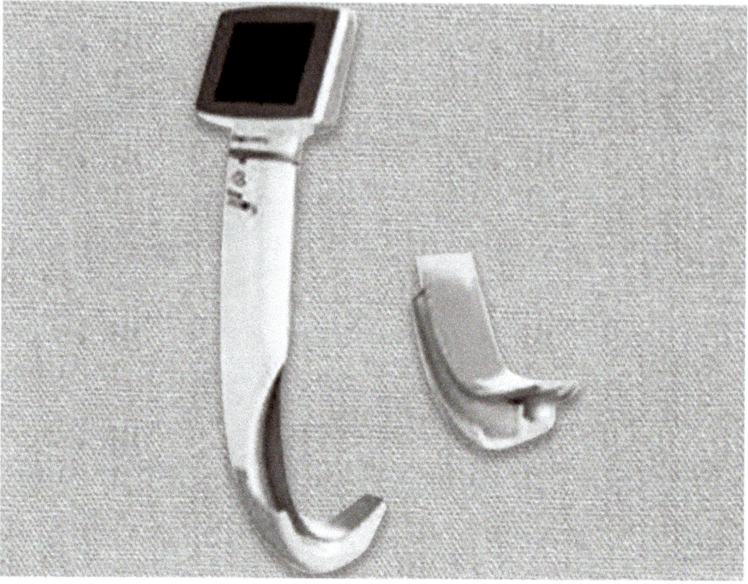

Fig. 32: King vision.

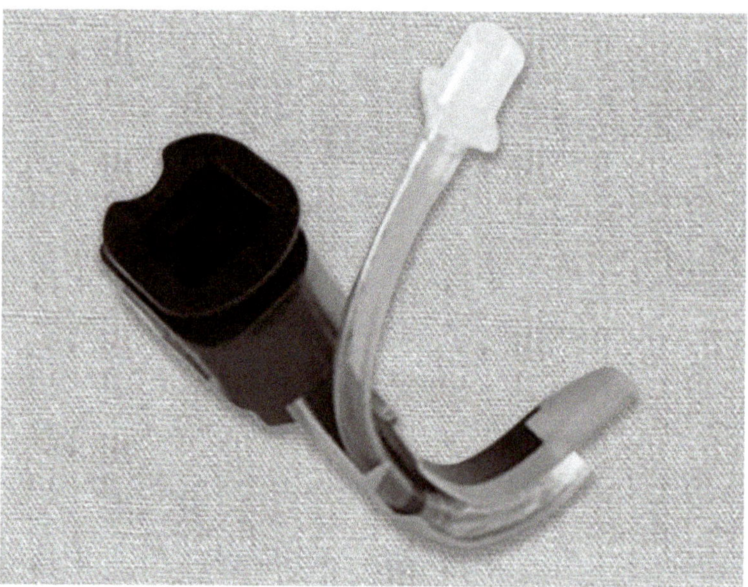

Fig. 33: Airtraq.

INTUBATING INTRODUCERS AND STYLETS

The introducers or stylets acts as a guide while passing ETT, especially in a difficult airway situation where the glottis is poorly visualized. Macintosh was the first one to make a mention of introducers back in 1949. This topic can be dealt upon four broad categories.

1. Intubating introducers
2. Tube exchangers
3. Stylets
4. Lighted stylets.

Intubating Introducers

Intubating introducers are commonly known as bougies. They are introduced first into the trachea and over which the ETT is rail roaded.

Eschmann Introducer

This introducer is a useful tool in situations where laryngeal opening cannot be visualized. It is made up of polyester core and resin covering. The curved tip facing anteriorly makes it easier to hook under the epiglottis. Once the tip crosses the glottis advance the bougie at a shallow angle to the patient. This allows clicking sensation which helps confirm the tracheal rings. The other way on confirming its tracheal position is by advancing further, which leads to slight deviation to right suggesting right main bronchus. There is a "Hold-up" at 30–35 cm mark. Checking for "hold-up" to be avoided as much as possible due to increase chance of trauma. Then rail road an endotracheal tube over the bougie and remove the bougie. Keep the laryngoscope in place while passing the ETT. At times jaw thrust helps in smooth placement of the tube.

Gum Elastic Bougie (Fig. 34)

This is good tool if epiglottis is visualized during laryngoscopy. On the other hand, it is better not to use this if the epiglottis is not visualized, as the successful intubation rate is unacceptably low. It is often called "Gum elastic bougie". However, it is neither made of gum nor elastic. And it is technically not a bougie, as bougie is generally a dilator.

Tube Exchanger (Fig. 35)

Tube exchanger are useful in difficult airway situation as it allows ventilation during this difficult period. Even though there are bougies which can be used as a tube exchanger, there are dedicated tube exchangers in the market such as Cook Airway Exchange Catheter and Sheriden Tube Exchanger. They are generally designed as a hollow tube with an attachable adapter for ventilation and also made flexible and straight like a bougie.

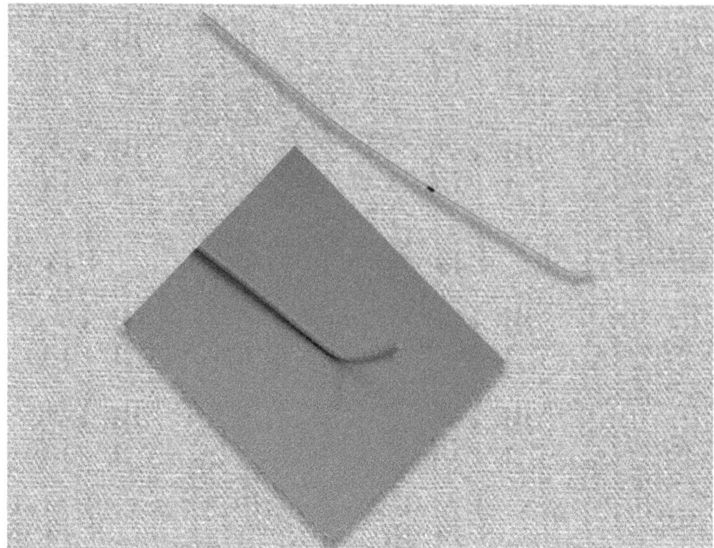

Fig. 34: Gum elastic bougie.

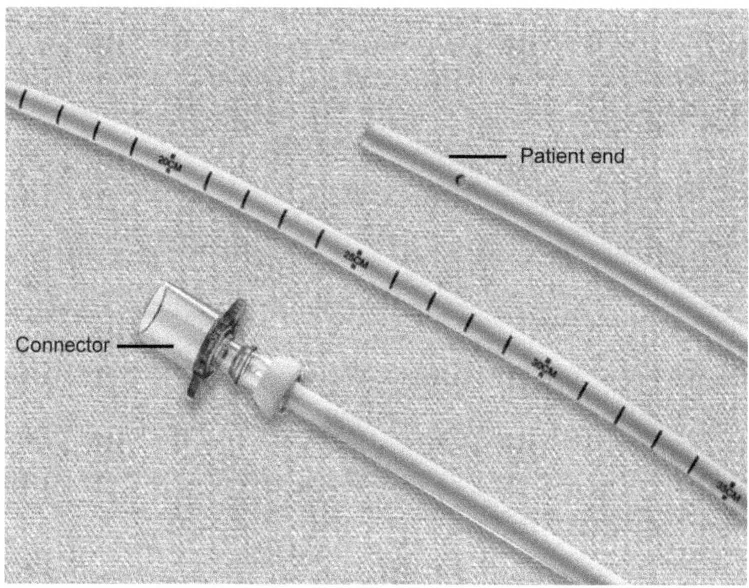

Fig. 35: Cook airway exchange catheter.

Stylets (Fig. 36)

Stylets are metal rods with a plastic covering which helps in making the ETT stiff or preshape it at the time of intubation. The stylet cannot be

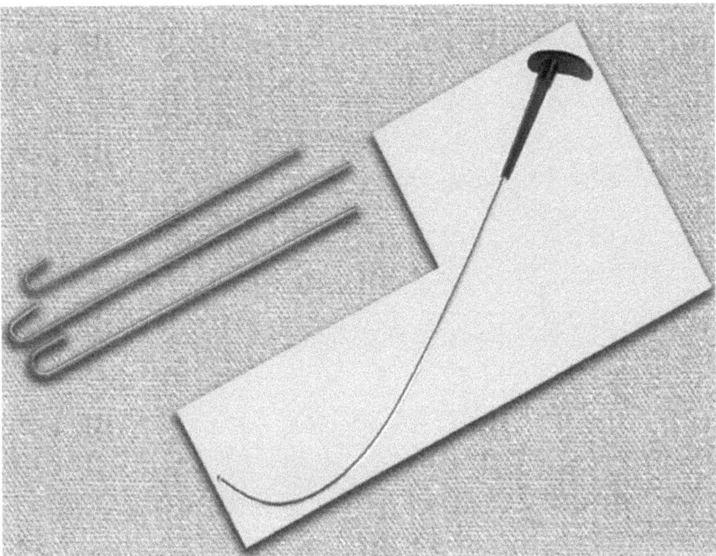

Fig. 36: Stylet.

used naked. It is usually passed through the ETT. To avoid make sure the tip of the stylet does not protrude beyond ETT tip. The ETT is generally made to assume "Hockey Stick" shape. However, it is the personnel using it may shape to his or her desire. An angle of 35° or less makes it less traumatic. Check the mobility of stylet within the ETT prior to intubation. The stylet should be removed once the tip of ETT enters the vocal cords.

Lighted Stylets (Fig. 37)

Lighted stylets uses principle of transillumination of soft tissue. The anterior position of trachea comes to its advantage. If the tip of the lighted stylet is past the glottis into trachea then there is a well-circumscribed glow of light below the thyroid prominence. If the tip is in esophagus then there is a diffuse glow or no glow. If the tip is in vallecula then there is a diffuse glow above thyroid prominence. This enables intubation without laryngoscopes.

Fiberoptic Lighted-Intubation Stylet (Benson Medical Industries Inc., Markham, Ont., Canada), the Flexilum (Concept Corporation, Clearwater, FL), the Tubestat (Concept Corporation), and the Fiberoptic Lighted Stylet (Fiberoptic Medical Products, Inc., Allentown, PA) are few of the earlier commercially available lighted stylets. They had certain limitations like poor illumination, short length, rigidity (making nasal intubation difficult), absence of connector to secure the ETT to the lighted stylet and most of them were single-use device.

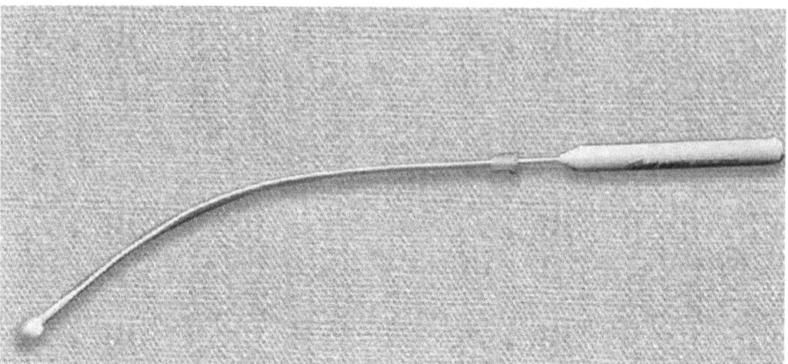

Fig. 37: Lighted stylet.

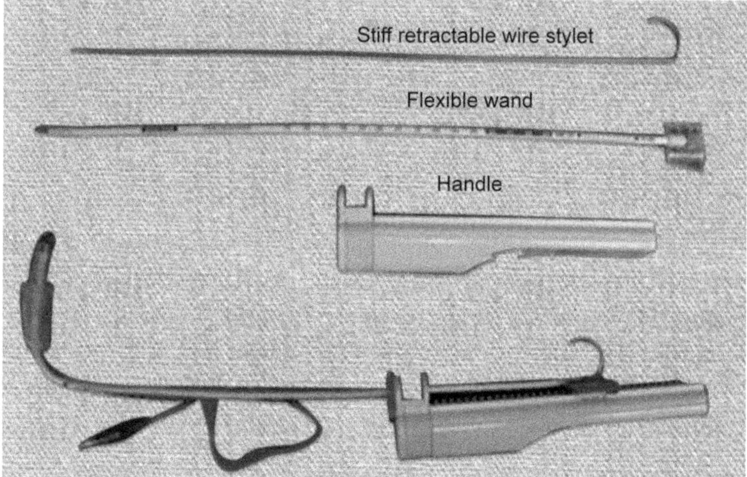

Fig. 38: Trachlight.

Trachlight

(Adapted from textbook of Benumof & Hagberg's airway management 2012)

Trachlight (Laerdal Medical Corp., Wappingers Falls, NY) (Fig. 38) was introduced in 1995 to overcome these limitation. It has three main parts—(i) a reusable handle, (ii) a flexible wand, and (iii) a retractable wire stylet. The handle encloses the power circuitory and batteries. The flexible wand allows the length to be adjusted. The retractable stylet helps maintaining the stiffness of ETT and thus increases ease of intubation. The light source is also more powerful.

The general complication of intubating introducers, tube exchangers, stylets and lighted stylets are few. They include laryngeal trauma, sore throat. However serious complications like tracheal, laryngeal and pharyngeal perforation and subluxation of cricoarytenoids are all rare complications.

CONCLUSION

The knowledge of airway equipments is so vital, especially during a difficult airway situation. The discovery of Laryngeal Mask Airway by Archie Brain led to discovery of various supraglottic airway devices. Over the years we have seen great many discoveries which have eased the intubation techniques like video laryngoscopes, lighted stylets, etc. Hope this chapter provided insight into these airway equipments.

5 Tracheal Intubation

Geetanjali S Verma

Tracheal intubation is the safest way to protect the airway, but the technique in itself can be hazardous when not practiced with precautions.

A golden rule to be followed is - "when in doubt, take it out"!

WHEN AND HOW

Geetanjali S Verma

The airway needs to protected for causes involving pathology, physiology or convenience.

INDICATIONS

Emergency	*Elective*
• Inability to maintain airway patency (GCS <8)	• Surgical procedures involving the head and neck/surgeries done in other positions than supine
• Inability to protect the airway against aspiration	• Positions that preclude manual airway support
• Ventilatory compromise or failure to adequately oxygenate pulmonary capillary blood	• Almost all situations involving neuromuscular paralysis (Botulism, Tetanus)
• Tracheobronchial toilet	• Surgical procedures involving the cranium, thorax, or abdomen
• Anticipation of a deteriorating course that will eventually lead to the inability to maintain airway patency or protection	• Procedures that may involve intracranial hypertension

CONTRAINDICATIONS

Absolute	*Relative*
Total upper airway obstruction, which requires a surgical airway	Anticipated "difficult" airway, in which endotracheal intubation may be unsuccessful, resulting in reliance on successful bag-valve-mask (BVM) ventilation to keep an unconscious patient alive
Total loss of facial/oropharyngeal landmarks, which requires a surgical airway	

PREPARATION

Prerequisites for Intubation

S – Suction
O – Oxygen
A – Airways
P – Position and preoxygenation
M – Monitoring equipments/Medications
E – $EtCO_2$

1. Skilled assistant
2. *Oral airway*: Guedel's airway of appropriate size or nasopharyngeal airway
3. *Face mask*: Well fitting, of appropriate size with Ambu bag
4. *Oxygen source*: Cylinder or pipeline
5. *Laryngoscope* of appropriate size with adequate illumination
   a. Miller (straight blade) #0, 1 for neonates
   b. Macintosh (curved blade) #0, 1 for neonates
      #2 - Young children
      #3 - Adults
      #4 - Large adults
   c. *Polio blade*: In case of short neck or obese patients
6. *Suction device*: To clear oral secretions
7. *Endotracheal tubes of appropriate size*: 1 size smaller and larger also to be available (with a syringe for inflation of cuff and tapes for fixation)
   a. Adult males - 8.5, 8
   b. Adult females - 7, 7.5, 8
   c. Young children - 6, 6.5, 7
   d. Children < 6 months - age/3 +3.5
   e. Children > 6 months - age/4 +4
8. *Good intravenous access*
9. *Drugs*
   a. For sedation - Fentanyl, Midazolam
   b. Neuromuscular blockers - Succinylcholine (in cases of emergency and anticipated difficult airway), non-depolarizing agents (Rocuronium, Vecuronium)

10. *Proper positioning of head*: Sniffing the morning air (avoid manipulation of cervical spine in trauma cases or those with suspected cervical spine injury)
11. *Adjuncts*: Stylets, bougie, Magill forceps
12. *Confirmation aids*: Stethoscope, saturation monitor, $EtCO_2$ monitor
13. *Difficult airway cart* (with surgical airway instruments and emergency drugs).

METHODS OF INTUBATION

1. Regular laryngoscopy and oral/nasal intubation
2. Blind nasal intubation
3. Retrograde intubation
4. Fiberoptic aided nasal/oral intubation (Refer chapter on fiberoptic intubation).

Regular Laryngoscopy and Intubation

Technique of Direct Laryngoscopy (Fig. 1)

The Macintosh and Miller blades of appropriate size and bright illumination are chosen. The tip of the Macintosh blade is inserted into the vallecula (the space between the base of the tongue and the pharyngeal surface of the epiglottis). Pressure against the hyoepiglottic ligament elevates the epiglottis to expose the larynx. The Miller blade is passed to include the

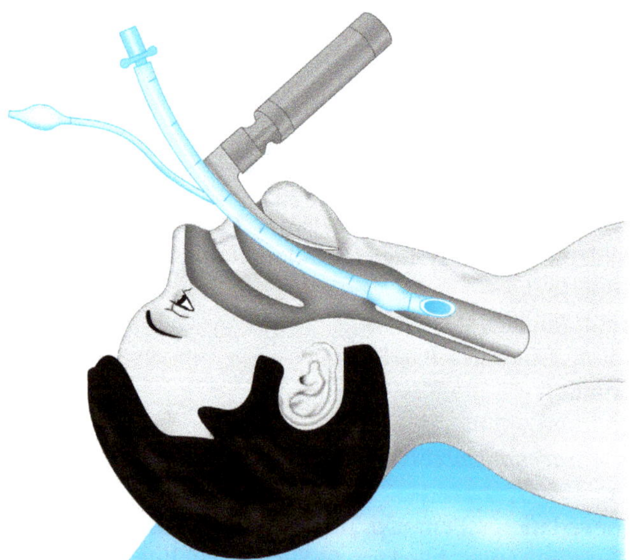

Fig. 1: The traditional method of oral intubation, first publicized by Kirstein in 1895, and still the most commonly used emergency airway management technique, is direct laryngoscopy.

epiglottis and the tip lies beneath the laryngeal surface of the epiglottis; the epiglottis is then lifted to expose the vocal cords. The Miller blade provides a better exposure of the glottic opening but provides a smaller room through the oro- and hypopharynx. Visualization of airway structures is easier if a sufficient distance is maintained between the operator's eyes and the patient's airway. Crouching too close to the mouth results in a narrowed visual depth of field.

After positioning the patient, the laryngoscope is held in the left hand (in right-handed individuals) and the fingers of the right hand are used to open the mouth gently (or assistant's help may be taken for it). The laryngoscope blade is introduced along the right corner of the patient's mouth avoiding the teeth and to enable the flange of the blade to keep the tongue to the left. The laryngoscope blade is advanced to expose the right tonsillar pillar and then advanced in the midline until the epiglottis comes in view. The tongue and pharyngeal soft tissues are lifted to expose the glottic opening. The direction of force is along the axis of the laryngoscope handle to pull it forward and upward. The blade should never be used as a lever, using the upper teeth or maxilla as the fulcrum. External pressure on the cricoid and/or thyroid cartilages may aid in visualization of the glottis for which assistant's help may be taken.

Oral Endotracheal Intubation

An appropriate-sized tube is chosen for the patient and the cuff is checked (for leaks) and lubricated with Lignocaine jelly before insertion. During insertion, the endotracheal tube is held in the operator's right hand and advanced through the oral cavity from the right corner of the mouth and then through the vocal cords (after visualization of cords). When the visualization of the glottis is poor, the tube can be directed anteriorly with the help of a malleable stylet. The end of the stylet should lie at least 1 cm proximal to the end of the endotracheal tube to reduce the chance of airway injury. The tip of the assembled stylet and endotracheal tube can be bent anteriorly into "hockey stick" curve. The tube is passed till the black line on the distal end passes the vocal cords. The markings on the tube in relation to the patient's incisors are noted. In adult males, the tube is generally inserted to about 23 cm at the incisors to position the tube tip an appropriate 4 cm above the carina. For females, the distance is about 21 cm.

Tube inserted too far will cause endobronchial intubation, while tubes that are not in far enough may be more at risk of accidental extubation. The endotracheal tube cuff is inflated to obtain a seal in the presence of 20–30 cm of H_2O positive airway pressure (also confirmed by keeping fingers over sterna notch to detect for leaks). The tube should be securely fastened with tapes. The entire attempt at endotracheal intubation should take no longer than 30 seconds.

Nasal Intubation

Indications

1. In the operating room for dental procedures and intraoral (e.g. mandibular reconstructive procedures or mandibular osteotomies) and oropharyngeal surgeries.
2. Securing the airway in patients with questionable cervical spine stability or severe degenerative cervical spine disease (using awake fiberoptic intubation technique), patients with intraoral mass lesions or structural abnormalities, and patients with limited mouth opening (e.g. trismus).

Contraindications

Absolute	*Relative*
• Suspected epiglottitis	• Large nasal polyps
• Midface instability	• Suspected nasal foreign bodies
• Coagulopathy	• Recent nasal surgery
• Suspected basilar skull fractures	• Upper neck hematoma
• Apnea or impending respiratory arrest (Any patient with advanced upper airway obstruction, who is apneic or having difficulties maintaining his or her airway, should not be subjected to any form of awake intubation)	• History of frequent episodes of epistaxis
	• Prosthetic heart valves (increased risk of bacteremia during the insertion)

Method (Fig. 2)

Patient may be intubated either awake or asleep. Once the endotracheal tube has passed into the nasopharynx, the breath sounds should be monitored. At each inspiratory effort, the tube is advanced while constantly monitoring breath sounds. If advancing the tube results in loss of or reduction in breath sounds, then the tube should be withdrawn till the breath sounds are maximally heard. The endotracheal tube can then be turned slightly and readvanced with each inspiratory effort. Successful tracheal intubation is detected by continued auscultation of distant breath sounds, some resistance as the tube passes through the vocal cords, the patient coughing, and the capnography reading and waveform.

If after repeated attempts of insertion of the endotracheal tube, it fails to enter the trachea, then the tube should be withdrawn to the point when

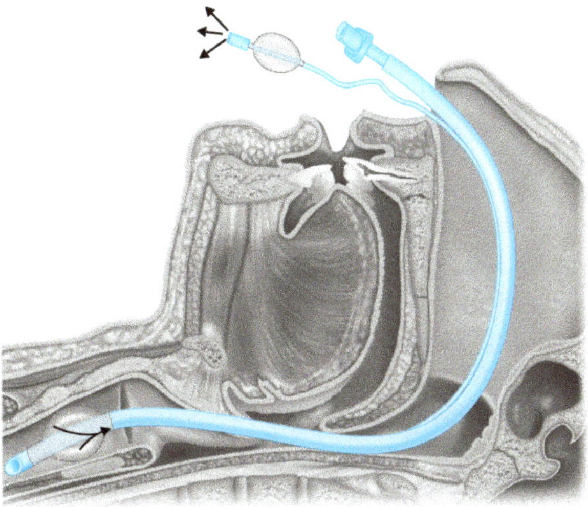

Fig. 2: Nasotracheal intubation.

the breath sounds are heard loudest. At this point, 10 mL of air can be introduced into the tube cuff (directing the tube tip anteriorly away from the posterior pharyngeal wall) and the endotracheal tube can be advanced a further 2 cm without loss of breath sounds. The cuff is then deflated and the tube advanced further into the trachea. Commonly, the tube tends to enter the esophagus. Extending the patient's neck or providing cricoid pressure tends to align the tube with the glottis and may increase the chances of the success.

Retrograde Intubation

Indications

1. Anticipated difficult intubation:
    a. To bypass existing tracheostomy for better surgical exposure
    b. Trismus
    c. Small mouth with protruding upper teeth
    d. Congenital anomalies - resulting in micrognathia, short neck, large tongue, limited neck movement and mouth opening, and cervical spine abnormalities
    e. Trauma - maxillofacial and cervical spine
    f. Tumor - tongue, mandible, floor of the mouth, pharynx and larynx
    g. Infection - retropharyngeal abscess, acute epiglottitis
    h. Bone and joint disorders - rheumatoid arthritis, ankylosing spondylitis, and unstable cervical spine
    i. Obstructive sleep apnea

j. Microstomia
k. Burns.
2. Failed intubation:
With blind nasal, direct laryngoscopic or fiberoptic scope guided technique.

Dedicated kits (Cook Retrograde Intubation Set, Bloomington, IN) are available for pediatric and adult use.

Retrograde guides that can be used: Vinyl plastic tubing, epidural catheters, long catheters inside needle, pulmonary artery catheter guidewire, straight guidewire, angiography catheter exchange guidewire, 'J' tipped guidewire, ureteral stent, nylon cord, surgical suture material, the Minitrach (Non Seldinger kit, Smith Medical International, Watford, UK) dilator.

Method (Fig. 3)

The supine patient is placed in the sniffing position (sitting position preferred for patients in respiratory distress). The oropharynx is topically anesthetized. An 18-gauge needle attached to a syringe containing 2 mL of 4% lidocaine is inserted through the cricothyroid membrane in a cephalad direction into the larynx. Aspiration of air confirms correct placement of the needle, and the local anesthetic is injected into the larynx. The guidewire is threaded through the needle into the pharynx. When the guide is passed upwards from the larynx, it may come out from the mouth, coil inside the pharynx or sometimes exit from one of the nostrils. When performed as an awake technique, the patient may be able to 'spit' the retrograde guide out of the mouth. Alternatively, when there is adequate mouth opening,

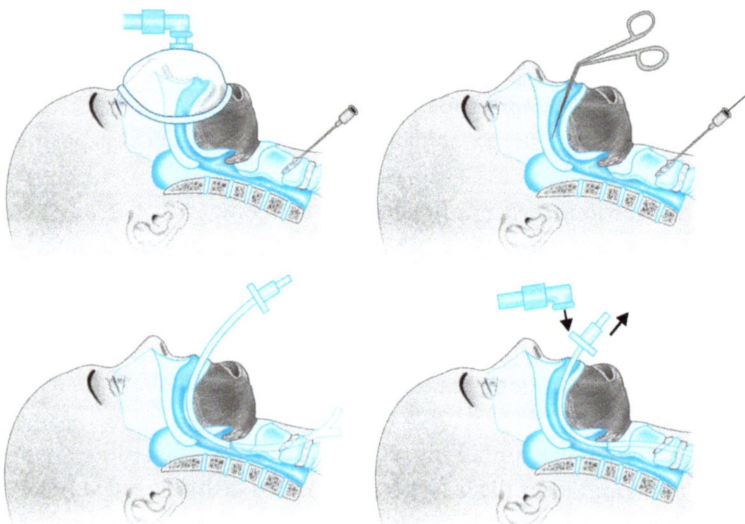

Fig. 3: Steps in retrograde intubation.

it may be picked up from the mouth or pharynx with fingers or a pair of forceps. A guide is passed over the wire through the mouth, cords, and into the trachea.

Then the endotracheal (ET) tube is advanced over the guide into the trachea. A fiberscope loaded with an ET tube can be advanced over the guidewire or next to the guidewire to assist retrograde intubation. A technique that involves passing the guidewire through the suction channel of the fiberscope has greatly improved the success rate of retrograde intubation.

COMPLICATIONS

Geetanjali S Verma

PREDISPOSING FACTORS FOR COMPLICATIONS

I. *Patient factors*:
   1. *Age*: More likely in infants and children (as they have a relatively small larynx and trachea and are more prone to airway edema)
   2. *Sex*: Common in adult women especially pregnant (airway edema)
   3. Difficult airway anatomy (congenital causes/acquired like burns)
   4. History of difficult airway management
   5. Emergency situations.

II. *Anesthesia related factors*:
   1. Skills of anesthetist
   2. Inadequate evaluation of airway
   3. Inadequate preoxygenation.

III. *Equipment related*:
   1. Use of inappropriately placed stylets
   2. Use of bougies
   3. Sterilization of plastic tubes with ethylene oxide may lead to production of toxic ethylene glycol if adequate time for drying has not been allowed
   4. Cuff related injuries might occur with the use of high-pressure cuffs or inappropriate use of low-pressure cuffs.

COMPLICATIONS

I. *During intubation (Immediate)*:
   a. Failed intubation
   b. Trauma to lips, teeth, tongue and nose
   c. Nasal, retropharyngeal, pharyngeal, uvular, laryngeal, tracheal, esophageal and bronchial trauma
   d. Cord avulsions, fractures and dislocation of arytenoids

   e. Noxious autonomic reflexes—Hypertension, tachycardia, bradycardia and arrhythmia, raised intraocular tension
   f. Laryngospasm
   g. Bronchospasm
   h. Airway perforation
   i. Esophageal intubation
   j. Bronchial intubation.

II. *Late*:
   a. Airway obstruction - mucous plug, dislodged tooth (foreign body)
   b. Aspiration - due to inadequate seal
   c. Disconnection and dislodgement of the tube
   d. Tension pneumothorax - with high positive pressures
   e. Trachea esophageal fistula.

III. *Post extubation:*
   a. Sore throat - most common
   b. Hoarseness
   c. Laryngeal edema
   d. Glottis and subglottic granulation tissues
   e. Tracheal stenosis
   f. Laryngomalacia
   g. Trachea esophageal fistula/trachea innominate fistula
   h. Nerve injury causing aspiration.

COMPLICATIONS ASSOCIATED WITH NASAL INTUBATION

1. *Epistaxis*: This is the most common complication, resulting from abrasion of the nasal mucosa when the tube is passed posteriorly. If bleeding is noticed but intubation could still be achieved, then it should be completed. An endotracheal tube in proper position allows tamponade of the bleeding and protects the airway. If repeated attempts are needed, then the tube should be withdrawn until the cuff is positioned to be inflated in order to tamponade the bleeding (usually in the post-nasal space). Another option is to withdraw the tube completely and pinch the nostrils together.
2. Damage to nasal cavity (avulsion of nasal polyps, fracture of the turbinates, septal abscesses)
3. Aspiration
4. Vagal stimulation
5. Laryngospasm
6. Vocal cord damage
7. Bacteremia from introduction of nasal flora to the trachea
8. Pneumothorax - rare.

COMPLICATIONS WITH RETROGRADE INTUBATION

1. Bleeding
2. Subcutaneous emphysema
3. Pneumomediastinum
4. Breath-holding
5. Catheter traveling caudad (displacement)
6. Trigeminal nerve trauma
7. Pneumothorax.

DETECTION OF COMMON COMPLICATIONS AND MANAGEMENT

1. *Failed intubation:*
   (refer to cannot intubate and CVCI algorithm).
2. *Autonomic reflexes:*
   Laryngoscopy and intubation produce reflex sympathetic stimulation and are associated with raised levels of plasma catecholamines, hypertension, tachycardia, myocardial ischemia, depression of myocardial contractility, ventricular arrhythmias and intracranial hypertension. It is aggravated by hypoxia and hypercarbia.

   Management: 100% oxygen.

   Deepen plane of anesthesia - adequate induction agents with analgesics and neuromuscular blocking agents in appropriate dosages.

   Prevention: Lidocaine 1–1.5 mg/kg IV given 90 seconds prior to laryngoscopy.

   Fentanyl 3–4 μg/kg given on induction.

   Others: Beta antagonists, sublingual Nifedipine or IV nitroglycerin.
3. *Esophageal intubation:*
   Detection: No chest rise on inspection.
   No breath sounds on auscultation (when in doubt, take it out!).
   $EtCO_2$ graph: Absent or decreasing slope.
   Management: Remove ETT immediately and reinsert.
4. *Laryngospasm/Bronchospasm*:
   Common in pediatric age group.

   Detection: Stridor or inadequate ventilation.
   Suprasternal, intercostal, subcostal retraction.
   Paradoxical movement of chest and abdomen.
   Decreased bag movement.
   Decreasing saturation on pulse oximetry.

   $EtCO_2$: Shark fin appearance (Fig. 4).

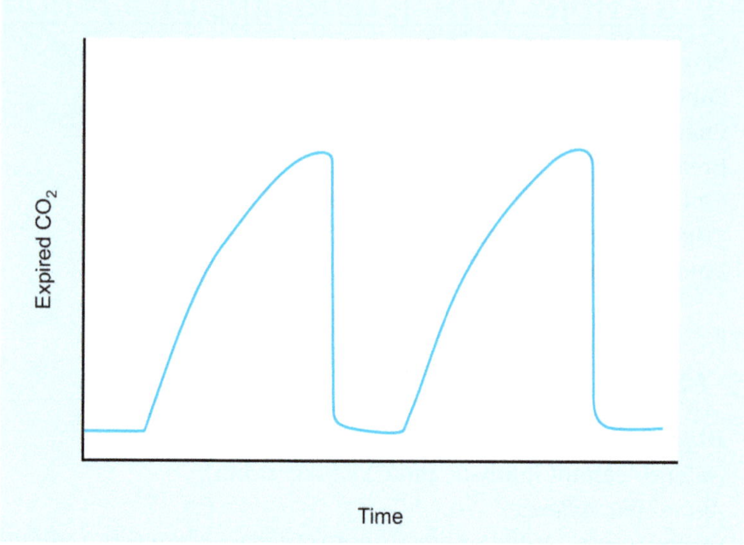

Fig. 4: Shark finn appearance in capnography.

Management: 100% oxygen continuous positive airway pressure (CPAP).

If not intubated, give jaw thrust and chin list to open airway.

Deepen plane of anesthesia with Propofol 0.25–0.8 mg/kg IV.

Succinylcholine 0.1–2 mg/kg IV.

Bronchospasm may be treated with bronchodilators (β1 agonists, Ketamine), steroids, anticholinergics.

5. *Endobronchial intubation:*

   Detection: Less chest movement on opposite side.

   Decreased air entry on opposite side.

   Fiberoptic bronchoscopy (confirmatory).

   Management: Withdrawal of ETT till bilateral air entry is equal.

6. *Perforation - tracheal, bronchial or esophageal:*

   Due to prolonged use of high pressure cuffs, multiple attempts on intubation, inappropriate tube size.

   Detection:
   - Esophageal - subcutaneous emphysema, neck pain, difficulty in swallowing, neck erythema and edema.
   - Airway perforation - subcutaneous emphysema, pneumothorax, pneumomediastinum.

   Management: Surgical intervention.

7. *Tension pneumothorax:*
   Detection: Decreased chest movements and breath sounds on the affected side.
   Increased airway pressures.
   Hypoxia and hypotension.
   X-ray: Confirmatory (but cannot be awaited, immediate management preceeds).

   Management: Immediate decompression with wide bore needle in 2nd intercostal space in mid-clavicular line on the affected side followed by intercostal drain insertion.
8. *Airway obstruction:*
   Causes: Mucous plug, foreign bodies (tooth), kinked tube.
   Detection: Inadequate ventilation (chest movements and breath sounds).
   Increased airway pressures on ventilator.
   Hypoxia.

   Management: Detect cause and treat.

   Prevention: Use of flexometallic tube to avoid kinking.
   Regular suctioning of tubes.
   Adequate humidification to prevent drying of secretions.
   Placement of oral airway to prevent biting of tube.
9. *Sore throat:*
   Treated by steam inhalation or nebulization of bronchodilators.
10. *Laryngeal edema*
    Causes: Too large a tube, trauma from laryngoscopy and/or intubation, excessive neck manipulation during intubation and surgery, excessive coughing or bucking on the tube, and present or recent upper respiratory infection.

    Detection: Diminished stridor may represent total airway obstruction and movement of air.

    Management: Warmed, humidified oxygen
    Nebulized racemic epinephrine (0.25 to 1 mL)
    IV dexamethasone (0.5 mg/kg-1 up to 10 mg)
    If obstruction is severe and persistent, reintubation must be considered.
11. *Nerve injury:*
    May be caused due to trauma during intubation or prolonged pressure of inflated cuff on the vocal cords.

    Detection: Stridor or hoarseness based on the degree and site of damage.

Vocal cord paralysis usually heals spontaneously over days to months
In case of life-threatening airway obstruction, reintubation to be done and may require tracheostomy.
Surgical repair of paralyzed cords.

12. *Tracheal stenosis:*
    Caused by over-sized tubes or over-inflated cuffs.
    Ischemia and eventual necrosis occur when the lateral tracheal wall pressure exceeds the capillary perfusion pressure of about 25 mm Hg.
    Prevention: Proper management of low pressure cuffs. Only high volume, low pressure cuffs must be used, and the cuff inflated to pressure not exceeding 25 mm Hg or 30 cm H_2O.
13. *Aspiration:*
    The presence of spontaneous ventilation, accumulation of fluid above the cuff, a head up position and the use of uncuffed tubes or cuff leakage increase the chances of aspiration.
    Detection: Tachycardia, tachypnea, hypoxemia, crepitations on auscultation, decreased breath sounds, egophony.
    X-ray: Multiple infiltrates (especially in basal regions).
    Management:
    Collect the tracheal aspirate and nasogastric aspirate and send for laboratory analysis and detect pH of aspirate.
    Protect airway with cuffed endotracheal tube.
    Prophylactic antibiotics may be started.
    Bronchodilators.

6 Fiberoptic Bronchoscope

Geetanjali S Verma

Developed in 1895 for removal of foreign bodies from the main stem bronchi. First performed by Gustav Killian in 1897. In 1968, Shigeto Ikeda introduced flexible fiberoptic bronchoscopy for clinical use.

COMPONENTS (FIG. 1)

1. *Eye piece*: Can be attached to a camera for display on screen.
2. *Diopter ring*: For focusing.
3. *Control lever*: Controls the tip. Permits movement only in a vertical plane. Two wires extend from the handle to the tip in the insertion cord (Moving the lever down, moves the tip up and moving the lever up, points the tip down). Side to side movement is accomplished by rotation of the body of the bronchoscope with the operator's wrist and shoulder.
4. *Working channel port*: For suction, local anesthetic instillation, oxygen delivery.
5. *Body*: Incorporates the eye piece, diopter ring, control level and working channel. Grasped by the operator's non-dominant hand.

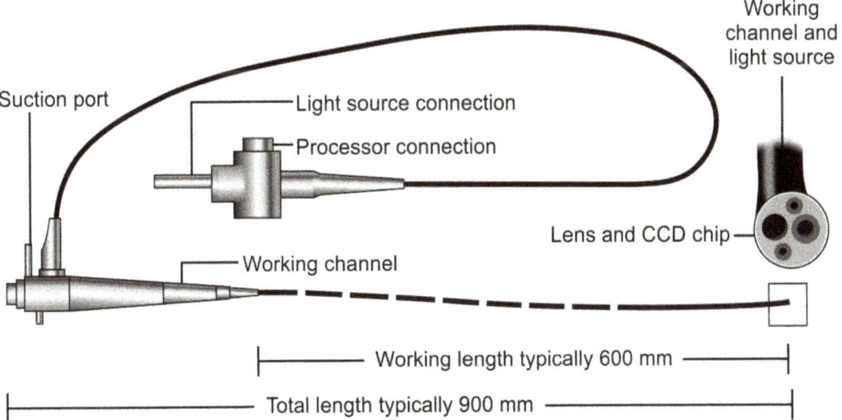

Fig. 1: Components of fiberoptic bronchoscope.

6. *Insertion cord*: Contains fiberoptic bundle for light and image transmission, tip bending control wires and working channel. Average length 600 mm (range 500–650 mm).
7. *Light source*: Can be a portable battery powered source or via a cable. Light source may be halogen, incandescent or LED.
8. Suction valve and port.

PHYSIOLOGY

Light travels at different velocities in different mediums. The effect of each substance on light velocity is indicated by the refractive index of the substance, which compares the velocity of the light through the substance with that through a vacuum. This difference in velocities has the effect of altering the direction of a light beam as it passes from one medium to another. If the light hits a glass-air interface at 90°, it will pass straight through, but at any other angle, as the light passes from the glass to the air, its direction will be altered. As the angle of incidence of the light is increased from the perpendicular, the greater the bending of the light as it emerges from the glass into the air. Eventually, there will be a point where the light is reflected back inside the glass, almost as if it had rebounded off a mirror. This is called 'total internal reflection' and occurs at the 'critical angle'. It becomes possible, therefore, to bounce light down the inside of a glass rod from one end to the other.

INDICATIONS

1. *Routine intubation*: For teaching purpose
2. *Difficult intubation/awake intubation*:
   a. History of difficult intubation
   b. Predictors of difficult intubation present-LEMON score
3. *Compromised airway*:
   a. Upper airway abnormality/cervical spine fracture
   b. Tracheal stenosis and compression
4. *Extension of neck to be avoided*:
   a. Unstable neck
   b. Vertebral artery insufficient
5. *High-risk of dental damage*:
   a. Poor, fragile, loose teeth
   b. Extensive dental restoration
6. *Diagnostic purposes*:
   a. Identification of indeterminate lung lesion, evaluation of recurrent or persistent atelectasis or pulmonary infiltrates

   b. Investigate cause of unexplained hemoptysis/persistent unexplained cough/localized wheeze
   c. Obtain specimens for cytologic, histologic and microbiologic evaluation (cell washings, biopsies)
   d. Evaluation of problems associated with endotracheal or tracheostomy tubes such as tracheal damage, airway obstruction or tube placement
7. *Therapeutic*:
   a. Removal of abnormal endobronchial tissue or foreign material by forceps, basket, or laser
   b. Retrieval of a foreign body (rigid bronchoscopy preferred)
   c. Therapeutic lavage
   d. Endobronchial laser surgery.

CONTRAINDICATIONS

Absolute

1. Untrained staff
2. Uncooperative patient
3. Lack of adequate facilities and personnel to care for the patient if an emergency occurs (such as cardiopulmonary arrest, pneumothorax, or bleeding)
4. Inability to adequately oxygenate the patient during the bronchoscopy.

Relative

1. Coagulopathy/bleeding diathesis
2. Severe obstructive airways disease
3. Severe refractory hypoxemia
4. Unstable hemodynamic status.

CHOOSING THE APPROPRIATE SIZE

When using a single-lumen endotracheal tube (8.0 mm ID), an adult fiberoptic bronchoscope should be used (5.0 mm outer diameter).

The internal diameter (ID) of the single-lumen endotracheal tube relative to the external diameter of the bronchoscope is an important consideration. Bronchoscopes in the non-intubated patient occupy only 10–15% of the cross-sectional area of the trachea. In contrast, a 5.7 mm bronchoscope occupies 40% of a 9 mm ID single-lumen endotracheal tube and 66% of a 7 mm ID single-lumen endotracheal tube.

LMA size (mm)	*ETT (mm)*	*FOB (mm)*
1	3.5	2.2
2	4.5	3.5
2.5	5	4.0
3	6 cuff	5.0
4	6 cuff	5.0

TECHNIQUE OF USAGE (FIGS. 2A TO C)

A systematic and complete fiberoptic bronchoscopy examination includes a clear view of the anterior wall (tracheal cartilage), posterior wall (membranous portion) of the trachea below the vocal cords and of the tracheal carina.

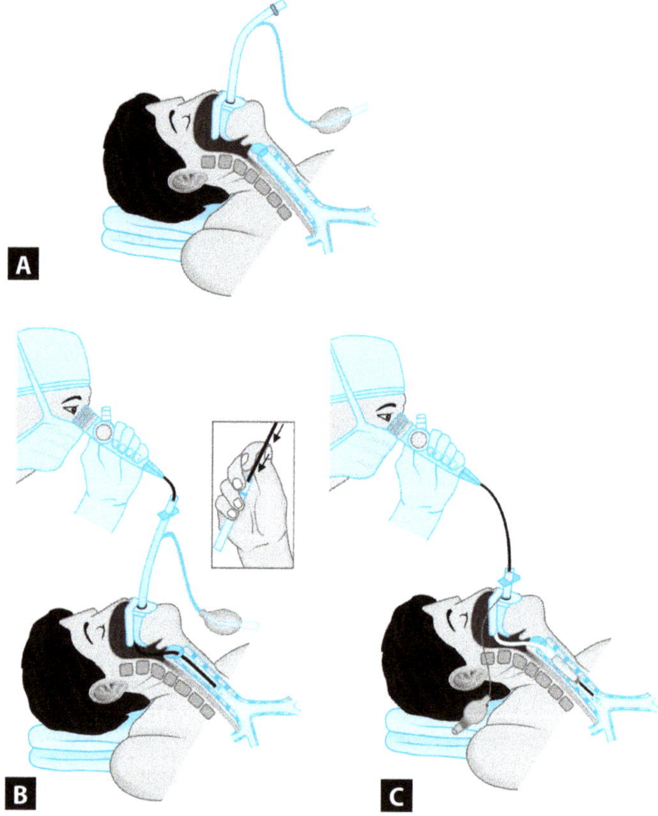

Figs. 2A to C: Fiberoptic orotracheal intubation in a conscious patient. (A) Ovassapian intubating airway and endotracheal tube (ET) position; (B) The bronchoscope is advanced through ET into midtrachea. Inset illustrates position of hand for holding tracheal ET and advancing the bronchoscope; (C) The ET is advanced over the bronchoscope into the trachea.
(*Source:* Ovassapian A: Fiberoptic Airway Endoscopy in Anesthesia and Critical Care. New York, Raven Press).

When advancing the bronchoscope through the right mainstem bronchus, a clear view of the bronchus intermedius should be seen, and at 3 o'clock the orifice of the right upper lobe bronchus should be seen. As the bronchoscope is advanced inside the take-off of the right upper bronchus, a clear view of the orifices is found: apical, anterior, and posterior segments (the only structure in the tracheobronchial tree that has three orifices).

After withdrawing the bronchoscope from the right upper bronchus, it is advanced distally into the bronchus intermedius in order to identify the middle and lower right lobe bronchi. The right middle bronchus has the shape of a letter D.

Once the complete examination has been performed on the right mainstem bronchus, the bronchoscope is withdrawn until the tracheal carina is seen again. Then the bronchoscope is readvanced into the left mainstem bronchus in which the bifurcation into left upper and lower lobe is visualized (Figs. 3A to D).

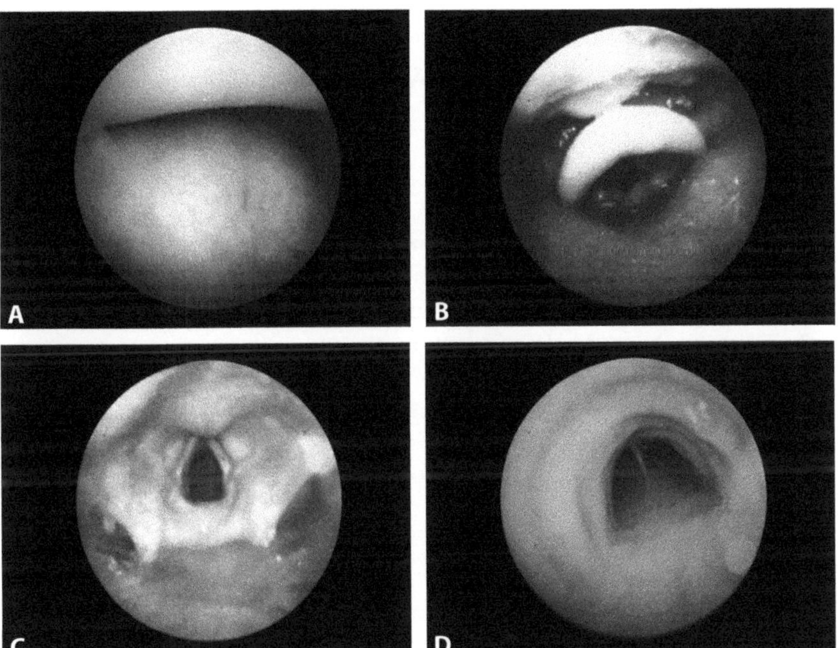

Figs. 3A to D: Bronchoscopic views during fiberoptic orotracheal intubation. (A) Pharyngeal surface of the Ovassapian airway is seen in white in the upper half of the picture. Soft palate is seen in the lower half of the picture; (B) The tip of bronchoscope is in oropharynx. Distal end of Ovassapian airway covering the base of the tongue. Epiglottis is in view; (C) The tip of bronchoscope passed beneath the tip of epiglottis. Glottis is in view; (D) The tip of the bronchoscope in lower third of the trachea. Carina is in view.
(*Source:* Ovassapian A: Fiberoptic Airway Endoscopy in Anesthesia and Critical Care. New York, Raven Press).

Advantages of fiberoptic intubation

Related to the Fiberoptic Bronchoscope

- Flexible instrument adaptable to airway anatomy
- Applicable for oral or nasal intubations
- Applicable to all age groups
- Excellent visualization of the airway
- Ability to apply topical anesthesia and insufflate oxygen during intubation
- Ability to integrate a video system

Related to the Intubation Technique

- High success rate in difficult intubation
- Prevention of unrecognized esophageal and endobronchial intubation
- Definitive check of endotracheal tube position
- Allows evaluation of the airway before intubation
- Less traumatic than rigid laryngoscopic intubation
- Less cardiovascular response during awake intubation (AI) than with rigid laryngoscopic intubation
- Excellent acceptance of AI by patients

COMPLICATIONS

1. Infection for healthcare workers or other patients
2. Cross-contamination of specimens or bronchoscopes
3. Epistaxis, hemoptysis and pneumothorax
4. Hypoxia and hypercapnia
5. Increased airway resistance
6. Laryngospasm, bronchospasm
7. Arrhythmias, hypotension
8. Localized trauma
9. Respiratory or cardiac arrest.

COMMON DIFFICULTIES

1. Poor vision due to: Inexperience, poorly focused eyepiece, film over the lens, fogging, secretions and blood, touching the mucosa (red out)
2. Bleeding
3. Coughing
4. Desaturation—respiratory depression due to drugs—excessive use of suction—endobronchial intubation—loss of airway
5. Laryngospasm and bronchospasm
6. Esophageal intubation

7. Failure to railroad the endotracheal tube ('hang ups')—use the nasal approach—use the correct size endotracheal tube (not too large, not too small)—if hang-up occurs - pull back and twist the endotracheal tube and do some external digital manipulations.

Causes of failure of fiberoptic intubation
• Lack of expertise
• Presence of secretions and blood
• Fogging of the objective and focusing lenses
• Poor topical anesthesia
• Decreased space between epiglottis and the posterior pharyngeal wall
• Distorted airway anatomy
• Passage of fiberoptic bronchoscope through the Murphy's eye
• Inadequate lubrication of a tightly fitting fiberoptic bronchoscope.

CARE AFTER BRONCHOSCOPY

1. Patient monitoring
   a. Level of consciousness
   b. Medications administered, dosage, route and time of delivery
   c. Subjective response to procedure
   d. *Vitals*: BP, heart rate, rhythm, SpO_2
   e. *During mechanical ventilation*: Tidal volume, peak inspiratory pressure, adequacy of inspiratory flow
   f. Lavage volumes (delivered and retrieved)
   g. Site of biopsies and washings and analysis requested of each
2. Send specimens for analysis
3. Keep O_2 for at least 2 hours. Monitor SpO_2.
4. NPO for at least 2-4 hours (local anesthetic effect)
5. Clean equipment per department procedure—gas sterilization with ethylene oxide at temperatures <55°C (10-12 hrs), 30 min exposure to 2% glutaraldehyde
6. Provide outpatients with written as well as oral instructions.

Important notes during intubation
• Keep the insertion cord straight and taut.
• Oxygenate through any possible route
• Antifogging to telescopic lens
• Push fiberscope very slowly and gently
• Identify the first land mark 'the epiglottis'

Contd...

Contd...

- Advance the fiberscope to the laryngeal opening
- Advance the fiberscope until it enters the subglottic space
- Identify the second landmark 'the trachea'
- Advance it down slowly till you see the third landmark 'the bifurcation'
- Advance the endotracheal tube with a gentle rotation motion
- Remove the fiberscope
- Verify the position and fix the endotracheal tube
- Connect the anesthesia circuit.

7 Surgical Airway

Deva Evu Subhas

INTRODUCTION

Surgical airway is generally last resort in gaining access to the airway. Beyond this, there is practically nothing much to offer. So, it becomes important that anesthesiologist should be trained in surgical airway techniques.

There are two main technique in achieving surgical airway access.

1. Cricothyrotomy
2. Tracheostomy.

HISTORIC ASPECTS

Surgical manipulation of the trachea for emergent airway control is one of the oldest invasive procedures documented. It was performed in ancient Egypt and India more than 3,000 years ago. Greek physician Galen (130–200 AD) has documented tracheostomy in his writings and also provided anatomic drawings of the airway. He based his anatomic knowledge on dissections of animals and assumed that the structures were identical in the human body. Galenic teaching persisted for more than 1300 years, until Andreas Wesele Vesalius (1515–1564 AD) published De Humani Corporis Fabrica, detailing the first correct description of human anatomy. He secretly conducted dissection of human cadavers and, published his landmark work in seven volumes. He gave a detailed description of tracheostomy—control of the airway with the use of a cane or reed and assisted ventilation of the lung. He allegedly performed a tracheostomy and experimentally inflated the lungs of a dead Spanish nobleman, which outraged the medical and clerical communities.

Chevalier Jackson, a laryngologist at the Jefferson Medical School in Philadelphia, described the surgical procedure for tracheostomy in 1909 and brought in standardization of technique. Later he published his 30 years of observation of his patients which revealed high incidence of laryngeal and subglottic stenosis. His technique was known as high tracheostomy which was later given up.

In 1969, Toye and Weinstein described a technique for percutaneous tracheostomy. The technique involved inserting a needle into the trachea and dilating the resultant needle tract to allow placement of a breathing catheter. Later various techniques for PDT was described by Ciaglias, Griggs using Seldinger technique.

CRICOTHYROTOMY

Cricothyrotomy is the access of airway through the space between inferior border of thyroid cartilage and superior border of cricoid cartilage.

Based on the urgency of clinical situation they can be classified as emergency or elective.

Based on the technique used it is classified as follows:
- Needle cricothyrotomy
- Percutaneous dilatation cricothyrotomy
- Open or surgical cricothyrotomy.

Anatomical Consideration (Fig. 1)

Cricothyroid membrane (CTM) is the membrane covering the space between thyroid cartilage and cricoid cartilage. The CTM is roughly around 10 mm long and 22 mm wide. The CTM consists of a central anterior triangular portion (i.e. conus elasticus) and two lateral parts. The thicker and stronger conus elasticus narrows above and broadens below, connecting the

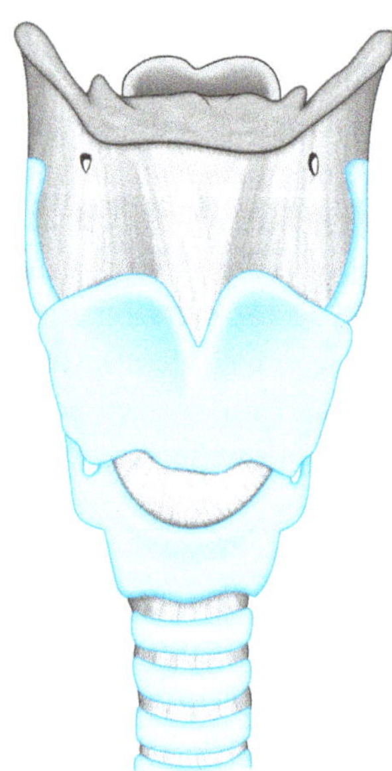

Fig. 1: Anatomy of larynx depicting cricothyroid membrane.

thyroid to the cricoid cartilage. It lies subcutaneously in the midline. The superior cricothyroid vessels crosses the midline at upper third of CTM. So, it is suggested to make incision at lower third to avoid bleeding.

Vocal cords usually lie 1 cm above the cricothyroid space, they are not commonly injured, even during emergency cricothyrotomy. The anterior jugular veins run vertically in the lateral aspect of the neck and are rarely injured, but tributaries may occasionally course over the cricothyroid space and be damaged during the procedure. Characteristically, the CTM does not calcify with age and lies immediately underneath the skin.

The CTM is identified by running the finger vertically down along the laryngeal prominence. And the first indentation or the dip felt is the CTM. It is roughly one to one and half finger breadths below the laryngeal prominence. The cricoid cartilage is palpated below the CTM. It is important to note these landmarks because entering the thyrohyoid space could be disasterous.

Indications

- For airway management when orotracheal or nasotracheal intubation and fiberoptic approaches have failed.
- In emergency room where endotracheal intubation is impossible or contraindicated such as maxillofacial trauma, cervical spine injury, head neck and multiple trauma.
- Immediate relief of upper airway obstruction.
- In the operating room and in the ICU, the technique is indicated when conventional methods of intubation fail and in whom other techniques of airway access are difficult or impossible to perform.
- Cricothyrotomy can also be used as an alternative to tracheostomy in patients with recent sternotomy to avoid communication with the mediastinal tissue planes.
- Emergency cricothyrotomy has largely replaced emergency tracheostomy.

Contraindications

The absolute and relative contraindications are rare. However, there are situations where it should be avoided.

- It should be done with caution in pediatric age group (<10 years) as the larynx is small with less fibrous supporting tissue.
- It should be completely avoided in age group less than 6 years unless a wire can be placed within cricothyroid space and placement within trachea confirmed.
- To be avoided in a patient who has been intubated for a prolonged period (some say 3 days and some suggest 7 days). These patients seem to be at high-risk for subglottic stenosis.

- Complication rates are high in the hands of inexperienced physician. Hence to be avoided.
- Patients with preexisting laryngeal disease such as cancer or inflammation are associated with high morbidity when cricothyrotomy is performed.
- Distortion of neck anatomy can make the procedure impossible.
- Bleeding diathesis predisposes to bleeding renders the procedure dangerous.

NEEDLE CRICOTHYROTOMY

Needle cricothyrotomy is performed using a wide bore needle or catheter on needle technique. This is more of a temporary solution for oxygenation at times of emergency. This technique is preferred in pediatric age group less than 10 years compared to surgical cricothyrotomy.

Technique

- Needle cricothyrotomy should be performed with universal precautions and sterile technique. Prepare the skin with povidone-iodine solution and infiltrate skin with local anesthetic if time permits.
- Hold the trachea in place and provide skin tension with the thumb and middle finger of the non-dominant hand placed on either side of the trachea. Palpate the cricothyroid membrane with index finger (Fig. 2).
- Hold a 3 to 10 mL syringe half-filled with saline attached to the over-the-needle IV catheter in the dominant hand.

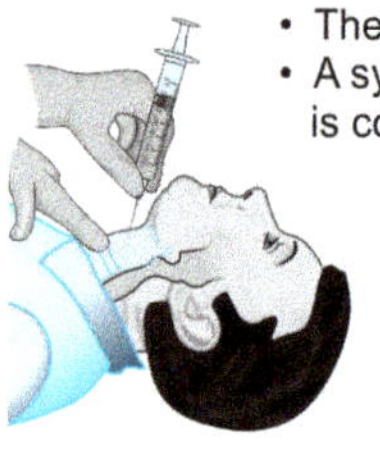

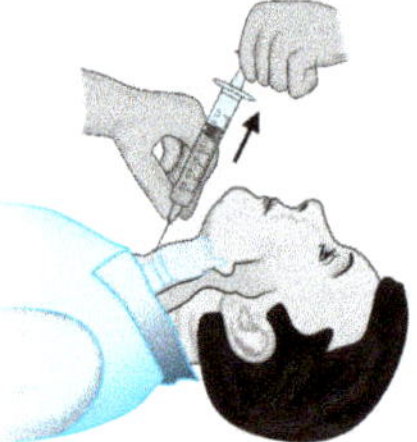

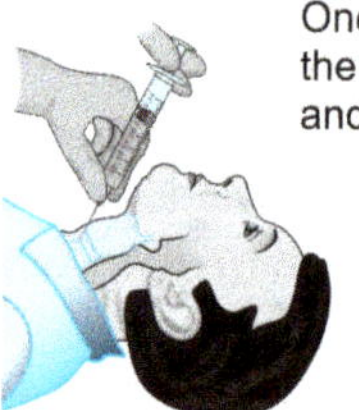

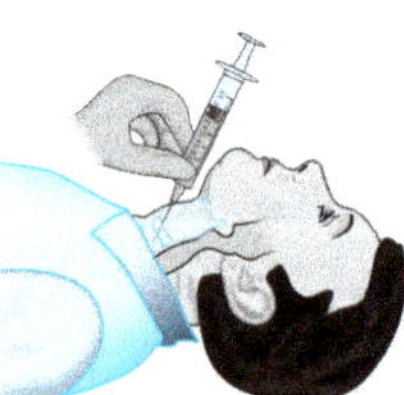

Fig. 2: Needle cricothyrotomy.

- Place the catheter in the midline of the neck at the inferior margin of the cricothyroid membrane (to avoid the cricothyroid blood vessels located superiorly and laterally). Direct it caudally (toward the feet) at an angle of 30° to 45°.
- Puncture the skin and subcutaneous tissue. Advance the catheter while continuously applying negative pressure on the syringe, until air bubbles are seen, confirming intratracheal placement.
- Advance the catheter forward off the needle until its hub rests at the skin surface. Remove the syringe and the needle.
- Reattach the syringe to the catheter and again aspirate for air to confirm that the catheter remains in the trachea.
- Hold the catheter firmly in place at all times or delegate an assistant to do this to reduce the chance of kinking or dislodgement, even after it has been secured with suture material.

Once the catheter is place ventilation is initiated by one of the following ways:

Percutaneous Transtracheal Jet Ventilation (Fig. 3)

Transtracheal jet ventilation is performed through needle cricothyrotomy. This is a temporary support, it can be continued for a period of maximum 45 minutes. By then all effort has to be made to establish a definitive airway.

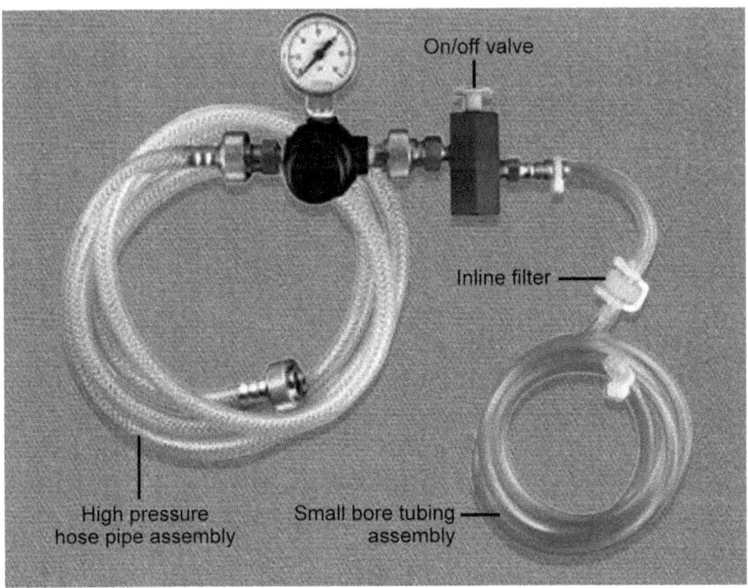

Fig. 3: Jet ventilator.

Bag-Valve-Mask Connector Options

If a bag-valve-mask will be used for patient ventilation, then it should connect to the catheter using one of the following improvised adapters:
- Three mL Luer lock syringe with plunger removed with 7.5 mm ID endotracheal tube connector (bag-valve-mask connector).
- 3.0 mm ID endotracheal tube connector attached directly to the catheter (bag-valve-mask connector).
- 2.5 mm ID endotracheal tube connector attached to cut off IV tubing with Luer lock end connected directly to the catheter.

Oxygen Tubing Connector Options

If oxygen tubing will be used to connect to the oxygen source, then the clinician may use one of the following options:
- Direct connection of oxygen tubing to catheter
- Y connector (oxygen tubing)
- Three-way stopcock (oxygen tubing).

The knowledge about connector option is important because the wide bore needle or catheter does not come with a connector that can be attached to a bag for ventilation. This connection has to be established using equipment which are readily available. It is important to make sure there is option for adequate exhalation. Most of the time the air escapes out through the vocal cords and nose.

PERCUTANEOUS DILATATION CRICOTHYROTOMY

This technique is based on Seldinger technique where the cricothyrotomy canula is rail roaded over a guidewire following dilatation. There are airway kits available which comprises complete set of equipment needed for the procedure. They all carry written instruction of the steps to be followed for their own kit. However, the fundamental steps and principle seems to be the same.

Basic steps in percutaneous dilatation cricothyrotomy:
- Position the patient in supine position and the neck to be extended if possible.
- Prepare the table and layout the kit.
- Prepare skin with povidone iodine and use local anesthetic if time permits.
- Identify the CTM as mentioned earlier.
- Make a horizontal or vertical skin incision (this step can be done following guidewire placement).
- Attach the introducer needle with syringe half filled with saline. Enter the airway through the lower one-third of CTM using the introducer.

Enter the airway at 45° angle to the plane of neck and the tip facing caudally.
- The position of introducer in the trachea is confirmed by aspiration of air into the syringe.
- If the introducer has a catheter over it then push the catheter in and pull out the needle. Depending upon the type of introducer the guide wire can be passed directly through the introducer or through the catheter.
- Once the guidewire is in place remove the introducer needle or the catheter.
- Introduce the dilator over the guide wire and dilate to the level mentioned in the kit. Lubricant can be used to enhance the fit and placement of emergency airway catheter.
- Advance the airway access assembly over the guidewire, making sure the proximal end of the guidewire is always in sight. Use in and out motion to advance the catheter until it is in position.
- As the airway catheter is advanced the dilator and guidewire is removed simultaneously.
- If the airway catheter is cuffed then inflate the cuff.
- Secure the airway catheter with tracheostomy tape strip in standard fashion.
- Using its standard 15- to 22-mm adapter, connect the emergency airway catheter to an appropriate ventilatory device.

There are variety of airway kits made available by different manufacturers. They are as follows:
- Melker (Cook)
- Pertrach (Pulmodyne)
- Quicktrach (VBM Medizintechnik)
- Portex cricothyrotomy kit
- Nu-Trake (Smith medicals).

OPEN OR SURGICAL CRICOTHYROTOMY

This is a surgical technique by which an airway access is obtained through CTM using scalpel and dissection of tissue. There are two commonly used techniques:
1. No-drop technique
2. Rapid four step technique.

No-Drop Technique

This is the traditional surgical cricothyrotomy (Fig. 4). Steps are as follows:
- *Preparation*: Positioning of the patient in supine position. Prepare the neck with appropriate aseptic solution if time permits. Layout the equipment. Infiltrate the skin with local anesthetic if possible.

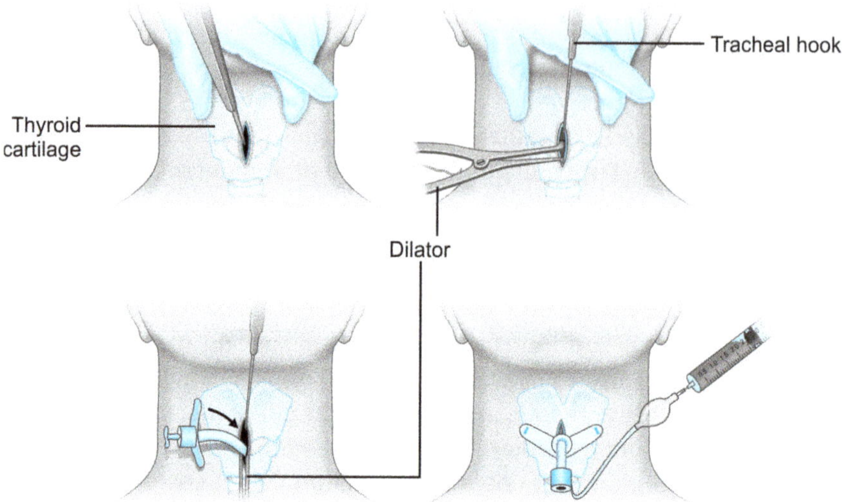

Fig. 4: Surgical cricothyrotomy.

- *Identification of landmark*: The CTM is identified as mentioned earlier. The operator should be positioned on the same side of the patient as the operator's dominant hand (i.e. the hand that will be used to make the incision). The non-dominant hand is used to fix the tracheal cartilage firmly (with the thumb and long finger). The index finger used to identify the CTM.
- *Vertical skin incision*: The operator uses the dominant hand to make a generous vertical incision in the midline (at least 2 cm) with its center over the CTM. The incision can be extended in an obese patient or if there is difficulty in identifying CTM. The incision should go through subcutaneous tissues down to, but not into, the thyroid and cricoid cartilages.
- *Confirmation of membrane location*: While the thumb and long finger are continuing to fix the thyroid cartilage the index finger is inserted into the wound to feel the CTM. The index to be kept in the wound feeling the lower border of the larynx (i.e superior border of CTM).
- *Horizontal incision on the CTM*: The index finger may be withdrawn just prior to incision or left in the wound to serve as a guide. The CTM should be incised horizontally for a distance of 1 to 2 cm preferably at the lower half of the membrane to avoid the superiorly placed cricothyroid artery and vein. At this point bleeding might obscure the view, however there is not enough time to control bleeding. It is better to achieve the airway access and then control bleeding. Sometime placing the index finger through CTM helps to identify the correct location.

- *Insertion of tracheal hook*: Tracheal hook is inserted transversely through the incision. When it is well within the airway, it is turned in cephalad direction. The hook is applied against the inferior border of larynx. This is handed over to an assistant who will be holding it up without letting it go until airway catheter is placed. Hence, the name 'No-Drop' technique.
- *Dilation of the opening with dilator*: Once the tracheal hook is stabilizing the larynx the operator can free his non-dominant hand. The opening is dilated with Trosseaus dilator in rostral caudal direction as this offers maximum resistance. The trosseaus dilators are left in place and transferred to non-dominant hand. Dominant hand needs to be free for introducing tracheostomy tube.
- *Insertion of tracheostomy tube*: Tracheostomy tube should be ready with obturator in place. With prongs of dilator in place, the tracheostomy tube is inserted between the prongs, following their natural curve. As the tracheostomy tube is advanced the dilator is rotated to 900 counter clockwise so that it moves out of the way. The dilator is gently removed as the tube is being advanced, just before it is seated in its final position.
- *Cuff inflation and securing the tube*: The cuff should be inflated and the obturator to be removed. Insert the inner tube if there is one. Secure the tube with twill or with a padded fastener that goes around the neck and attaches to the neck plate of the tube.
- *Confirmation of tube position*: The tube position confirmed using end tidal carbon dioxide. If there is concern that the tube is placed outside the trachea, a nasogastric tube may be gently inserted. In the airway the tube advances easily, but resistance is met if the tube is in a false passage. A chest radiograph will help ruling out barotrauma. The hook to be removed only after confirming the position of the tube. Care to be taken while removing the hook as to avoid accidental extubation.

Rapid Four-step Technique

The rapid four-step technique (RFST) is an attempt to simplify the cricothyrotomy procedure by using a horizontal stab incision through the skin and membrane simultaneously, followed by tracheal hook traction applied caudad at the cricoid ring. Cadaveric studies have shown that it is easy to learn and much faster in achieving access to airway.

Advantages

- Less equipment is necessary (it is performed with a scalpel, hook and tracheostomy tube).
- It may be performed independently.
- The operator is positioned at the head of the bed, similar to the stance for performance of orotracheal intubation.

The incidence of acute complication is more with RFST compared to traditional no-drop technique. The stab incision increases incidence of trauma to posterior trachea and esophagus. RFST is better avoided in patient in whom landmark identification is difficult. The preparation prior to the procedure is pretty much same for both the techniques.

RFST is performed in following manner:

- *Landmark identification*: The landmark identification is exactly same as the traditional technique. The position of the operator alone changes. The operator stands on the head end similar to that of endotracheal intubation. If the landmarks are not identified it is better to go for a vertical incision.
- *Horizontal stab incision*: Once the landmark is confidently identified make a horizontal incision using 20 blade. The stab incision is made around 1.5 cm wide and through the skin and CTM. The blade is left in the airway until the tracheal hook is secured.
- *Stabilization of larynx with tracheal hook*: Introduce the tracheal hook parallel to the blade and then turn it caudally to control cricoid ring. The tracheal hook is used to apply gentle traction on the cricoid ring to lift the airway up toward the surface of the skin and to provide modest stoma dilation. The direction of force on the hook is reminiscent of the 'up and away' direction. The chance of trauma to the cricoid can be reduced by using double tined hooks.
- *Insertion of tracheal tube*: The tracheal tube is gently inserted into the airway while the traction on the cricoid ring is maintained. Once the tube is inside the trachea the cuff is inflated and the tube is secured after confirming the position. All these steps are similar to that of the traditional technique.

Complications

Immediate

- Hemorrhage
- Tube misplacement
- Subcutaneous emphysema
- Esophageal trauma and intubatioin
- Laceration of thyroid
- Injury to vocal cords and larynx
- Mediastinal emphysema
- Hypoxia and death.

Delayed

- Tracheomalacia/tracheal stenosis
- Infection/mediastinitis
- Bleeding
- Fistulae
- Scarring
- Displacement.

TRACHEOSTOMY

Tracheostomy is an invasive procedure by which access to airway is achieved through the cervical trachea. It can be done by either of the following ways:

- Percutaneous dilatation tracheostomy (PDT)
- Open tracheostomy.

Indications

Airway Maintenance

- Upper airway obstruction
- Inability to protect the airway.

Prolonged Ventilation

- Prolonged dependence on mechanical ventilation (actual or anticipated)
- Secretion management
- Permanent or long-term airway access in traumatic or neurological diseases.

Contraindications

Absolute

- Patient refusal.
- Children <16 years of age (small, mobile and compressible airway).
- Anatomical anomalies, e.g. anterior neck mass, large goiter.
- Bleeding disorder/coagulopathy with high-risk of active bleeding.
- Infection at site.

Relative

- Known or suspected difficult intubation, i.e. possible difficulty in managing the airway during the procedure.
- Difficult landmarks/anatomy, e.g. obesity, short neck (cricoid <3 cm above sternal notch), high or aberrant (cervical) innominate artery, previous neck surgery distorting relevant anatomy.

- Unstable cervical spine injury.
- Platelet count < 50 × 10^9 per liter (or severe platelet dysfunction).
- INR > 1.5, activated partial thromboplastin time (APTT) >50 or prolonged prothrombin time.
- Therapeutic unfractionated heparin infusion, especially when also on antiplatelet drugs.

There is no absolute contraindication when it comes to surgical tracheostomy, especially when it comes to emergency tracheostomy. The contraindications mentioned above are primarily for PDT. However for an elective tracheostomy bleeding disorder and infection can be considered as contraindication. Some authors mention carcinoma larynx waiting for laryngectomy as one of the absolute contraindication for elective tracheostomy because of increased incidence of stomal metastasis.

PERCUTANEOUS DILATATION TRACHEOSTOMY (FIG. 5)

Percutaneous dilatation tracheostomy (PDT) uses Seldinger technique followed by dilation to achieve access to the airway. Four techniques have been described based on the way dilatation is done.

1. *Ciaglias multiple dilator technique*: It is a Seldinger based technique where graded dilatation of the trachea is achieved using multiple dilators.

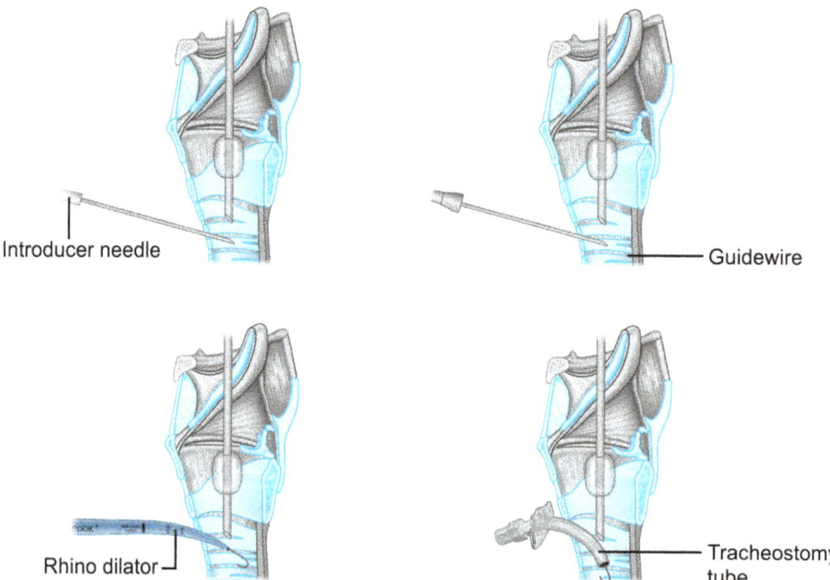

Fig. 5: Technique of percutaneous dilatation tracheostomy.

2. *Griggs technique*: Similar to Ciaglia but involves a single step dilatation of trachea using modified Howard-Kelly forceps.
3. *Single graduated dilator technique*: It is a modification of Ciaglia's with single-graded dilator replacing the multiple dilators.
4. *Balloon dilatation technique*: This is one of the newer techniques where a pressurized balloon is used instead of rigid curved dilators. There is decreased incidence of trauma to posterior tracheal wall and esophagus. However, the duration of procedure and bleeding increases with this procedure as compared to other techniques.

Insertion Technique

- Position the patient in supine position with head extended by placing a rolled towel or pillow under the scapulae.
- Prepare the skin using appropriate antiseptic solution. The skin and subcutaneous tissues are infiltrated with 2% lidocaine and a 1 : 100,000 solution of epinephrine one or two finger breadths below the previously palpated and marked cricoid cartilage.
- Make a 1.5 cm wide horizontal incision. The subcutaneous tissue is dissected us in a blunt hemostat.
- The endotracheal tube (ETT) can be withdrawn after placing a fiberoptic bronchoscope (FOB) at the tip.
- The extent to which the ETT to be withdrawn is determined using transillumination. Stop withdrawing the ETT at the point where maximum transillumination is seen through the skin incision.
- FOB can be left *in situ*, so that rest of the procedure can be done under vision.
- The 16- or 17-gauge introducer needle is inserted between the first and second or second and third tracheal rings. The entry into airway can be confirmed by aspiration of air into the syringe.
- The catheter is left in place after removing the introducer needle.
- Guidewire is inserted through the catheter.
- Catheter is replaced by a dilator (depending on the set used). The tracheal stoma is widened enough to allow the tracheal tube.
- The dilator is replaced by the preloaded tracheostomy tube, which is advanced into the trachea.
- The guidewire and dilator assembly is removed together.
- Connect the tracheostomy tube to the ventilator and then remove the ETT.

OPEN TRACHEOSTOMY

Open tracheostomy involves placement of a tracheostomy tube into the trachea by dissection and incision of the trachea under direct vision. This may be performed in the operating room (OR) or in the ICU.

Technique

- Position the patients in supine position with head in extension using a rolled towel or pillow under the scapulae.
- Prepare the skin using appropriate antiseptic solution. The skin and subcutaneous tissues are infiltrated with 2% lidocaine and a 1: 100,000 solution of epinephrine along the line of incision.
- Make a vertical incision about 3 cm long starting just inferior to the cricoid cartilage. Some advocate horizontal incision. Dissect the subcutaneous tissue and cauterize the fat to aid exposure and to prevent fat necrosis later.
- Dissect through the platysma until the midline raphe between the strap muscles is identified.
- Palpate for innominate artery along the inferior border of the wound. Also ligate and cauterize anterior jugular vein and smaller vessels.
- Separate the strap muscles and retract laterally until the pretracheal fascia and thyroid isthumus is exposed.
- Retract the isthumus superiorly exposing the trachea. Sometime it requires transecting the isthumus.
- By this stage make sure good hemostasis is achieved so as to prevent aspiration of blood while opening the trachea.
- After blunt dissection of the pretracheal fascia identify the tracheal ring. Preferably second tracheal ring.
- One of 2 types of tracheal entry is usually used. These are complete removal of the anterior part of one of the tracheal rings to create the stoma, and creation of a flap with the severed part of the ring. Prior to making the tracheal incision the endotracheal tube needs to be withdrawn so that the tip of ETT stays above the incision.
- Silk stay suture can be placed through the tracheal wall on each side and taped to the neck skin on either side. This facilitates tube replacement should it dislodge in the immediate postoperative period.
- With help of gentle traction on stay sutures tracheostomy tube is inserted into the stoma.
- Inflate the cuff and secure the tube after confirming the position using end tidal CO_2.
- Connect the tracheostomy tube to the ventilator and then remove the ETT.

Complications

Intraoperative Complications

- Hemorrhage
- Loss of airway or premature extubation

- Pneumothorax
- Tracheal-esophageal fistula or posterior tracheal wall injury
- Hypoxia and ventilation problems
- Hypotension
- Cardiopulmonary arrest
- Recurrent laryngeal nerve injury.

Postoperative Complications

Early:

- Hemorrhage
- Stomal infection
- Pneumothorax and subcutaneous emphysema
- Tube obstruction.

Late:

- Displaced tracheostomy tube or unplanned decannulation
- Granuloma
- Subglottic stenosis
- Stomal infection or infection of lower respiratory tract
- Tracheocutaneous fistula.

8 Confirmation Techniques of Secured Airways

Geetanjali S Verma

CLINICAL

a. Direct visualization using laryngoscopy/fiberoptic scope
b. *Chest lift*: Bilateral
c. Moisture/fogging on ETT
d. *Sound*: Gurgling on PPV implies esophageal intubation
e. *Auscultation*: Apex, midaxillary, epigastric.

END TIDAL CO_2 DETECTORS

a. *Capnography (Figs. 1 and 2)*
   In low cardiac output states like shock, cardiac arrest or inadequate chest compressions, $PetCO_2$ may not be detected.
   False positive seen in: If a patient has had carbonated beverages, if mouth-to-mouth ventilation has been attempted.
b. *Fenum end tidal CO_2 detector (Fig. 3)*
   In presence of CO_2 detection, the color changes from purple to yellow. Not useful in cardiac arrest.

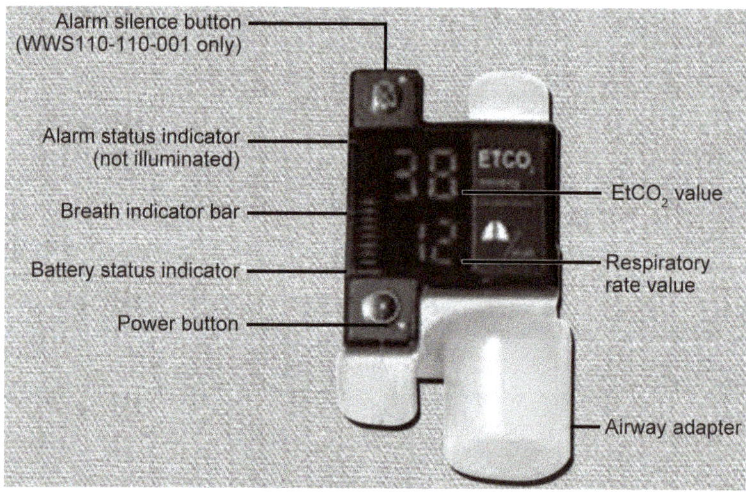

Fig. 1: Capnograph showing $EtCO_2$ and respiratory rate.

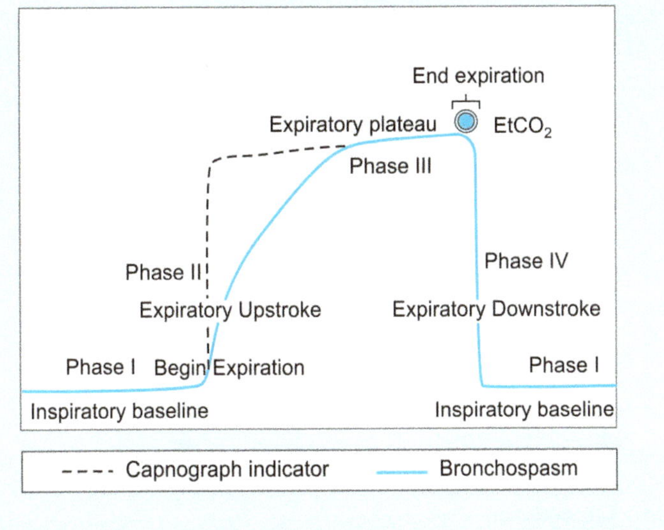

Fig. 2: Four phases of capnography.

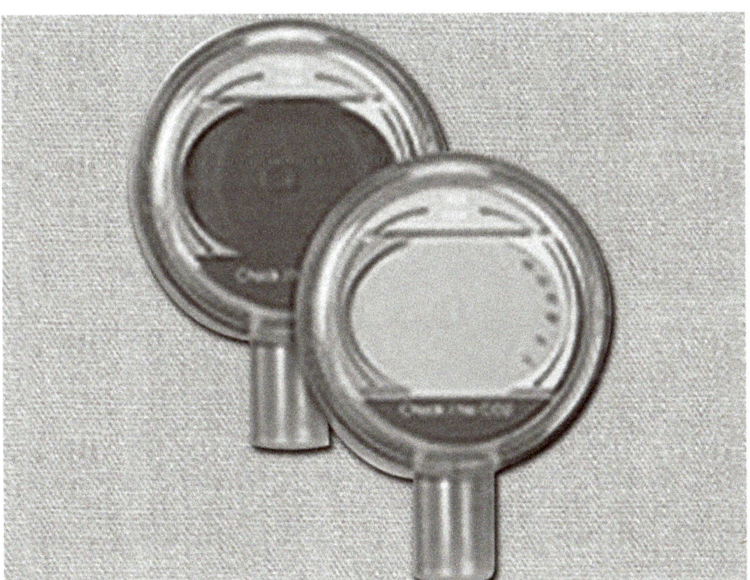

Fig. 3: Fenum end tidal CO_2 detector.

c. *LED CO_2 detector (Fig. 4)*
   If no CO_2 detected, an audible alarm rings.
d. *Thiopentone test*
   0.25% thiopentone used—exhaled gas bubbled through the solution of thiopentone—if CO_2 present, there is precipitation due to acidic media.

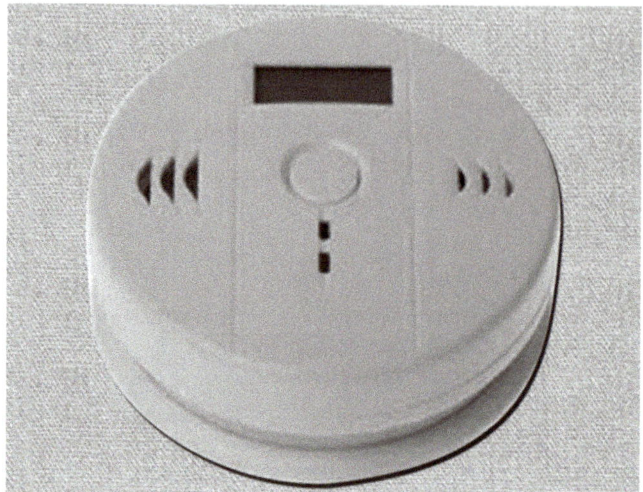

Fig. 4: LED CO_2 detector.

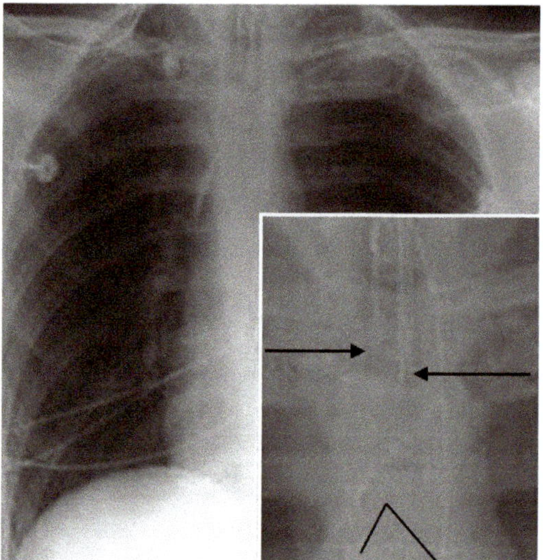

Fig. 5: Chest X-ray showing ETT in situ.
Ideal position: With the neck in neutral position, a distance of 5–7 cm above the carina is acceptable for adults.

e. *Bromothymol blue test*
   10% bromothymol blue used which changes color from reddish blue to greenish yellow when exposed to CO_2.

CHEST X-RAY (FIG. 5)

It helps in detecting the position and depth of ETT.

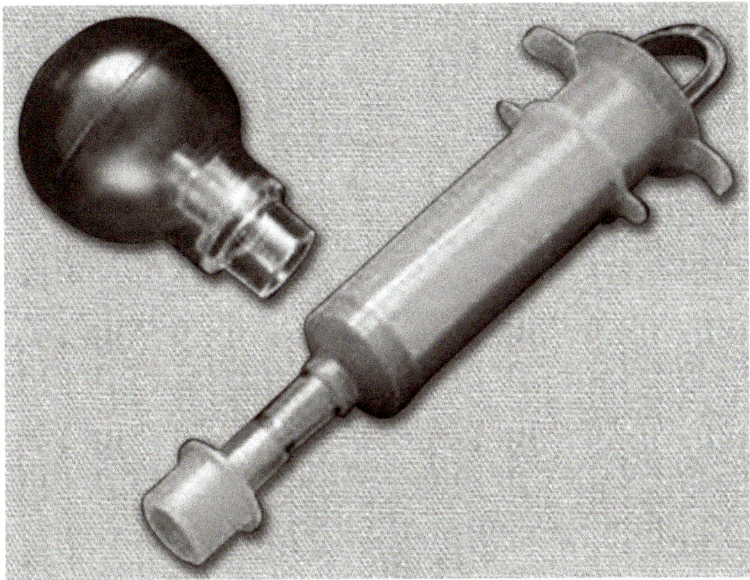

Fig. 6: Esophageal detector device with a bulb and syringe.

ESOPHAGEAL DETECTOR DEVICE (FIG. 6)

Attach esophageal detector device (EDD) to ETT while maintaining ETT placement by using pincer grip to stabilize tube.

Evaluate ETT Placement

Bulb test: Allow bulb to self-expand; if bulb expands in < 5 sec, the ETT is in the trachea, ventilate and clinically check placement.

If bulb expands slowly (>5 sec) tracheal intubation is questionable clinically check placement.

If bulb remains collapsed or gastric contents obtained, the ETT is in the esophagus-remove the ETT immediately and ventilate with BVM device.

Syringe test: Syringe—retract plunger over 2-3 seconds.

If air fills syringe completely, the ETT is in the trachea ventilate and clinically check placement.

If resistance and no air enters the syringe, or if gastric contents obtained, the ETT is in the esophagus—immediately remove the ETT and ventilate with BVM device.

OTHERS

a. Sonomatic confirmation of tracheal intubation device (by soundwave resonance) (Fig. 7).

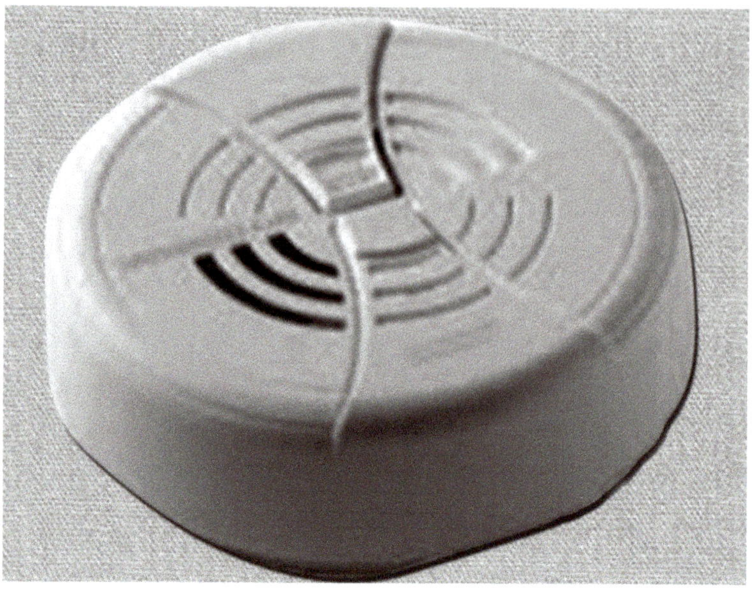

Fig. 7: Sonomatic device for tracheal intubation.

b. Fiberoptic bronchoscopy
c. Lightwand
d. Ultrasound of airway.

VERIFICATION OF DEPTH OF INSERTION OF TUBE

1. *Reference marks on ETT*: Usually 22–23 cm mark in men and the 20–21 cm mark in women of average adult size at inscisor level.
2. *Direct visualization of cuff of tube*: Since the length of the trachea is 10 to 13 cm in an average adult, placing the upper end of the cuff of a tube (size 7 or 8 inside diameter) 2 cm below the vocal cords positions the distal end of the tube approximately 4 cm from the carina (mid-trachea level).
3. Prevention of ETT displacement after intubation.

Precautions to Prevent Tracheal Tube Displacement

The laryngoscope blade should be gently removed after intubation while securing the tube in position.

The tube should be taped or anchored carefully in place.

An oropharyngeal airway (or a bite block) placed adjacent to the tube can minimize the movement of the tube inside the mouth and prevent its dislodgement, especially during coughing.

The head should be kept in neutral position unless head extension or flexion is needed for the surgical procedure.

9 One Lung Ventilation

Geetanjali S Verma

INDICATIONS

Absolute	*Relative*
Isolation of lung Infection/abscess/hemorrhage	Facilitation of surgical exposure Pneumonectomy, upper lobectomy, thoracic aortic aneurysm, mediastinal exposure, esophageal resection
Controlled ventilation Fistula/cyst/bulla/trauma	Post-CPB status after removal of totally occluding chronic unilateral pulmonary emboli
Unilateral lavage	Severe hypoxemia due to unilateral lung pathology
Video and robotic-assisted thoracoscopic surgery	

PREOPERATIVE WORK UP

Spirometry, PFT, chest-X ray, CT/MRI chest, ABG.

Predictors for high risk of one lung anesthesia
Poor exercise tolerance
Pulmonary hypertension
FVC<50% predicted
FEV_1<50% predicted or <2 liters
MBC<50% predicted
RV/TLC>50%

PHYSIOLOGY

LATERAL DECUBITUS POSITION (FIG. 1)

In this position, blood flow is determined by gravity (60% to dependent lung). Anesthesia in lateral decubitus position causes preferential ventilation

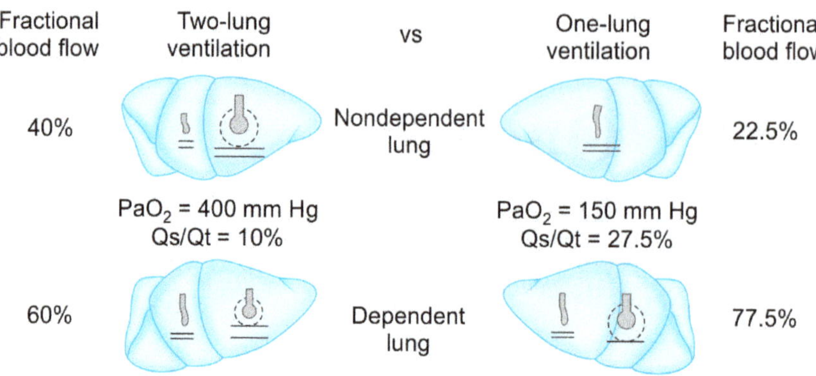

Fig. 1: Schematic representation of two-lung ventilation (TLV) versus one-lung ventilation (OLV). Typical values for fractional blood flow to the nondependent and dependent lungs, as well as PaO_2 and [Q with dot above]s/[Q with dot above]t for the two conditions, are shown. The [Q with dot above]s/[Q with dot above]t during two-lung ventilation is assumed to be distributed equally between the two lungs (5% to each lung). The essential difference between two-lung ventilation and OLV is that, during OLV, the nonventilated lung has some blood flow and therefore an obligatory shunt, which is not present during two-lung ventilation. The 35% of total flow perfusing the nondependent lung, which was not shunt flow, was assumed to be able to reduce its blood flow by 50% by hypoxic pulmonary vasoconstriction. The increase in [Q with dot above]s/[Q with dot above]t from two-lung to OLV is assumed to be due solely to the increase in blood flow through the nonventilated, nondependent lung during OLV.

of nondependent lung. Compliance and FRC of dependent lung are reduced by weight of mediastinum contents, elevated diaphragm and suboptimal positioning. This produces V/Q mismatch.

PULMONARY BLOOD FLOW

When the nondependent lung is collapsed, HPV (Table 1) will increase pulmonary vascular resistance and decrease lung blood flow in this area. If no complicating factors exist, HPV should decrease blood flow to that lung by approximately 50%. Consequently, the nondependent lung should be able to reduce its blood flow from 40 to 20% of the total, and the nondependent/dependent lung blood flow ratio during OLV should be 20%/80%

In atelectasis, all the blood flow to the nonventilated lung is shunt flow. Therefore, OLV creates an obligatory right-to-left transpulmonary shunt that was not present during two-lung ventilation. If no shunt existed during two-lung ventilation (ignoring the normal 1 to 3% shunt flow due to the bronchial, pleural, and the besian circulation), an ideal total shunt flow of 20% would be expected during OLV. PaO_2 with fractional inspired

O_2 concentration (FiO_2) equal to 1 should be approximately 280 mm Hg if hemodynamic and metabolic states are normal. Clinically, PaO_2 (FiO_2 = 1) ranges from 150 to 250 mm Hg.

Ventilation perfusion changes in lateral decubitus position

	Dependent	*Nondependent*
Ventilation	Reduced	Increased
Perfusion	Increased	Reduced
Pulmonary blood flow	80%	20%

Table 1: Hypoxic pulmonary vasoconstriction (HPV)

First noted by Von Euler and Liljestrand in 1946

- Autoregulatory mechanism
- To improve oxygenation and prevent V/Q mismatch

Low FiO_2/hypoventilation/atelectasis
↓
Decreased
PaO_2 ↓
Stimulates redox-based O_2 sensor (mediates Ca-K channels and causes release of Ca)
↓
Pulmonary artery smooth muscle vasoconstriction in hypoxic region
↓
Diverts blood to ventilated lung/decreases shunt flow

Drugs inhibiting HPV: Inhalational agents, nitroglycerin (vasodilators), β agonists/antagonists, Ca channel blockers

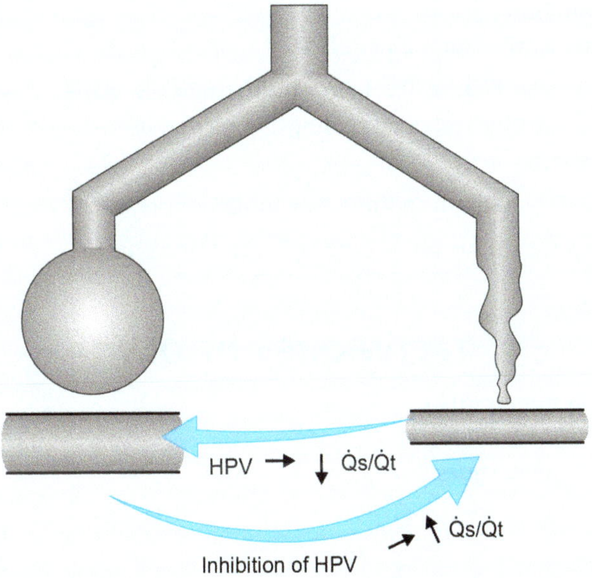

PRINCIPLES OF USING OLV

1. Delaying initiation until after the patient to turned to the lateral decubitus position while still allowing sufficient time for the nondependent lung collaps.
2. Confirming correct positioning of the double-lumen tube by fiberoptic bronchoscopy.
3. Using high-inspired O_2 concentrations (100%) to decrease the risk of systemic hypoxemia.
4. Using a large tidal volume of approximately 10 mL/kg and adjusting respiratory rate to keep $PaCO_2$ at approximately 40 mm Hg.
5. Continuously monitoring oxygenation using pulse oximetry.
6. Continuously monitoring ventilation by noting changes in end tidal CO_2 concentrations and peak inspiratory pressures.

Recruitment maneuver

A sustained pressure of approximately 35 cm H_2O, (above the tidal ventilation range) is applied for a period of 30–60 seconds in order to inflate lung units.

After this maneuver, increasing the tidal volume or PEEP is not necessary because the subsequent lung volumes should be maintained.

A successful maneuver will result in improved oxygenation, reduced end-tidal CO_2, and improved compliance.

INITIATING OLV

- Start with FiO_2 0.33
- Vt 6-8 mL/kg
- Peak airway pressure <25 cm H_2O.

Then increase FiO_2 to 0.5 before initiating OLV clamp Y connector to non-dependent lung and open sealing cap on that lumen - can cause airway pressures to rise.

Adjust Vt and ventilation to limit Paw to <35 cm H_2O.

Check with surgeon for other lung collapse (Flowchart 1).

TECHNIQUES OF OLV

1. Double lumen tubes
2. Bronchial blockers
3. Single lumen tubes.

Flowchart 1: Lung separation in a patient with a difficult airway.

Lung separation in a patient with a difficult airway

Recognized

Proper preparation

Awake intubation

Unrecognized

Mask ventilation

Failed laryngoscopy tracheal intubation

Fiberoptic bronchoscopy video laryngoscopy

Single-lumen tube

Relative indications

Use single-lumen tube

Absolute indications

Bronchial blocker

One-lung ventilation

Tube exchanger with laryngoscopy

Double-lumen tube, univent

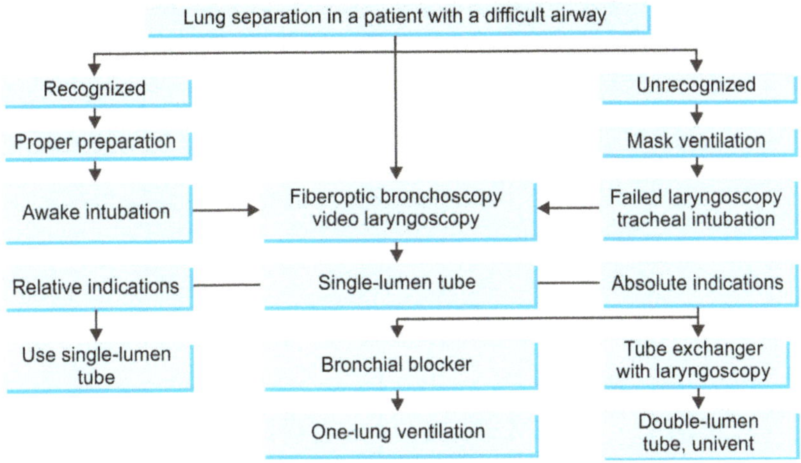

(LMA: Laryngeal mask airway).

DOUBLE LUMEN TUBES

Robertshaw, Carlens, White		
Robertshaw	Left and right sided	No carinal hook
Carlens	Left sided	Carinal hook present
White	Right sided	Carinal hook present

Material: PVC

Sizes: 28, 35, 37, 39, 41 F (1F = 3.14* external diam (mm) or 1F = (4*internal diam) +2)

Commonly used: adult female - 37F, adult male - 39F

Depth of insertion: 37F = 27cm, 39F = 29cm, 41F = 31 cm

Insertion Technique

1. *Choosing the tube*:
   a. Size
   b. Right or left sided: A left-sided DLT is preferable for most procedures because the origin of the right upper lobe (RUL) approximately 0.5 to 1.0 cm below the carina complicates placement of a right-sided tube. A right-sided DLT is indicated in case of large exophytic lesions within the left mainstem bronchial, tight left mainstem bronchus stenosis, distortion of the left mainstem bronchus by an adjacent tumor or a thoracoabdominal aneurysm, and tracheobronchial disruption (Fig. 2).

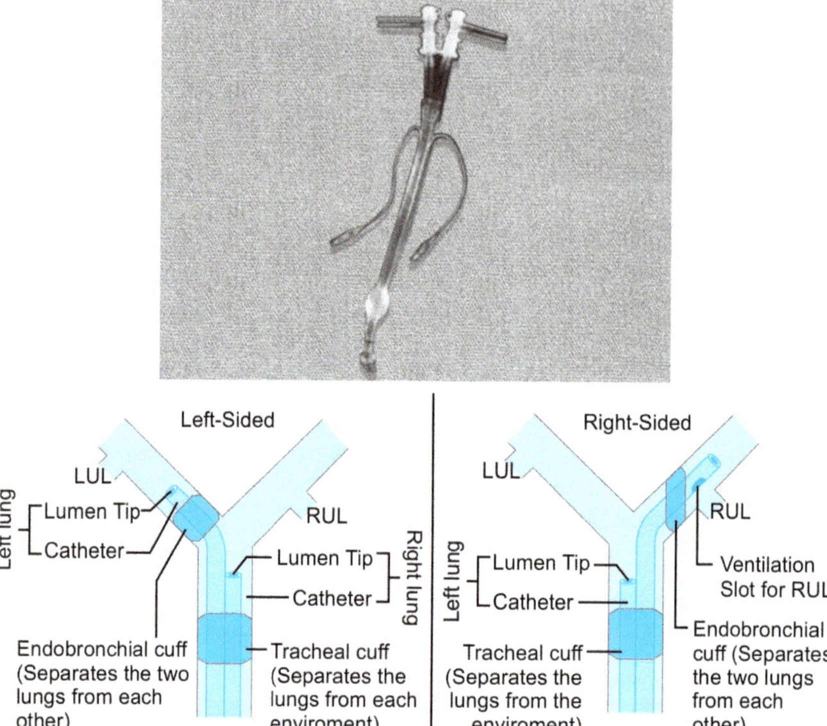

Fig. 2: Essential features and parts of left-sided and right-sided double lumen tubes. (RUL: Right upper lobe; LUL: Left upper lobe). (*From Benumof JL: Anesthesia for Thoracic Surgery. Philadelphia, WB Saunders*)

2. *Insertion (Figs. 3 and 4)*

   The DLT has 2 curves—anteroposterior, and a 2nd curve of the bronchial tube (left or right).

   Prior to insertion of a DLT, check the patency of both tracheal and endobronchial balloons.

   Insertion is often aided by the use of a stylet, with an anterior curve applied to the bronchial lumen.

   Standard laryngoscopy is done, and when the tip of the bronchial lumen is just through the laryngeal inlet (just past the vocal cords), the stylet can be removed. A 70° to 90° rotation of the tube is then performed in the direction of the bronchus to be intubated (clockwise rotation for a right-sided tube or counter-clockwise for a left-sided tube). The tube is advanced until resistance is felt, avoiding excess force.

   The tube is connected to the anesthetic circuit, and the tracheal cuff inflated until there is no air leak, and bilateral chest movement and air entry is confirmed by auscultation. Note the peak airway pressures. The tracheal lumen is opened, and the fresh gas flow to it clamped. The bronchial cuff is inflated (1–2 mL of air), until no air leak is felt

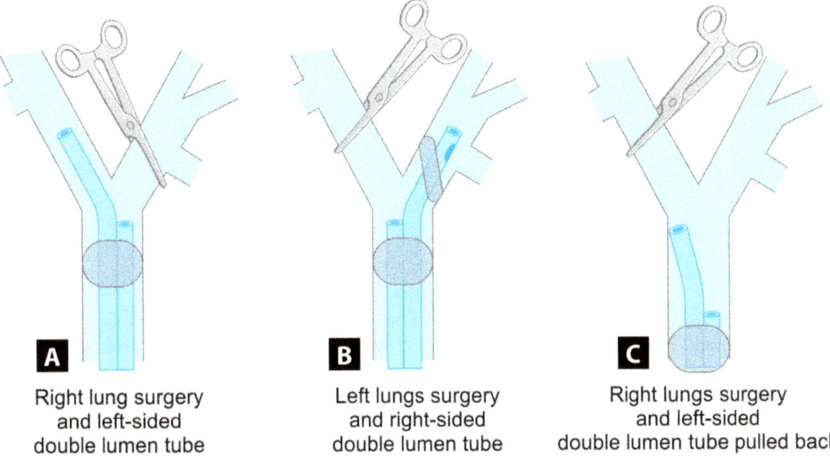

Figs. 3A to C: Use of left-sided and right-sided double-lumen tubes for left and right lung surgery (as indicated by clamp). When surgery is going to be performed on the right lung, a left-sided double-lumen tube should be used (A). When surgery is going to be performed on the left lung, a right-sided double-lumen tube may be used (B). However, because of uncertainty about the alignment of right upper lobe ventilation slot to the right upper lobe orifice, a left-sided double-lumen tube can also be used for left lung surgery (C). If left lung surgery requires a clamp to be placed high on left mainstem bronchus, the left endobronchial cuff should be deflated, the left-sided double-lumen tube pulled back into the trachea, and the right lung ventilated through both lumens (use double-lumen tube as a single-lumen tube).
(From Benumof JL: Anesthesia for Thoracic Surgery. Philadelphia, WB Saunders).

at the tracheal opening during ventilation. Auscultation is used to ensure good air entry at the apex and base of the lung unilaterally, and confirmed deflation of the contralateral lung. Airway pressures noted. There should be a rise of no more than 8 to 12 cm H_2O in peak airway pressure. Ventilate both lungs again. The bronchial lumen is opened, and its fresh gas flow inlet clamped. Tracheal ventilation is then initiated, which is confirmed by unilateral air entry on auscultation and unilateral chest expansion. *If there is a rise in airway pressure greater than 12 cm H_2O, or there is reduced air entry to the nonbronchial lumen it suggests the bronchial cuff is causing obstruction (by herniation across the carina) and needs to be inserted further.* The bronchial cuff is deflated and auscultation is repeated. If there is no difference in air entry or if there is NO change in airway pressures on deflation of the cuff it suggests the tube is abutting the carina or the tracheal portion of the tube is endobronchial, and the tube should be slightly withdrawn.

3. *Confirmation of placement*
   a. Auscultation.
   b. *Fiberoptic bronchoscopy (Fig. 5):* During bronchoscopy, the tracheal cartilaginous rings are anterior and the tracheal membrane is

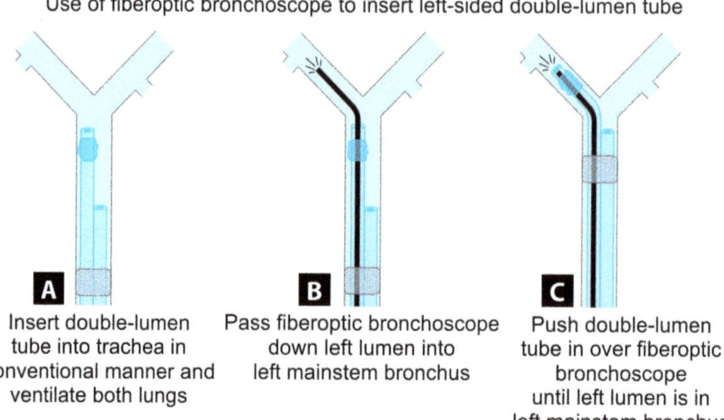

Figs. 4A to C: Double-lumen tube can be put into trachea in a conventional manner, and both lungs can be ventilated by both lumens (A). Fiberoptic bronchoscope may be inserted into left lumen of double-lumen tube through a self-sealing diaphragm in the elbow connector to the left lumen; this allows continued positive-pressure ventilation of both lungs through right lumen without creating a leak. After fiberoptic bronchoscope has been passed into the left mainstem bronchus (B), it is used as a stylet for left lumen (C); fiberoptic bronchoscope is then withdrawn. Final precise positioning of double-lumen tube is performed with fiberoptic bronchoscope in right lumen
(*From Benumof JL: Anesthesia for Thoracic Surgery. Philadelphia, WB Saunders*).

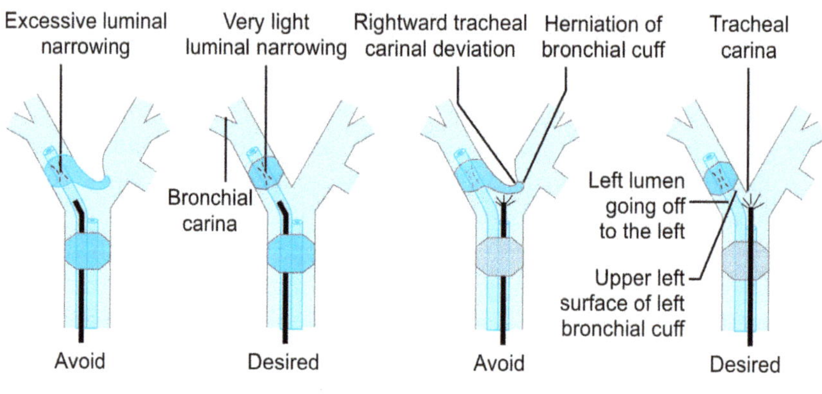

Fig. 5: Complete fiberoptic bronchoscopy picture of left-sided double-lumen tubes (both desired view and view to be avoided from both lumens). When bronchoscope is passed down the right lumen of the left-sided tube, the endoscopist should see a clear, straight-ahead view of the tracheal carina, the left lumen going off into the mainstem bronchus, and the upper surface of the blue left endotracheal cuff just below the tracheal carina. Excessive pressure in the endobronchial cuff, as manifested by tracheal carinal deviation to right and herniation of endobronchial cuff over carina, should be avoided. When bronchoscope is passed down left lumen of left-sided tube, endoscopist should see a very slight left luminal narrowing and a clear, straight-ahead view of bronchial carina in the distance. Excessive left luminal narrowing should be avoided.
(*From Benumof JL: Anesthesia for Thoracic Surgery. Philadelphia, WB Saunders*).

seen posterior. Therefore, the right and left sides can be discerned by the relation of the mainstem bronchi to the anterior cartilaginous ring and the posterior membrane. Also, looking for the RUL takeoff (which usually arises from the lateral aspect of right mainstem bronchus just below the tracheal carina) is a useful landmark (when the airway anatomy has been obscured by bleeding, edema, or radiation-induced changes, or it has been distorted by extrinsic compression). Left DLT position and depth are confirmed by inserting the FOB in the tracheal lumen. The entire right mainstem bronchus should be visible and the tracheal lumen orifice should be 1 to 2 cm above the tracheal carina. When properly positioned, the upper surface of the blue endobronchial cuff is visualized just below the tracheal carina in the left mainstem bronchus.

If a right DLT is used, correct positioning is confirmed both by visualization of the bronchial cuff in the right main bronchus and by visualization of the RUL orifice through a port on the lateral surface of the DLT

4. *Confirm position after positioning the patient again.*

Contraindications to DLT Use

1. Upper airway distortion-recessed jaw, bull nect, prominent teeth
2. Airway stricture/tumors
3. Small patients
4. Critically ill patients who cannot tolerate cessation of MV/PEEP for a short time

BRONCHIAL BLOCKERS

Single lumen tube with balloon tipped endobronchial catheter.

Advantages	*Disadvantages*
Facilitates OLV in patients with a difficult airway or where a DLT is contraindicated Can be placed through an existing single-lumen ETT in emergent situations	Inability to suction efficiently or intermittently ventilate the lung distal to the blocker without deflating the balloon Bronchoscope needed for positioning
Eliminates the need to change ETTs for postoperative mechanical ventilation	Difficulty in maintaining position in the right mainstem/isolating the RUL efficiently if the takeoff is close to carina
	Obstruction of the trachea if the bronchial blocker dislodges proximally or bilateral lung ventilation if the cuff is not inflated proper Risk of being stapled in the bronchial stump if not retracted at an appropriate time

Types:
1. Arndt wire guided endobronchial blocker
2. Fogarthy catheter
3. Univent tube.

ARNDT WIRE GUIDED ENDOBRONCHIAL BLOCKER (FIG. 6)

- Low pressure high volume cuffs, epileptical or spherical.
- Inserted through the ETT via a three-way connector (catheter, bronchoscopy, ventilation circuit) and are made with a guide suture loop at the tip that can be placed around a bronchoscope (to facilitate positioning). This suture loop is then removed, leaving an inner lumen that allows for suctioning, CPAP, or jet ventilation.

1. Patient is intubated with a 7.5 mm or larger standard endotracheal tube. If a smaller tube must be used, the pediatric Arndt blocker and an infant bronchoscope may be used.
2. Bronchoscopy is performed using a standard bronchoscope or the 3.2 mm scope. (to ensure no unanticipated endobronchial pathology). It is important not to have the endotracheal tube positioned too close to the carina as this may inhibit directing the blocker into the correct.
3. The 3.2 mm bronchoscope is lubricated and placed through the bronchoscopy adapter provided. The blocker is likewise placed through the appropriate port. Both are passed distal to the connector before the connector is placed in the circuit and the bronchoscope is passed through the loop at the end of the blocker.
4. The ventilation circuit is then disconnected from the patient and the bronchoscope, passed through the blocker loop is passed into the endotracheal tube.

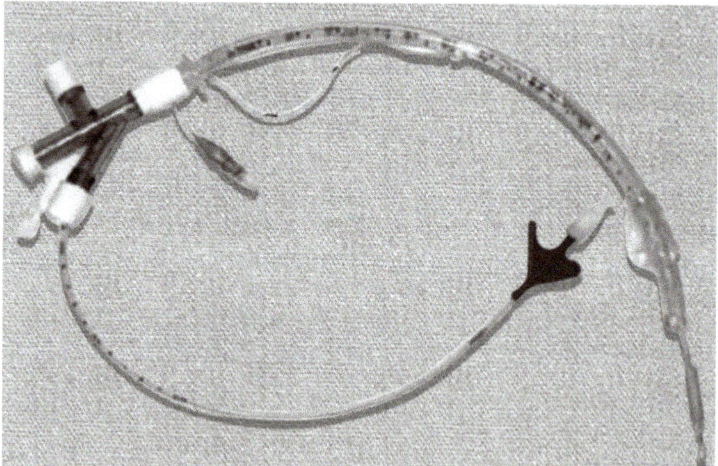

Fig. 6: Arndt wire guided endobronchial blocker.

5. The Arndt adaptor is connected to the ET tube and ventilation is resumed while bronchoscopy is performed.
6. The bronchoscope is passed fairly deep into the bronchus of the lung being operated upon or isolated.
7. The blocker is then slid into the bronchus and the scope is partial withdrawn so that the blocker is visualized.
8. The blocker is pulled back to the proximal mainstem bronchus and inflated with air under direct vision. A brief period of apnea is helpful at this point to allow the lung to deflate prior to obstruction. The blocker must be deep enough into the bronchus so that it does not herniate into the trachea when the balloon is inflated.
9. On the right side, the balloon should be placed at just below the take-off of the right upper lobe bronchus so that when the balloon is inflated, both the RUL bronchus and the bronchus intermedius are occluded.
10. The suture loop can then be removed from the blocker and the blocker secured in position by tightening the connector where the blocker enters.
11. Once the loop is removed, suction can be placed on the blocker which may help with lung collapse. This lumen can also be used for CPAP during the case should oxygen desaturation be a problem.

FOGARTY CATHETER

- 12 or 20 mL high pressure, low volume balloon (latex/nonlatex)
- Has a metallic stylet that aids in insertion/positioning
- Usually placed outside single lumen ETT and positioned with FOB
- If placed inside the ETT, a connector (like two swivel adaptors in series) is needed to facilitate insertion of both the catheter and the bronchoscope.

Placement

1. The tip of the Fogarty catheter is bent approx. 20° at the balloon. (The guide wire should be in place when this is done).
2. The patient is sedated and then intubated with the blocker and the ET tube at one laryngoscopy. The ET tube is secured to the face ensuring it is no lower than the midportion of the trachea. The blocker should be placed just deep enough to be in the trachea and is not secured at this point. A connector that allows for ventilation to proceed during bronchoscopy is used and a full bronchoscopy of the airway is performed. If the blocker is in one mainstem bronchus, it should be withdrawn into the trachea to allow full inspection of the airway.
3. With the scope at the end of the ET tube, the ET tube cuff is deflated and the blocker is placed into the bronchus of the lung to be isolated and operated upon. The catheter can be directed by twisting it and taking advantage of the angle at the tip.

4. The balloon is positioned in the same position as with the Arndt blocker and a test inflation is performed to ensure that the balloon occludes the bronchus but does not herniate back into the trachea. The proper amount of air should be recorded.
5. The ET tube cuff is then reinflated and the blocker is secured to the ET tube with tape. It is helpful to "tab" the tape so that it can be easily removed should repositioning be required.
6. The guidewire is removed from the Fogarty.
7. One lung ventilation is achieved by having a short period of apnea and then inflating the catheter balloon.

UNIVENT TUBE (FIG. 7)

Univent ID, mm	*Univent FG of single main lumen (marked on tube)*	*Univent OD, mm lateral/AP*	*Equivalent SLT OD, mm*	*Equivalent DLT, FG*
7.5	31	11.0/12.0	9.6	35
8.0	33	11.5/13.0	10.9	37
8.5	35	12.0/13.5	11.6	39
9.0	37	12.5/14.0	12.2	41

Data from MacGillvray RG: Evaluation of a new tracheal tube with a moveable bronchus blocker. Anaesthesia 43:687, 1988 and Slinger P: Con: The Univent tube is not the best method of providing one-lung ventilation. J Cardiothorac Vasc Anesth 7:108–112, 1993.

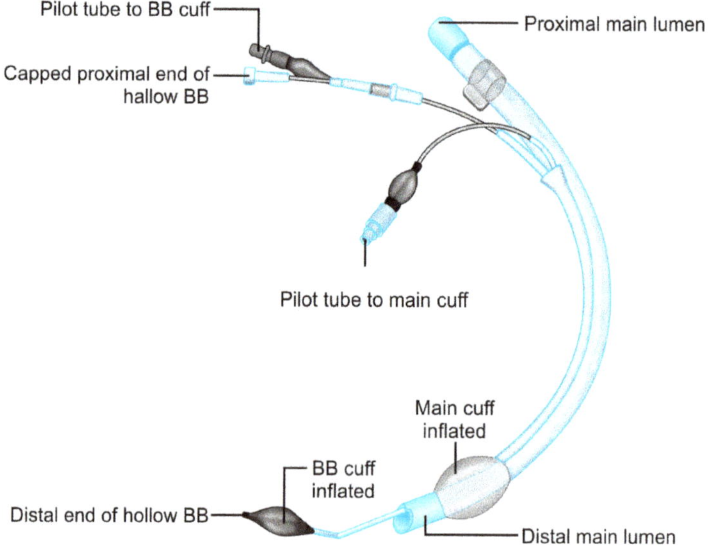

Fig. 7: Univent tube.

Placement (Figs. 8 and 9)

1. The patient is intubated with the Univent tube. The tube should be no lower than the midportion of the trachea.
2. Bronchoscopy of the airway is done.
3. The bronchoscope is pulled back to just distal to the end of the Univent tube and the balloon catheter is advanced into the desired mainstem bronchus. Positioning and inflation are the same as with the Arndt and Fogarty blocker.

SINGLE LUMEN TUBE

- Useful in small children.
- Usually, the normal endotracheal tube can be placed easily in right bronchus by advancing the depth. But, for intubating the left bronchus, the patient's head needs to be turned to the right and tube advanced with concavity facing posteriorly (Fig. 9).
- Effective in emergencies due to ease of placement (e.g. hemoptysis).

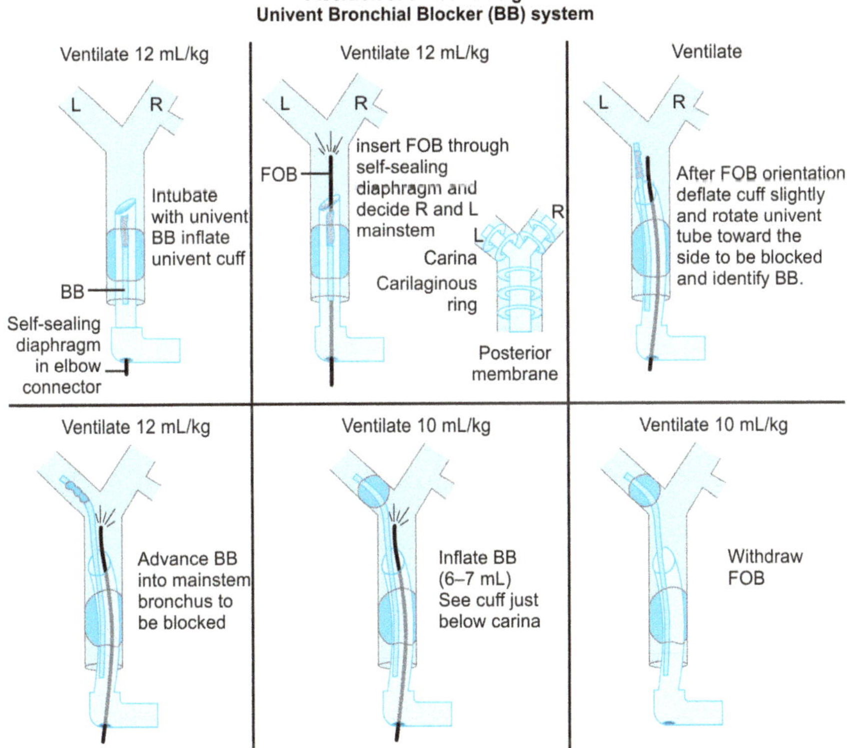

Fig. 8: The sequential steps of the fiberoptic-aided method of inserting and positioning the Univent bronchial blocker in the left mainstem bronchus. See text for full explanation. One- and two-lung ventilation is achieved by simply inflating and deflating, respectively, the bronchial blocker balloon.
(FOB: Fiberoptic bronchoscope; L: Left; R: Right).
(From Benumof JL: Anesthesia for thoracic surgery. Philadelphia, WB Saunders)

Lung separation with single lumen tube and left lung bronchial blocker inside of single lumen tube

Lung separation with single lumen tube and right lung bronchial blocker inside of single lumen tube

LL RL LL RL LL RL LL RL

LL RL LL RL LL RL LL RL LL RL LL RL

Fig. 9: Sequence for lung separation with single-lumen tube and bronchial blocker within the single-lumen tube. (A) Left lung bronchial blocker. (B) Right lung bronchial blocker. The bronchial blocker (Fogarty embolectomy catheter) is placed in the correct mainstem bronchus under fiberoptic vision.
(From Benumof JL: Anesthesia for Thoracic Surgery. Philadelphia, WB Saunders).

Flowchart 2: Plan at end of surgery

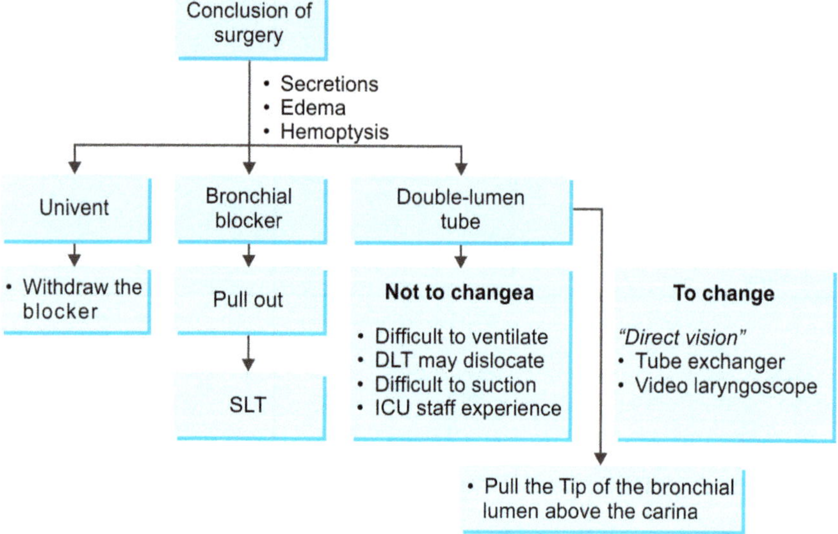

POSTOPERATIVE MANAGEMENT (FLOWCHART 2)

Bronchus of nonventilated lung suctioned and lung fully inflated.

Then, resume two lung ventilation.

Perform a chest X-ray to rule out pneumothorax, hemothorax, misplaced chest drain or collapse.

Pain relief: Thoracic epidural or paravertebral blocks.

COMPLICATIONS

DOUBLE LUMEN TUBES

1. *Malposition*

   Cause: Distal migration—associated with flexion of the neck; cephalad migration—by surgical manipulation, neck extension, or traction on an inadequately secured tube.

   Manifestation: Peak airway pressure suddenly increases, hypoxemia occurs, or inflation of the nonventilated lung is detected.

   Management: Confirm position by FOB, surgeon can manipulate manually.
2. *Trauma*: Ecchymosis of the mucous membranes, arytenoid dislocation, vocal cord rupture, tracheobronchial rupture.

   Cause: Forceful advancement against resistance, excessive pressure in either the tracheal or bronchial cuffs.

   Prevention: When use of a stylet is required for intubation of the trachea, it should be withdrawn before the bronchial lumen of the DLT is advanced into the mainstem bronchus; cuff pressure should be regularly monitored by palpation of the pilot balloon or by use of a calibrated device.

Others

1. Hypoxemia
2. Unable to ventilate
3. *High peak airway pressures*: Malposition, occlusion, pneumothorax.

IMPROVING OXYGENATION DURING OLV

Reconfirm proper tube placement after turning to the lateral decubitus position.

Increase FiO_2

Increase TV if too small or reduce TV if too large

Consider malposition of double-lumen tube or balloon reconfirm position of ETT with bronchoscope.

Optimize volume status, cardiac output, and hemoglobin content to improve O_2 delivery and prevent mixed venous O_2 desaturation; the latter will magnify the effect of any given degree of shunt on PaO_2.

Start nondependent lung CPAP with 5 cm H_2O; increase as needed.

Start dependent lung PEEP to follow, then match CPAP of nondependent lung.

Intermittent reinflation of the nondependent lung with positive pressure breaths with 100% FiO_2 every 5 minutes, as needed.

Reinstitute two-lung ventilation.

Clamping/ligation of the pulmonary artery of the nondependent lung.

10 Difficult Airways

Geetanjali S Verma

DEFINITIONS

As per ASA (American Society of Anesthesiologists) literature (See Flowchart 1 at the end of chapter).

Difficult Airway

The clinical situation in which a conventionally trained anesthesiologist experiences difficulty with face mask ventilation of upper airway, difficulty with tracheal intubation or both.

Descriptions of Difficult Airway

1. *Difficult face mask or SGA ventilation*: It is not possible for the anesthesiologist to provide adequate ventilation because of one or more of the following problems: inadequate mask or SGA seal, excessive gas leak, or excessive resistance to ingress or egress of gas. Signs of inadequate ventilation include—absent or inadequate chest movement, absent or inadequate breath sounds, auscultatory signs of severe obstruction, cyanosis, gastric air entry or dilatation, decreasing or inadequte oxygen saturation, absent or inadequate $EtCO_2$ and spirometry measures and hemodynamic changes associated with hypoxemia (hypertension, tachycardia, arrhythmia).
2. *Difficult SGA placement*: SGA placement requires multiple attempts in the presence or absence of tracheal pathology.
3. *Difficult laryngoscopy*: It is not possible to visualize any portion of the vocal cords after multiple attempts at conventional laryngoscopy.
4. *Difficult tracheal intubation*: Tracheal intubation requires multiple attempts in the presence or absence of tracheal pathology.
5. *Failed intubation*: Placement of endotracheal tube fails after multiple attempts.

COMPONENTS OF PREOPERATIVE AIRWAY EXAMINATION

(Anesthesiology 2013, V 118; no. 2)

Airway examination component	*Nonassuring findings*
Length of upper incisors	Relatively long
Relationship of maxillary and mandibular incisors during normal jaw closure	Prominent overbite
Relationship of maxillary and mandibular incisors during voluntary protrusion of mandible	Cannot bring mandibular incisors anterior to maxillary incisors
Interincisor distance	< 3 cm
Visibility of uvula	Not visible when tongue is protruded with patient in sitting position *(MPC < 2)
Shape of palate	Highly arched or very narrow
Compliance of mandibular space	Stiff, indurated, occupied by mass or on resilient
Thyromental distance	<3 ordinary finger breadths
Length of neck	Short
Thickness of neck	Thick
Range of motion of head and neck	Patient cannot touch tip of chin to chest or cannot extend neck

DIFFICULT AIRWAY PATHOLOGIES

Congenital Pathologies

1. *Hypoplastic mandible (micrognathia)—difficult intubation*
   Pierre Robin sequence
   Treacher Collins
   Hemifacial microsomia (Goldenhar syndrome).
2. *Midface hypoplasia—difficult bag-mask ventilation*
   Apert syndrome
   Crouzon syndrome
   Pfeiffer syndrome
   Saethre-Chotzen syndrome.
3. *Macroglossia—difficult bag-mask ventilation and difficult intubation*
   Hurler's/Hunter's syndrome (mucopolysaccharidoses)
   Beckwith-Wiedemann syndrome
   Down's syndrome.

Acquired Pathologies

1. *Chronic obstruction*:
   Tonsillar hypertrophy
   Glottic web
   Hemangioma
   Subglottic stenosis.
2. *Acute obstruction*:
   Infection (epiglottitis, retropharyngeal abscess)
   Foreign body aspiration
   Trauma.
3. *Poor mouth opening or mobility of jaw, neck*
   Temporomandibular joint disease, e.g. infection
   Spinal fusion
   Burns contractures
   Measles stomatitis.

Basic Preparation for Difficult Airway Management

1. Availability of equipment for management of difficult airway
2. Informing the patient or responsible person with a known or suspected difficult airway of the risk and procedures pertaining to airway management
3. Assigning and acertaining presence of an individual to provide assistance when a difficult airway is encountered
4. Preanesthetic preoxygenation by mask: 3 minutes or 4 vital capacity breaths
5. Administration of supplemental oxygen throughout the process of difficult airway management - by face mask/nasal cannulae/LMA/insufflation of oxygen

IDENTIFYING DIFFICULTIES IN CONGENITAL PATHOLOGIES

Geetanjali S Verma

APERT SYNDROME

- Autosomal dominant (AD) disorder
- Caused by fibroblast growth factor receptor- 2 gene mutations
- *C/f*: Midfacial hypoplasia, craniosynostosis, high arched or narrow palate with or without cleft, high forehead, flat occiput, syndactyly
- *Occasionally*: Choanal stenosis or atresia, cervical spine fusion
- *Abnormal tracheal cartilage*: Prone to trauma during suctioning and reduced ability to clear secretions.

BECKWITH-WIEDEMANN SYNDROME

- Sporadic/autosomal dominant inheritance
- Insulin like growth factor gene 2 involved

- *C/f*: Macroglossia, macrosomia, omphalocele, visceromegaly, exophthalmos, malocclusion, mandibular prognathism and underdevelopment.

CROUZON SYNDROME

- Autosomal dominant disorder
- Caused by fibroblast growth factor receptor- 2 gene mutations
- *C/f*: Premature craniosynostosis of coronal, sagittal and lambdoid sutures, maxillary hypoplasia, hypertelorism, shallow orbits
- *Occasionally*: Cleft lip/palate, tracheobronchomalacia, hearing loss.

DOWN'S SYNDROME (TRISOMY 21)

- *C/f*: Small chin, macroglossia (predisposing to OSA), flat and wide face, short neck, instability of the atlantoaxial joint, high arched palate, adenoid and tonsillar hypertrophy
- *Others*: Excessive joint flexibility, extra space between big toe and second toe, abnormal patterns on the fingertips and short fingers, hip dislocations
- Slanted eyes, flat nasal bridge, poor muscle tone, single crease of the palm
- Prevention of postoperative respiratory compromise: CPAP.

GOLDENHAR SYNDROME

- Anomalies of 1st and 2nd brachial arch
- *C/f*: Hypoplasia of malar, maxillary and mandibular regions, hypoplasia of facial musculature, lateral cleft like extension of corner of mouth, anomalies of tongue, microtia, cleft lip/palate.

KLIPPEL FEIL SEQUENCE

- *Cause*: Intrauterine disruption of subclavian or vertebral arteries and failure of normal segmentation of cervical spine
- Short neck, limited head movement, low hairline.

PFEIFFER SYNDROME

- Type 1: AD
- Type 2, 3: sporadic
- FGFR1, 2 mutations
- *C/f*: Craniosynostosis, mild syndactyly, broad thumb and great toes, mandibular hypoplasia and proptosis, shallow orbits
- *Occasionally*: Laryngomalaia, tracheomalacia, bronchomalacia, upper cervical vertebral fusion.

PIERRE ROBIN SYNDROME

- *C/f*: Micrognathia, glossoptosis, cleft soft palate
- Neuromuscular dysfunction of lingual and pharyngeal musculature
- *Anesth*: Prone position, nasopharyngeal airway helpful.

TREACHER COLLINS SYNDROME

- AD, TCOF1 gene
- *C/f*: Malar hypoplasia, downslanting palpebral fissures, zygomatic hypoplasia, mandibular hypoplasia, malformation of external ear, lower eyelid colobomas, small mouth opening, high-arched palate, cleft lip/palate, pharyngeal hypoplasia
- *Anesth*: FOB/SGA.

MANAGING ANESTHESIA

Geetanjali S Verma

Consider the following before planning to take up the case:

1. Signs suggesting congenital or acquired abnormality?
2. Condition of the patient—Well settled? Respiratory distress? In extremis?
3. Upper respiratory tract infection?
4. What are the surgical requirements—is an endotracheal tube mandatory?
5. Do you have help?
6. Do you have the appropriate equipment/experience/personnel?
7. Do you have ENT cover if necessary?

INVESTIGATIONS REQUIRED

1. Measurement of oxygen saturation with a pulse oximeter is essential.
2. Arterial blood gases: To assess severity and progress of respiratory distress.
3. Respiratory function tests: To differentiate extrathoracic from intrathoracic obstruction.
4. Plain X-ray, CT scan or MRI: To diagnose of the cause or site of obstruction, or bony or soft tissue abnormalities.
5. A sleep study may be useful to assess the severity of sleep apnea (not routine). Overnight pulse oximetry may be more practical.
6. It may be possible to visualize the larynx using nasoendoscopy if the child is cooperative.

PATIENT PREPARATION

- Starvation times must be strictly adhered to prior to elective surgery.
- A variety of premedication drugs are available:
  - EMLA/Ametop cream to aid early intravenous cannulation
  - Midazolam—0.5 mg/kg PO, max dose 20 mg (sedatives may diminish genioglossus tone and worsen obstruction if present)
  - Atropine (0.02 mg/kg—max 500 mg PO) or glycopyrrolate (0.05 mg/kg IV)
  - H_2 blockers such as ranitidine and/or metoclopramide may be given to those patients felt to be at risk for gastric aspiration.
- IV access.

SETTING UP A PLAN

Inhalation induction is usually our technique of choice in children with a difficult airway.

Effective preoxygenation can be difficult in children so inhalational induction should be carried out with an FiO_2 of 1.0 to maximize safety. Inhalational induction may be slow, and airway obstruction may occur or worsen due to the loss of airway tone as anesthesia deepens. This can generally be resolved by careful positioning, opening the mouth, gentle application of jaw thrust, the use of an oro/nasopharyngeal airway or the application of 10 to 15 cm H_2O of CPAP. As the depth of anesthesia increases the child's ventilation can be gradually assisted and controlled.

Once controlled mask ventilation has been demonstrated, neuromuscular blockade may be an option, depending on planned technique of intubation.

In rare cases, for example measles stomatitis or burns contractures causing severe neck flexion, surgical release of soft tissues may be carried out under a combination of ketamine sedation and local anesthesia to facilitate intubation by conventional means.

Suggested Contents of Difficult Airway Cart

1. Rigid laryngoscope blades of alternate design and size from the routinely used; this may include a rigid fiberoptic laryngoscope
2. Video laryngoscope
3. Tracheal tubes of assorted sizes
4. Tracheal tube guides: stylets, ventilating tube changer, light wands, forceps, bougies
5. SGA: LMA, ILMA of assorted sizes
6. Flexible fiberoptic intubation equipment
7. Equipment suitable for emergency invasive airway access
8. Exhaled CO_2 detector.

TECHNIQUES FOR DIFFICULT AIRWAY MANAGEMENT

Difficult intubation	*Difficult ventilation*
Awake intubation	Intratracheal jet stylet
Blind intubation (oral/nasal)	Invasive airway access
Fiberoptic intubation	SGA
Intubating stylet or tube changer	Oral and nasopharyngeal airways
SGA as an intubating conduit	Rigid ventilating bronchoscope
Laryngoscope blades of varying design and size	2 person mask ventilation
Light wand	
Video laryngoscope	

STRATEGY FOR INTUBATION

1. Assessment of likelihood and anticipated clinical impact of six basic problems that may occur alone or in combination.
   a. Difficulty with patient cooperation or consent
   b. Difficult mask ventilation
   c. Difficult SGA placement
   d. Difficult laryngoscopy
   e. Difficult intubation
   f. Difficult surgical access.
2. Consideration of relative clinical merits and feasibility of four basic management choices:
   a. Awake intubation vs intubation after induction of general anesthesia
   b. Noninvasive vs invasive techniques for initial approach to intubation
   c. Video-assisted laryngoscopy as initial approach to intubation
   d. Preservation vs ablation of spontaneous ventilation.
3. Identification of primary or preferred approach to
   a. Awake intubation
   b. Patient who can be adequately ventilated but is difficult to intubate
   c. Life-threatening situation in which the patient cannot be ventilated or intubated.
4. Identification of alternative approaches that can be used if primary approaches fail or is not feasible.
5. Confirmation of tracheal intubation using capnography or $EtCO_2$ monitoring.

Flowchart 1: Difficult airway algorithm.

American Society of Anesthesiologists®

DIFFICULT AIRWAY ALGORITHM

1. Assess the likelihood and clinical impact of basic management problems:
   - Difficulty with patient cooperation or consent
   - Difficult mask ventilation
   - Difficult supraglottic airway placement
   - Difficult laryngoscopy
   - Difficult intubation
   - Difficult surgical airway access.
2. Actively pursue opportunities to deliver supplemental oxygen throughout the process of difficult airway management.
3. Consider the relative merits and feasibility of basic management choices:
   - Awake intubation *vs.* intubation after induction of general anesthesia
   - Non-invasive technique *vs.* invasive techniques for the initial approach to intubation.
   - Video-assisted laryngoscopy as an initial approach to intubation
   - Preservation vs. ablation of spontaneous ventilation.
4. Develop primary and alternative strategies:

Awake intubation

Airway approached by noninvasive intubation

Invasive airway access[(b)*]

Succeed*

Fail

Cancel case[(c)]

Consider feasibility of other options[(a)]

Invasive airway access[(b)*]

Intubation after induction of general anesthesia

Initial intubation attempts unsuccessful

Initial intubation attempts successful*

From this point onwards consider:
1. Calling for help
2. Returning to spontaneous ventilation
3. Awakening the patient

Face mask ventilation adequate

Face mask ventilation not adequate

Consider/attempt SGA

Nonemergency pathway ventilation adequate, intubation unsuccessful

SGA adequate*

SGA not adequate or not feasible

Alternative approaches to intubation[(c)]

If both face mask and SGA ventilation become inadequate

Emergency pathway ventilation not adequate, intubation unsuccessful

Call for help

Successful intubation*

Fail after multiple attempts

Emergency noninvasive airway ventilation[(e)]

Invasive airway access[(b)*]

Consider feasibility of other options[(a)]

Awaken patient[(d)]

Successful ventilation*

Fail

Emergency invasive airway access[(b)*]

***Confirm ventilation, tracheal intubation, or SGA placement with exhaled CO_2.**

a. Other options include (but are not limited to): surgery utilizing face mask or supraglottic airway (SGA) anesthesia (e.g., LMA, ILMA, laryngeal tube), local anesthesia infiltration or regional nerve blockade. Pursuit of these options usually implies that mask ventilation will not be problematic. Therefore, these options may be of limited value if this step in the algorithm has been reached via the emergency pathway.

b. Invasive airway access includes surgical or percutaneous airway, jet ventilation, and retrograde intubation.

c. Alternative difficult intubation approaches include (but are not limited to): video-assisted laryngoscopy, alternative laryngoscope blades, SGA (e.g., LMA or ILMA) as an intubation conduit (with or without fiberoptic guidance), fiberoptic intubation, intubating stylet or tube changer, light wand, and blind oral or nasal intubation.

d. Consider repreparation of the perfect for awake intubation or cancelling surgery.

e. Emergency non-invasive airway ventilation consists of a SGA.

11

Extubation

Geetanjali S Verma

PLANNING A NORMAL EXTUBATION

Initial Plan

- Deep extubation
- Awake extubation
- Deep replacement of tracheal tube with LMA.

Other Preparations

- Patient position plan: Sniff position preferred during extubation followed by lateral/recovery position (to prevent tongue fall)
- Bite block in place
- Throat pack removed
- Preoxygenation
- Secretions aspirated from pharynx/trachea.

Essentials

Continuous administration of oxygen
Continued ventilation
Strategy to facilitate reintubation

ADVERSE RESPONSES TO EXTUBATION

CVS: Hypertension, tachycardia, dysrhythmias

CNS: Increase in IOP and ICP

RS: Laryngospasm/bronchospasm, cough reflex, airway obstruction causing negative pressure pulmonary edema.

PREVENTION OF ADVERSE RESPONSES

1. Complete reversal of neuromuscular blockade
2. Avoidance of sedative premedications and inhalational anesthetics a while prior to planning extubation

3. Sevoflurane may be preferred to isoflurane or halothane (rapid excretion)
4. Remifentanil preferred to fentanyl/morphine (short acting)
5. N_2O may be used but requires 3 minute oxygenation postextubation inorder to prevent diffusion hypoxia
6. Lignocaine (1–1.5 mg/kg 90 seconds prior) may be given prior to extubation to avoid hemodynamic fluctuations
7. β-blockers may also be used to blunt hemodynamic responses.

Complications of Routine Extubations

Failed extubation
Hypoxia
Hypoventilation
Pulmonary toilet
Obstruction
Unintended extubation
Tube entrapment
Hemodynamic changes
Tachycardia or other dysrhythmias
Hypertension
Increased intraocular pressure
Coughing, breath-holding
Laryngospasm
Negative-pressure pulmonary edema
Tracheal or laryngeal trauma
Laryngeal edema
Arytenoid dislocation
Vocal fold paralysis
Laryngeal incompetence
Pulmonary aspiration

IDENTIFYING HIGH-RISK EXTUBATIONS

1. Airway obstructions
   - Postcervical spine surgery
   - Maxillofacial injury
   - Tracheomalacia
   - Cervical cord compression.
2. Pulmonary causes
   - Depressed neurological status
   - Neuromuscular impairment, malnutrition
   - Central sleep apnea
   - Diaphragmatic dysfunction.

3. Inability to protect airway
   - Laryngeal incompetence due to injury
   - Neurological depression
   - Neuromuscular weakness.
4. Difficult airway
   - Previous airway history
   - Damage to airway
   - Rheumatoid arthritis
   - Cricoarytenoid arthritis.
5. Difficult access to airway
   - Oromaxillofacial fixation
   - Limited cervical spine mobility (halo fixation, cervical collar, cervical fusion, ankylosing spondylosis)
   - Smoke, chemical inhalation
   - Burns.

SIMPLE ALGORITHM FOR PLANNING EXTUBATION

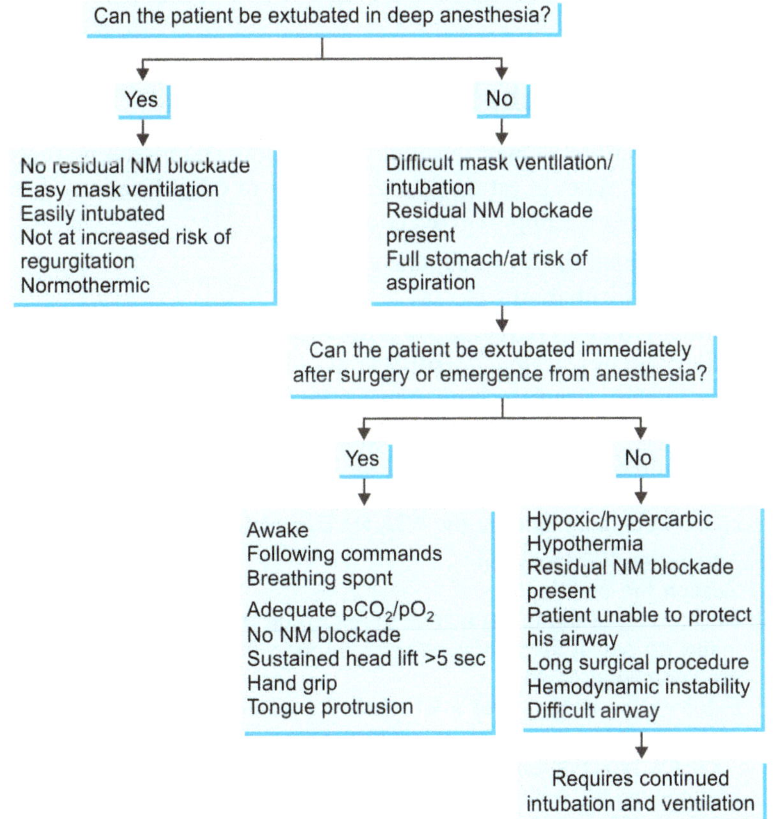

EXTUBATION OF HIGH-RISK PATIENTS

Involves 4 crucial steps:

1. Planning
2. Preparation
3. Performing the extubation
4. Postextubation care.

Planning Extubation

Review the patient's medical notes for airway problem and general risks factors and surgical conditions, previeous extubation problems should be reviewed.

Consider operative problems: Massive fluid resuscitation, burns, inhalational injuries, subglottic stenosis, laryngotracheobronchitis, cervical spine injury, halo traction vertebra).

Current and past medical illnesses: CVS, pulmonary, renal, hepatic, coagulopathy, sepsis.

Review current ventilatory requirements: FiO_2, PEEP, MV, secretions, ETT tolerance during awake state) and vital signs, mental and neurologic status before extubation.

Preparing for Extubation

Optimize the cardiovascular, respiratory, metabolic, temperature and neuromusclar block. Plan to extubate in the theater or other location where all the monitoring and equipment available.

Decide to extubate by the systematic approach.

a. Standard extubation
b. Extubation and evaluation via a fiberoptic bronchoscope (FOB)
c. Extubation by placement of supraglottic airway (SGA) for airway patency, oxygenation, ventilation and pathway for potential reintubation
d. Extubation over an airway excange catheter (AEC)
e. Postpone extubation or surgical airway.

Recommended Technique by the ASA for Extubation of the Difficult Airway

1. Administer 100% oxygen.
2. Suction the oropharynx.
3. Deflate cuff of the endotracheal tube for cuff leakage check.
4. Insert an airway exchange catheter through the endotracheal tube to a predetermined depth.
5. Extubate the patient over a jet ventilation catheter.
6. Apply oxygen by facemask or insufflation through a jet ventilation catheter.
7. Tape the proximal end to the patient's shoulder to stabilize it.
8. Remove the jet ventilation catheter after 30 to 60 minutes if no obstruction appears.

Standard Extubation

- Perform laryngoscopy/bronchoscopy: If edema present, give 2 doses of corticosteroids prior to extubation and extubate.
- Leak test may be performed to rule out tracheomalacia/edema (deflate cuff of tracheal tube prior to extubation and listen for a audible leak—If present, it is a normal response. Absence of the leak indicates edema/tracheomalacia).
- Extubation should be performed in an awake patient after breathing 100% oxygen to maximize oxygen stores.
- Helium, noninvasive ventilation and CPAP may reduce the risk for reintubation.

Extubation Over the FOB

In a spontaneously breathing patient extubation over a fiberoptic bronchoscope is a useful to brief evaluation of the airway, observe the periglottic functions, injury, mucosal integrity and surrounding pharyngeal tissues.

When significant abnormalities are noted, a decision can be made to maintain the current situation, extubate or elective surgical way.

The down side of the FOB needs skill, cannot leave in the airway for long because heaviness of the equipment, not effective oxygen supply because of the narrow diameter and does not have distance marker.

If required, reintubation can be facilitated using an Aintree intubation catheter which jackets the flexible bronchoscope.

Extubation over Supraglottic Airway

This technique is considered in suspected pharyngeal paralysis or tube entrapment. Adequate depth of anesthesia is very important to avoid laryngeal spasm in patients with irritable airways, smokers and asthmatics.

Not useful with periglottic injury, risk of regurgitation and in whom reintubation would be difficult.

The following sequence for LMA exchange extubation:

- Administer 100% oxygen
- Maintain deep plane or neuromuscular blockade
- Laryngoscopy and do suction under direct vision
- Insert deflated intubating LMA or LMA behind the tracheal tube and confirm the position
- Deflate tracheal tube and remove tube with maintaining the positive pressure
- Administer oxygen through the LMA and emergence from anesthesia.

Extubation over the Tracheal Tube Exchange Catheter: (Reversible Tracheal Intubation)

This strategy is very useful for patients expected to be difficult to reintubate.

Cook airway exchange catheter are 85 cm long, hollow catheter with 15 mm connector for jet or manual ventilation and respiratory monitoring. Its also have depth marker and radiopaque. This device is inserted into tracheal tube before extubation. Catheters external diameter of 3.7 and 4.7 mm compatible with 4 and 5 mm of ETT.

Air exchange catheters are well-tolerated by awake patients, who can breathe around them. Insufflation of oxygen at low pressure or positive pressure ventilation by intermittent application of high pressure is possible. Using PPV—the lowest pressure that produces acceptable tidal volume (judged by movement of chest and upper abdomen) should be used. The next inspiration should not be started until the chest returns to its preinspiration position. Expiratory resistance should be overcome by jaw thrust and head extension, augmented by oropharyngeal airway or LMA.

Severe cases may require a small dose of muscle relaxant to "break" the spasm along with reintubation.

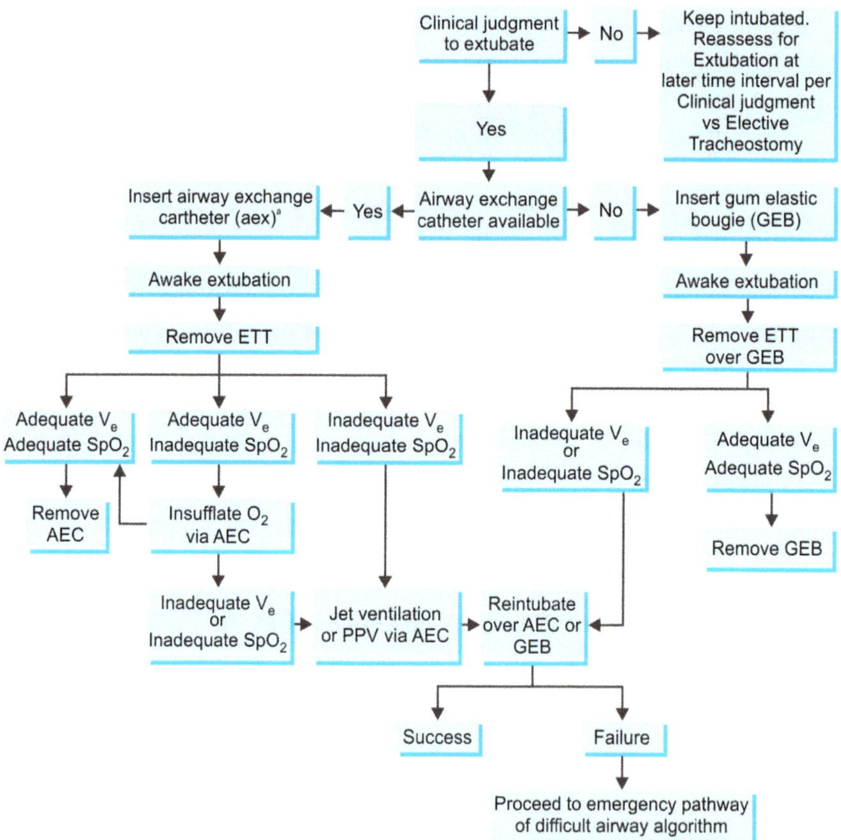

Postpone Extubation

At any time, airway threat is so severe the extubation should be postponed for few hours or few days is most appropriate course of action. Time delay reduces the airway edema and need to take consideration of future operative schedule as well. Transfer the patient to a critical care unit and write clear instruction of the reintubation plan.

Elective Tracheostomy

Tracheostomy gives rapid postoperative emergence without fear of extubation failure or failure to intubate. The anesthetist and surgeon should discuss these problems in patients with preexisting airway problems, extented tumors, swelling and edema. The surgical tracheostomy indicated if there is anticipated postoperative airway deterioration, problem in rescue the airway and longer duration of airway compromise.

FOLLOW-UP AFTER DIFFICULT AIRWAY MANAGEMENT

American Society of Anesthesiologists (ASA) guidelines recommend that anesthesiologists should document the presence and nature of difficult airway, inform the patient and evaluate and arrange appropriate management of complications.

Documentation

1. Document the presence and nature of airway difficulty in medical record:
   a. The description should distinguish between difficulties in face-mask or SGA ventilation and difficulties in intubation.
   b. Description of various airway management techniques used and their beneficial or detrimental role in management of airway.
2. Inform the patient or responsible person of the airway difficulty encountered—for facilitating delivery of future care.
   Notification systems include a written report or letter to the patient, a written report in medical chart, communication with patients surgeon or primary caregiver, a notification bracelet or an equivalent identification device or chart flags.
3. Evaluate and follow up patient for potential complications of difficult airway management.
   These include edema, bleeding, tracheal and esophageal perforation, pneumothorax and aspiration.
   The patent should be advised of the potential signs and symptoms (sore throat, pain and swelling of face and neck, chest pain, subcutaneous emphysema and difficulty swallowing) associated with management of difficult airway.
   See guidelines discussed in DAS algorithms

AIRWAY ALERT FORM

Name ....

Date of Birth ....

Hospital Number ....

Home Address ....

Telephone ....

Fax ....

Email ....

To the Patient

Please keep this letter safe and show it to your doctor if you are admitted to hospital.

Please show this letter to the anesthetic doctor if you need an operation.

This letter explains the difficulties that were found during your recent anesthetic and the information may be useful to doctors treating you in the future.

To the GP

Please copy this letter with any future referral.

Summary of Airway Management

Date of operation:

Type of operation:

		Reasons/comments
Difficult mask ventilation?	Yes/No	
Difficult direct laryngoscopy?	Yes/No	
Difficult tracheal intubation?	Yes/No	
Laryngoscopy grade	1/2/3/4	

Equipment used:

Other information:

Is awake intubation necessary in the future?

Follow-up care (tick when completed)

- Copies of letter
- One copy to patient
- One copy to GP
- One copy in case notes
- One copy in anesthetic department
- Spoken to patient
- Anesthetic chart complete
- Information on front of case notes
- Medic alert or difficult airway
- Society referral (specify)

Name of anesthetist: Grade: Date:

If you require further information please contact the Anesthetic Department.

12 Ventilation Strategies

Geetanjali S Verma

INDICATIONS/DECIDING THE NEED

1. Inadequate oxygenation
   a. Respiratory failure
   b. Hypoxemia (PaO_2 < 55 mm Hg)
   c. ARDS
   d. Hypotension/CVS collapse.
2. Inadequate ventilation
   a. Respiratory muscle fatigue
   b. Bradypnea/apnea with respiratory arrest
   c. Tachypnea.
3. To protect the airway
   a. Comatose/obtunded paticnts
   b. Proposed surgery on airway/head and neck
   c. Neuromuscular diseases: myasthenia gravis, GBS, spinal cord injuries, muscular dystrophy
   d. Trauma to airway.

MODES OF VENTILATION

Geetanjali S Verma

BASIC CLASSIFICATION

1. Invasive/noninvasive
2. Controlled/assisted
3. Pressure controlled/volume controlled/both.

NONINVASIVE VENTILATION

Indications	*Contraindications*
Increased dyspna—moderate to severe	Respiratory arrest (absolute)
Tachypna (>24 bpm in obstructive, >30 min^{-1} in restrictive)	Unable to fit mask (absolute)

Contd...

Contd...

Indications	*Contraindications*
Signs of increased work of breathing, accessory muscle use and abdominal paradox	Relative: Medically unstable—hypotensive shock Uncontrolled cardiac ischemia or arrhythmia Uncontrolled copious upper gastro-intestinal bleeding Agitated, uncooperative Unable to protect airway Swallowing impairment Excessive secretions not managed by secretion clearance techniques Multiple (i.e. two or more) organ failure Recent upper airway or upper gastro-intestinal surgery
Acute or acute on chronic ventilatory failure: >6.0 kPa, pH <7.35	
Hypoxemia: PaO_2/FiO_2 ratio <200	

Application

- Using nasal or face mask, secured with straps
- Patient seated in 30°–90° position
- Suction airway prior to application of mask.

Continuous Positive Pressure Ventilation (CPAP) (Fig. 1)

- Delivers air at a constant pressure during inspiration and expiration. (Provides positive airway pressure throughout all phases of spontaneous ventilation).
- The patient must be able to breathe spontaneously.
- Prevents alveolar collapse and facilitates oxygen delivery to pulmonary capillaries. It increases the functional residual capacity and opens collapsed alveoli, which, in turn, enhances gas exchange and oxygenation.
- Mainly used for hypoxemic respiratory failure (acute pulmonary edema).
- CPAP reduces left ventricular transmural pressure (thereby increasing cardiac output). Hence, it is very effective for treatment of acute pulmonary edema.
- Pressures usually are limited to 5–15 cm H_2O.

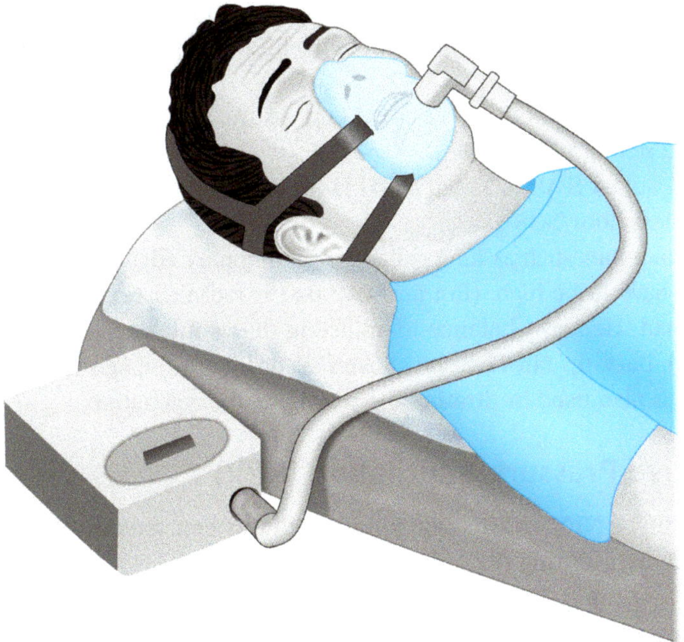

Fig. 1: Continuous positive pressure ventilation device using face mask.

Bilevel Positive Airway Pressure

- Pressure-limited ventilation.
- Predetermined inspiratory pressure is delivered, which can cause different tidal volumes, depending on the resistance of the respiratory system.
- Leak compensation present.
- It is preferred for most short-term applications because pressure-limited modes are better tolerated than volume-limited modes.
- 3 types:
  - *Pressure support*: The ventilator delivers air at a set pressure during inspiration each time a patient initiates a breath.
  - *Pressure control*: The ventilator automatically delivers a set number of breaths per minute at a set pressure.
  - *Bilevel positive airway pressure*: The ventilator delivers different pressures during inspiration and expiration. If necessary, this mode can fully ventilate the patient.
- *Provides 2 levels of positive pressure*: Inspiratory positive airway pressure (IPAP) and expiratory positive airway pressure (EPAP). (required in patients with respiratory fatigue or failure).
- During exhalation, pressure is variably positive. Airflow in the circuit is sensed by a transducer and is augmented to a preset level of ventilation.

Cycling between inspiratory and expiratory modes may be triggered by the patient's breaths or may be preset. BiPAP helps in improving patient comfort.

- *Initial IPAP settings*: 10–12 cm H_2O pressure.
- *EPAP settings*: 5–7 cm H_2O.
- Then adjust IPAP to 15–20 cm H_2O (depending upon the response over the next hour/SOS).
- In conditions such as lung collapse or pulmonary edema, the initial EPAP may have to be high. (But an EPAP that is too high can lead to reduced preload. Hence, a balance in adjusting the ventilatory settings is desirable). Back-up rates can be chosen according to the age of the patient.
- FiO_2 is also used in titrating the response to oxygenation.

Negative Pressure Ventilation (NPV)

The prototype NPV was the iron lung, which was first used in 1928 but most famously used during the polio epidemics of 1950s.

HFO: Designed to provide negative pressure during inspiration and positive pressure during expiration, creating controlled ventilation, including high-frequency chest wall oscillation.

Monitoring of the Patient

1. Conscious level
2. Chest wall motion
3. Accessory muscle recruitment
4. Patient ventilator synchrony
5. Vital signs
   a. Respiratory rate
   b. Exhaled VT (flow, volume, pressure waveform for poor synchrony)
   c. Heart rate
   d. Blood pressure.
6. Gas exchange
   a. Pulse oximetry
   b. Arterial blood gas (baseline, then, every 2 hours or as per institution protocol).

Complications

1. *Inadequacy*: Due to increased secretions/obtunded mentation/ill fitting masks
2. *Skin*: Necrosis at application sites of masks
3. Eye irritation

4. Congestion of nasal sinuses
5. Pain
6. Distension of stomach—aerophagia and vomiting/aspiration (prevention: nasogastric tube insertion).

INVASIVE VENTILATION

Controlled	*Supported*	*Combined*
VC	PS	VC-VS
PC	VS	PC-PS
PRVC		PRVC-VS
		SIMV: VC+PS PC+PS PPRVC+PS

Initiating Ventilation

Mode	*Indication*	*Characteristics*	*Advantages*	*Disadvantages*	*Initial settings*
Assist control/ VC (Figs. 2 and 3)	Total ventilator support may be needed for a sedated or paralyzed patient. Helps decrease the work of breathing in patients with unusually high minute ventilation (severe metabolic acidosis) Not used for weaning	Vent delivers a preset tidal volume with a constant flow during a preset inspiratory time at a preset frequency Patient may initiate additional breaths but these breaths will be delivered at the preset tidal volume	Guarantees the preset rate and tidal volume	High peak pressures may cause lung injury	Adults: AC: 12 Vt: 600 cc PEEP 5 FiO_2: 50% Pediatrics: Weight/ Age Dependent

Contd...

Contd...

Mode	*Indication*	*Characteristics*	*Advantages*	*Disadvantages*	*Initial settings*
PC	Used to limit peak pressures and improve oxygenation in patients with noncompliant lungs such as ARDS and in neonatal ICU for RDS Not used for weaning	Vent delivers a breath with a decelerating flow during a preset inspiratory time, at a preset pressure and preset frequency Patient may initiate additional breaths but these breaths will be delivered at the preset pressure and inspiratory time No preset tidal volume so volumes may vary with changes in lung compliance, i.e. if the lungs become less compliant (stiffer), tidal volume will decrease vice versa if the lungs become more compliant (more elastic) the tidal volumes will increase	Helps protect noncompliant lungs against further injury such as over distension or prevent barotraumas by controlling peak pressures Guarantees a minimum rate Ability to manipulate inspiratory time while guaranteeing adequate flow	No guaranteed minimum volume May require increased sedation for patient comfort especially if using long inspiratory times	PC 25 Frequency 16, I:E 1:1 PEEP 10 FiO_2: 80%

Contd...

Contd...

Mode	*Indication*	*Characteristics*	*Advantages*	*Disadvantages*	*Initial settings*
PRVC	Combines the advantages of volume control and pressure control while eliminating the disadvantages Control mode so not used in weaning	Control mode where ventilator delivers a preset tidal volume and frequency during a preset inspiratory time with decelerating flow Ventilator will vary the inspiratory pressure control level to deliver the breath at the lowest possible pressure to guarantee the preset tidal volume and minute volume Ventilator monitors inspiratory pressures and changes breath by breath if needed until preset tidal volume is obtained	Combines the advantages of volume control and pressure control while eliminating the disadvantages Control mode so not used in weaning	Minor for a control mode	PRVC 14 Vt: 650 PEEP 5 FiO_2: 40%

Contd...

Contd...

Mode	*Indication*	*Characteristics*	*Advantages*	*Disadvantages*	*Initial settings*
SIMV (Figs. 5 and 6)	Allows patient to breathe in a more natural manner and help maintain their PCO_2 Allows for weaning by simply decreasing the frequency as the patient improves SIMV in conjunction with pressure support may be used with a full face mask (covers nose and mouth) for noninvasive ventilation – an option for short-term support	Breaths are delivered the same as in volume control but the number of control bpm is limited to the preset frequency Patient may take spontaneous breaths between the control breaths without assistance (or with augmentation if pressure support is used)	Guarantees preset tidal volume and frequency Allows patient to breathe spontaneously between controlled breaths May be used as a weaning mode	Risk of lung injury due to high peak airway pressures	SIMV 10 Vt: 700 mL PEEP 5 FiO_2: 30% or SIMV 12 Vt: 600 mL PS 5 PEEP 7.5 FiO_2: 50%
PS (Fig. 4)	If the respiratory drive is intact, may be used as the primary mode of ventilation Commonly used in conjunction with SIMV to augment the spontaneous breaths May be used in a noninvasive manner using a full face mask Most commonly used mode in weaning	Support mode where vent delivers breaths with preset pressure kept constant during inspiration with a decelerating flow Patient triggers all breaths	Patient determines respiratory rate and inspiratory time Tolerated better than other modes since it most closely duplicates normal breathing	No preset tidal volume or frequency to guarantee ventilation	PS 10 PEEP 5 FiO_2: 50% or PS : titrate for VT between 450–500 mL PEEP 5 FiO_2: 35%

Contd...

Contd...

Mode	*Indication*	*Characteristics*	*Advantages*	*Disadvantages*	*Initial settings*
VS	If patient is able to spontaneously breathe and achieve the preset tidal volume they may do so without any support If the patient effort falls short of the tidal volume, the ventilator will add support to reach the preset volume Breath-to-breath process to guarantee the set volume is at the lowest possible pressure level	Support mode where ventilator delivers a preset tidal volume at a constant pressure with decelerating flow but pressure may vary from breath-to-breath depending on patients need	Patient determines respiratory rate and inspiratory time Provides backup mode and frequency in case of apnea: if the patient becomes apneic, the vent will automatically switch to PRVC Guarantees preset tidal volume and minute volume	May reduce respiratory drive if tidal volume is set too high Requires thorough knowledge and understanding to optimize settings	VS 550 mL, PEEP 5 O_2: 40%

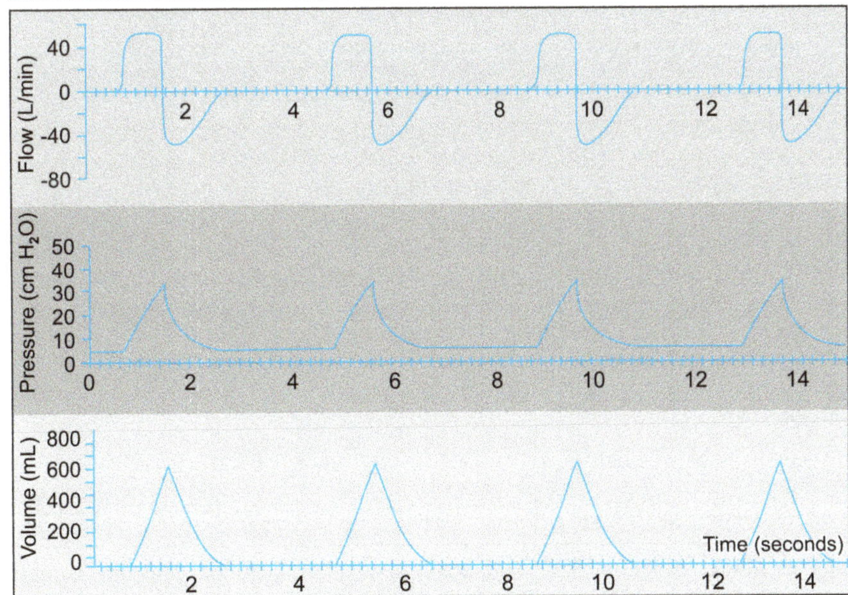

Fig. 2: Flow, airway pressure, and volume waveforms during volume-targeted square wave flow, control mode ventilation. Note that there are no negative airway pressure deflections indicating patient's effort.

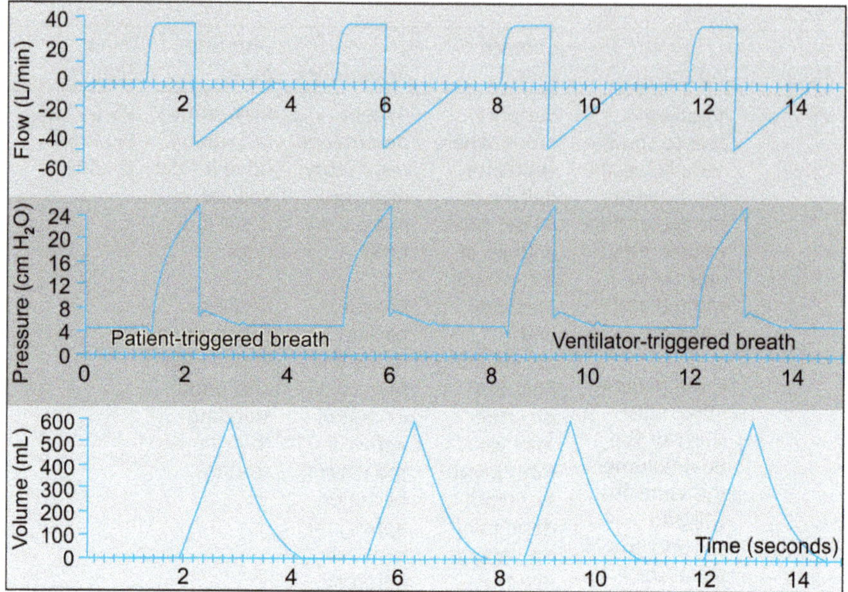

Fig. 3: Airway pressure, flow, and volume waveforms during volume-targeted, square wave flow, assist/control ventilation. Note the negative airway pressure deflection at the start of each breath.

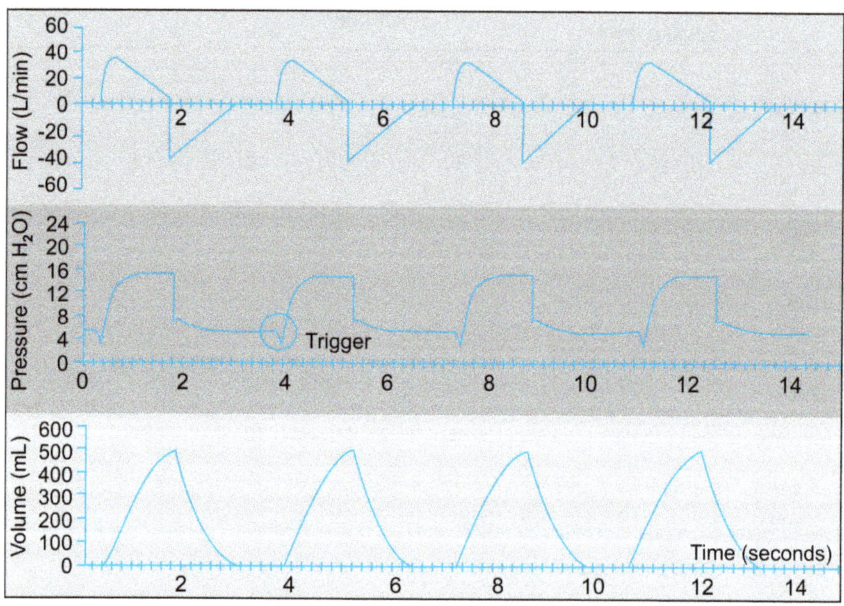

Fig. 4: Airway pressure, flow, and volume waveforms during pressure support ventilation. Note that every breath is patient triggered.

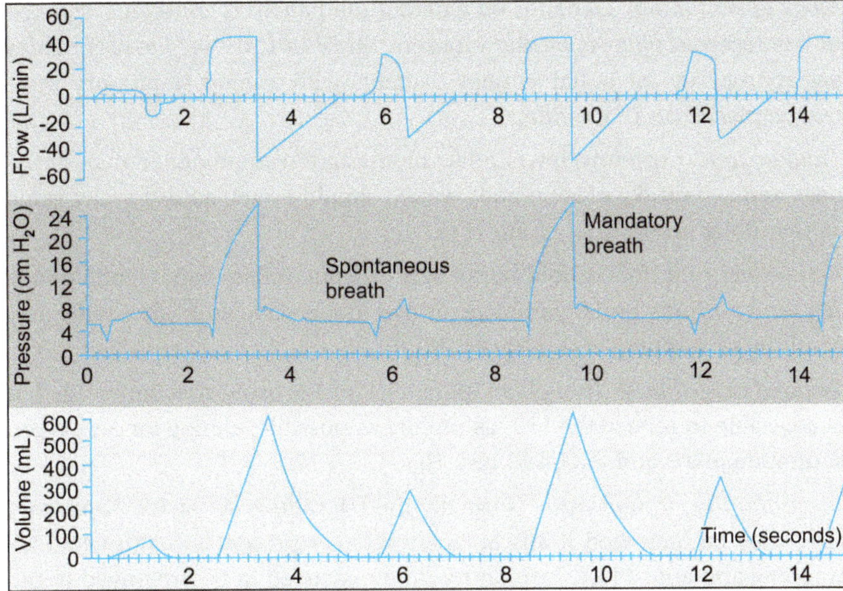

Fig. 5: Airway pressure, flow, and volume waveforms during synchronized intermittent mandatory ventilation.

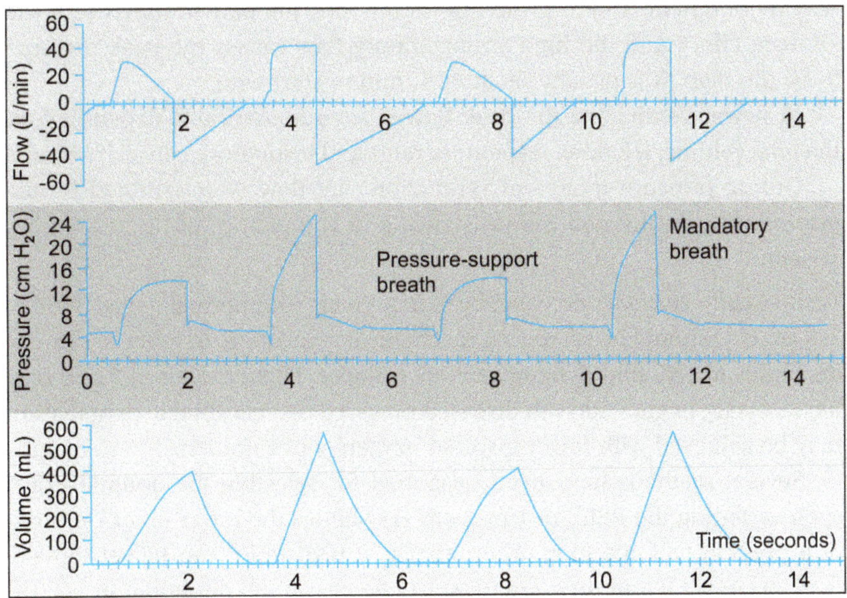

Fig. 6: Airway pressure, flow, and volume waveforms during synchronized intermittent mandatory ventilation with pressure support applied to the nonmandatory breaths.

Mode of ventilation: Depends on whether the patient is conscious, sedated or has received neuromuscular blockers. SIMV or CMV (+/- assist) modes are appropriate for initial settings. Patients with a good respiratory drive can be placed on PSV mode.

Tidal volume: Currently, lower tidal volumes are recommended than in the past, and 5-8 mL/kg of ideal body weight should be set, adjusting the value so that Pplat is less than 35 cm H_2O.

Respiratory rate: This should be set at 8–10 bpm, unless hyperventilation is required for intracranial pathology or metabolic acidosis. Higher rates may result in air trapping and intrinsic PEEP.

Inspired oxygen level: Though an initial FiO_2 of 1 is usually recommended, it is advisable to reduce the FiO_2 as rapidly as possible, aiming for an oxygen saturation >90% and PaO_2 >60 mm Hg.

Inspiration/expiration ratio: Normally the I/E ratio is set at 1:2. Expiratory time may be increased if airway obstruction is present so as to avoid air trapping and auto-PEEP. Inspiratory time may need to be prolonged in the setting of severe ARDS so as to equal or even exceed expiratory time (inverse ratio ventilation).

Inspiratory flow rate: Inspiratory peak flow rate may need to be set in some ventilators when volume control ventilation (VCV) is being used. It should be set at 4 times the desired minute volume so that the patient's inspiratory flow requirement is met. If the flow is too low, the patient needs to make an extra effort, and too high an inspiratory flow causes the peak pressure to be too high. It is usually set at 60 L/min to start with.

In newer ventilators, the peak flow is set automatically, depending on the tidal volume, I/E ratio, respiratory rates and inspiratory pause, if present.

During pressure modes of ventilation, the flow is determined by the inspiratory pressure and the resistance and compliance of the respiratory system.

Positive end-expiratory pressure: Even in patients with normal lungs, PEEP of 3-5 cm H_2O should be set during mechanical ventilation, in order to prevent decreases in FRC and dynamic airway collapse. Higher levels of PEEP may be necessary in patients with diseased lungs, so that acceptable oxygenation may be achieved with lower inspired oxygen concentrations.

Several methods have been described for selecting the optimal PEEP, such as setting the PEEP at 1 or 2 cm H_2O above the lower inflexion point of a pressure/volume loop. Alternatively, a high PEEP can be set initially (e.g. 20 cm H_2O) and then progressively decreased till desaturation occurs. At this point, a recruitment maneuver is done and the PEEP is set about 2 cm H_2O higher.

Sensitivity: If pressure triggering is used, the trigger sensitivity is set at -2 cm H_2O initially, keeping in mind that the presence of intrinsic PEEP increases the effort required by the patient if an adequate level of extrinsic PEEP is not set. Modern ventilators provide the option of flow-triggering which needs less effort from the patient.

Newer Modes of Ventilation

Pressure-regulated Volume Control

The PRVC and VS are true dual modes of ventilatory support. Each targets both a maximum pressure and VT and each readjusts gas delivery on the basis of the previously delivered breath.

The PRVC is essentially PA/C with a volume target. Here, the clinician sets a maximum peak pressure, the targeted VT, inspiratory time, sensitivity, FiO_2, PEEP, and rise time. VS is essentially pressure support where the clinician sets a maximum peak pressure, the targeted VT, sensitivity, FiO_2, PEEP, rise time (and in some ventilators inspiratory termination criteria). In both of these modes, the ventilator initially provides a test breath at a low pressure, then calculates the peak pressure necessary to deliver the tidal volume. Subsequently, the necessary pressure level is delivered either in a single jump to the calculated pressure or by a second test breath and then a jump to the calculated pressure.

A specialty of these modes is that if the targeted VT is not provided on a given breath, the peak pressure is adjusted on the next breath from 1 to 3 cm H_2O to achieve the targeted VT. Theoretically, the peak pressure could be adjusted every breath if the VT is not on target. Airway pressure can increase to the maximum level set or can decrease to baseline (PEEP/CPAP). That is, positive pressure could be eliminated if the patient were capable of inspiring spontaneously the delivered VT without ventilatory support.

There are limited data indicating the effectiveness of PRVC and VS.

The PRVC can be applied without concern in patients not triggering the ventilator. With this controlled setting, PRVC very adequately adjusts gas delivery to maintain both targeted volume and pressure. Of potential concern with both PRVC and VS is the patient with a strong ventilatory demand. If a patient's ventilatory demand is increased by fever, hypoxemia, or anxiety and the patient can exceed the targeted VT, the ventilating pressure may be reduced inappropriately to zero. In this setting, both modes should be cautiously applied.

Airway Pressure Release Ventilation (APRV)

The APRV and bilevel ventilation are modes of ventilation that are a unique mix of SIMV and inverse ratio pressure control ventilation. APRV was first

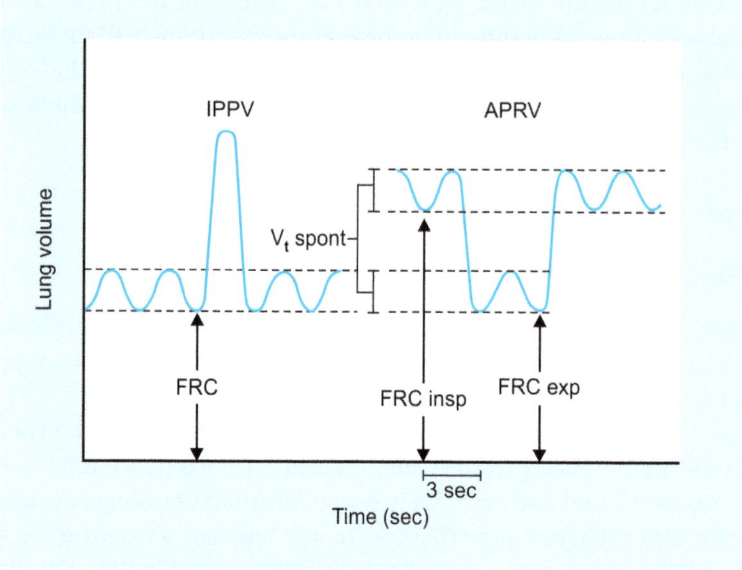

Fig. 7: Theoretical spirometric tracing depicting change in lung volume that would occur in a patient with a mechanical IPPV breath compared with the change that would occur with an APRV breath. IPPV—intermittent positive pressure ventilation; APRV—airway pressure release ventilation. Inspiratory lung volume is the lung volume during spontaneous inspiration with continuous positive airway pressure during APRV—Expiratory lung volume is the lung volume during release of Paw during APRV, that is, lung volume after mechanical expiration. Expiratory lung volume is similar to functional residual capacity (FRC) during IPPV. FRC is the passive expiratory lung volume during APRV and is greater than FRC during IPPV. *(From Stock MC, Downs JB, Frolicher DA: Airway pressure release ventilation. Crit Care Med)*

described by Stock and coauthors as the application of two levels of CPAP. At both levels the patient is allowed to breath spontaneously. Some authors recommend limiting the time at the low CPAP level to avoid complete exhalation by the patient causing air trapping and auto-PEEP as well as avoidance of spontaneous breathing at this level. Others allow complete exhalation with the lower CPAP level set as one would set PEEP. Essentially, the low CPAP level is set to treat hypoxemia and the higher CPAP level to assist the patient's spontaneous breathing in CO_2 elimination. As with other modes, the VT created by movement from a high to low CPAP level should be limited (Fig. 7).

The advantages of APRV are better distribution of ventilation and improved cardiac output because the patient is spontaneously breathing and creating a large decrease in intrathoracic pressure with each breath.

The disadvantages are patient-ventilator dyssynchrony and increased work of breathing. Dyssynchrony is observed primarily when the patient is trying to exhale and the ventilator moves from the lower to the higher CPAP level or when the patient is inhaling and the ventilator goes from the high to the low CPAP level. Spontaneous breathing during APRV can result in markedly high pleural pressure changes with each breath, exceeding 10 cm H_2O. This indicates high effort and work by the patient. This increased work is in part responsible for the increase in cardiac output observed with APRV.

Automatic Tube Compensation

This mode of ventilation has been referred to as electronic extubation. Essentially, the ventilator determines the amount of pressure needed to overcome the resistance to gas flow through the endotracheal tube. In order to do this, resistive features of various types and sizes of artificial airways are programmed into the ventilator. The clinician must indicate the airway type and size. During inspiration, the ventilator can instantaneously monitor the flow demand of the patient. Knowing these two factors, the ventilator can calculate the amount of pressure (pressure = resistance × flow) needed to overcome the resistance of the artificial airway at any flow rate.

With this mode, pressure is applied only when inspiratory flow is generated, that is, high flow, high pressure and low flow, low pressure. At the end of the breath the pressure decreases if the patient's inspiratory flow demand decreases. As a result, automatic tube compensation (ATC) is less likely to cause overdistention than pressure support because it does not force a ventilatory pattern. ATC gives control of ventilatory support to the patient. If the patient's ventilatory demand decreases, the applied pressure decreases. There is no set variable except the percentage of ATC. That is, the clinician sets the percentage of the resistance that is to be overcome during inspiration, 100% or a lower level. Thus, the patient may choose a ventilatory pattern with 200 mL VT and a rate of 40/min or 600 mL VT and a rate of 15/min.

WEANING MECHANICAL VENTILATION

Geetanjali S Verma

PREREQUISITES

- Reversal of primary problem causing need for ventilation
- Patient awake and responsive
- Good analgesia, ability to cough
- Reducing or minimal doses of inotropic support
- Ideally—functioning bowels, absence of abdominal distension
- Normalizing metabolic status
- Adequate hemoglobin concentration.

Ventilatory Indices for Successful Weaning

Minute ventilation	<10 liter min–1
Vital capacity/weight	>10 mL kg–1
Respiratory frequency	<35 bpm
Tidal volume/weight	>5 mL kg–1
Maximum inspiratory pressure	<–25 cm H_2O
Respiratory rate/tidal volume	<100 liter–1
PaO_2/FiO_2	>200 mm Hg (26.3 kPa)

Terminate spontaneous breathing trial if:

Respiratory rate	>35 bpm
SpO_2	<90%
Heart rate	>140 beats min–1 or change by >20%
Systolic blood pressure	>180 or <90 mm Hg
Agitation	
Sweating	

Anxiety or signs of increased work of breathing (paradoxical breathing, intercostal retraction, nasal flaring).

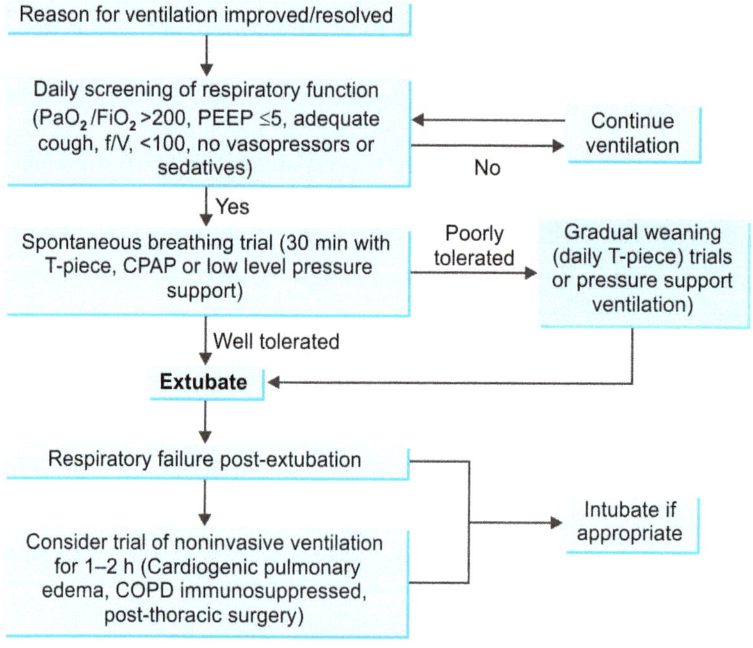

COMPLICATIONS

Mechanical

a. *Trauma/injuries*: Lips, tongue, teeth, oropharynx, larynx
b. Endobronchial intubation
c. Esophageal intubation
d. Severe hypoxia
e. Severe hypotension.

CVS

a. Decreased CO due to PPV
b. Hypotension.

Respiratory

a. *Barotrauma*: Lung injury associated with high alveolar pressures (>35–40 cm H_2O), presentation ranges from asymptomatic pulmonary interstitial emphysema (PIE), through subcutaneous emphysema, pneumomediastinum; to tension pneumothorax.
b. *Volutrauma*: Refers to lung injury due to overstretching of alveoli because of excessive tidal volumes, which leads to release of inflammatory mediators that have both pulmonary and systemic effects, increasing morbidity and mortality. When nonhomogeneous pulmonary pathology is present, tidal volume delivered by the ventilator is preferentially delivered to the more compliant, relatively normal areas of the lung. Thus normal alveoli are overstretched, and the remaining normal lung is damaged, further increasing lung injury and damage. Repeated closing and reopening of alveoli (recruitment and collapse) is another factor which causes damage due to shear stress and loss of surfactant. The release of inflammatory mediators can cause damage to remote organs such as the liver and kidney.

   Barotrauma is due to high alveolar pressures while volutrauma is related to high transalveolar pressure gradient.
c. Tracheal stenosis.
d. *Auto PEEP*: This is the positive pressure which develops in the alveoli at the end of expiration due to incomplete emptying of alveoli, either due to airway obstruction due to secretions, bronchospasm or airway closure; or else if expiratory time is too short. This cannot be detected at the ventilator end of the tube but causes increased work of breathing and progressive over-distension of the lungs, if not corrected.
e. Laryngeal edema.

Inflammatory Cytokines

Increased IL 4, TNF a (increased catecholamine release/decreased CO).

Oxygen Toxicity

High inspired oxygen concentrations ($FiO_2 > 0.5$) cause cellular damage due to free radical formation. In addition, high FiO_2s are also associated with absorption atelectasis. Hence, it is important to set the lowest FiO_2 possible, aiming for SaO_2 >90%.

a. Tracheobronchitis
b. Absorptive atelectasis
c. Hypercarbia
d. Diffuse alveolar damage.

GI

a. Aspiration
b. Erosive esophagitis
c. UGI bleed
d. Decreased motility of stomach and small intestine
e. Reduced portal venous blood flow
f. Abdominal distension.

Renal

In response to decreased CO.

Neuro

a. PEEP reduces CPP.

Others

a. VAP.

Ventilator Associated Pneumonia (VAP):

Early-onset pneumonia (VAP ≤ 5 days) commonly results from aspiration of endogenous community-acquired pathogens such as Enterobacteriaceae, *Staphylococcus aureus*, *Streptococcus pneumoniae*, *Haemophilus influenzae* and *Candida sp.* with endotracheal intubation and impaired consciousness being the associated main risk factors.

Late-onset pneumonia (VAP ≥ 5 days) is followed by aspiration of oropharyngeal or gastric secretions containing potentially drug-resistant nosocomial pathogens, e.g. nonfermenters (*Pseudomonas* spp. and *Acinetobacter* spp.)

Contd...

Contd...

The diagnostic criteria of a radiographic infiltrate and at least one clinical feature (fever, leukocytosis, or purulent tracheal secretions) have high sensitivity but low specificity (especially for VAP).

The clinical pulmonary infection score (CPIS) scoring system grades the severity of pneumonia and this includes six features. Each of these six features scores on a scale from 0 to 2, as follows:

Temperature (Celsius):	>36.5 and <38.4 = 0 >38.5 and <38.9 = 1 >39.0 or <36.5 = 2 •
White blood cell count:	>4,000 and <11,000 = 0 <4,000 or >11,000 = 1 <4,000 or >11,000 and band forms >50% = 2•
Tracheal secretions:	None or scant = 0 Nonpurulent = 1 Purulent = 2 •
PaO_2/FiO_2:	0 = >240 or acute respiratory distress syndrome (ARDS) 2 = ≤ 240 and no ARDS
Chest radiograph:	No infiltrate – 0 Diffuse (or patchy) infiltrate = 1 Localized infiltrate = 2 •
Pathogenic bacteria cultured from tracheal aspirate:	Rare or light quantity or no growth = 1 Moderate or heavy quantity (with same growth on Gram stain) = 1

CPIS score serves as tool to limit antibiotic abuse. VAP is less severe if CPIS score is less than or equal to 6 and prolonged course of antibiotics is unnecessary.

Components of VAP bundle:

a. 30–45% head elevation
b. Chlorhexidine mouth care
c. Selective gut decontamination
d. Stress ulcer prophylaxis
e. Daily wake tests/sedation vacation
f. Use of subglottic secretion drainage (SSD) endotracheal tube
g. Closed suction systems (CSS)
h. Heat and moisture exchangers (HMEs)
i. Early weaning
j. Hand washing.

Empirical therapy is broadened to include

(i) Either an antipseudomonal cephalosporin (cefepime or ceftazidime), an antipseudomonal carbapenem (imipenem or meropenem), or a β-lactam/β-lactamase inhibitor (piperacillin-tazobactam) plus
(ii) An antipseudomonal fluoroquinolone (ciprofloxacin or levofloxacin) or an aminoglycoside (amikacin, gentamicin, or tobramycin) plus linezolid or vancomycin.

13 Airway Management in Airway Surgeries and Airway Fires

Geetanjali S Verma

AIRWAY MANAGEMENT

Aims of Anesthetic Technique Used

1. Simple to use
2. Provide complete control of airway with no risk of aspiration
3. *Control ventilation*: Adequate oxygenation and CO_2 removal
4. Smooth induction and maintenance of anesthesia
5. Clear and motionless surgical field
6. No time restrictions for surgeon to be imposed
7. Devoid of risk of airway fire and hemodynamic instability
8. *Safe emergence*: No laryngospasm, bucking or coughing
9. Pain-free, comfortable, alert patient at emergence.

Two Types of Airway Control

	Closed system	*Open system*
Technique	Cuffed endotracheal tube used with protection of lower airway	No cuffed endotracheal tube used; spontaneous ventilation or jet ventilation or insufflation techniques +/- muscle paralysis
Advantages	• Routinely used by anesthetists • Good control of airway • Controlled ventilation • Minimal pollution by volatile agents	• Laser safety • Complete laryngeal visualization: better for surgeons • Reduced risk of trauma imposed by use of endotracheal tubes

CLOSED SYSTEM

Laser Tubes

- Used especially for laser surgeries.
- Most commonly used: all metal Norton tube (no cuff).

- Three types of tapes may be used to prevent risk of airway fires:
  a. Aluminum foil with adhesive backing
  b. Copper foil with adhesive backing
  c. Plastic tape thinly coated with metal on one side and adhesive on the other (never use lead foils!)

When using tubes for laser surgeries, keep the following in mind:
- Keep inspired oxygen concentrations at the minimal level required to maintain adequate saturations.
- Air preferred to N_2O use.

Microlaryngoscopy Tubes

- These have small internal (4–5 mm) and external diameters and have long length.
- High volume, low pressure cuffs.
- Not suitable for laser surgeries.

OPEN SYSTEM

Spontaneous Ventilation and Insufflation Techniques

Useful in removal of foreign bodies, evaluation of airway dynamics and removal of uncompromised glottic and supraglottic lesions.

The patient is induced with Sevoflurane and 100% oxygen and maintained with oxygen and inhalational agents or Propofol infusion. Oxygen administration may be done by a small catheter introduced into nasopharynx and placed above the laryngeal opening or a cut tracheal tube placed from nasopharynx till beyond the soft palate or through a nasopharyngeal airway or through the side arm of laryngoscope/bronchoscope.

Depth of anesthesia may be assessed by rate and depth of respiration, pupil size, eye reflexes and vital signs.

Limitations with this technique include: lack of airway control, soiling of airway and pollution of operating room with volatile agents use.

Jet Ventilation

a. *Supraglottic jet ventilation*

   Gas emerges in the supraglottis by attachment of a jetting needle to the rigid suspension laryngoscope.

   Limitations of this technique include:
   - Misalignment of suspension laryngoscope to the glottic inlet, leading to poor ventilation and gastric distension
   - Blood, smoke, debris blown into distal trachea

- Movement and vibration of vocal cords interfering with operating field
- $ETCO_2$ cannot be measured
- Barotrauma, pneumomediastinum, pneumothorax and subcutaneous emphysema.

b. *Subglottic jet ventilation*

It involves the placement of a small (2–3 mm diameter) catheter or tube through the glottis into the trachea.

Reduced driving pressures required, minimal cord movements and good surgical view.

More risk of barotrauma than in supraglottic ventilation and risk of airway fire.

c. *Transtracheal jet techniques*

It involves the placement of a specifically designed percutaneous transtracheal catheter through the cricothyroid membrane or trachea.

It may be placed under local or general anesthesia.

The risks of barotrauma, blockage, kinking, infection and failure to site the catheter exist.

AIRWAY FIRE

It is a feared complication of laser use during airway surgeries. Incidence is noted to be 0.5–1.5%.

All of the elements to support a fire are found in the setting of laser surgery for airway: (Fig. 1) oxygen (supports combustion, along with N_2O), combustible material (endotracheal tube), and an ignition source (laser).

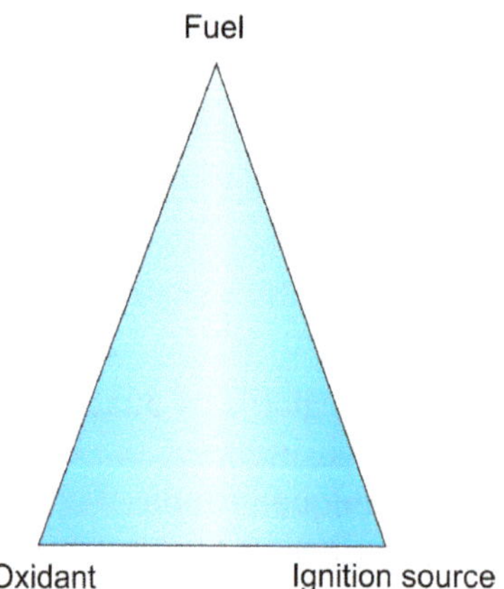

Fig. 1: Elements of fire.

Precautions to be taken:

1. Consider a tubeless technique using spontaneous ventilation, apneic techniques, or jet ventilation.
2. Use an appropriate laser endotracheal tube, such as metal, Mallinckrodt®, Xomed®, Sheridan®, or Red Rusch®.
3. Reduce inspired oxygen as tolerated by the patient to <30%, ideally 21%.
4. Use either air or helium to dilute the oxygen; N_2O supports combustion.
5. Fill the endotracheal tube cuff with a saline–dye mixture or lidocaine jelly.
6. Completely soaked gauze should be placed within and around the airway to reduce ignition risk.
7. Use H_2O-based ointments; petroleum-based ointments are flammable.
8. Limit the duration and intensity of laser exposure; continuous mode allows heat buildup.
9. Maintain a ready source of water in case of fire (multiple 60-mL filled syringes).

Strategies to reduce the incidence of fire:

a. Reduction of flammability of endotracheal tube (Oxidant)
   i. By taping with aluminium or copper foils or use of metal tubes.
   ii. The cuffs may be inflated with colored saline or lignocaine jelly to detect cuff leakage/rupture.
b. Removal of flammable materials (Oxidant) from airway by using a metallic venturi jet ventilation cannula or intermittent extubation with or without apnea
c. Reduction of available oxygen (Fuel) content to the minimum required for adequate oxygen saturation.

MANAGEMENT OF AIRWAY FIRE

1. Stop ventilation. Inform surgeon.
2. Disconnect the oxygen source and flood the airway with water.
3. Remove the burned endotracheal tube and examine the airway.
4. Mask ventilate the patient and reintubate.
5. Survey the extent of injury using a flexible bronchoscope.
   If the fire was of interior blowtorch type, gentle bronchial lavage may be indicated, followed by fiberoptic assessment of more distal airways. Patient's face and oropharynx must be assessed and chest X-ray must be obtained.
6. Monitor the patient for 24 hours in high dependency unit (HDU).
7. Administer steroids to reduce inflammation and edema.
8. Provide antibiotics and ventilatory support if indicated.
   Pulmonary damage due to heat or smoke inhalation may necessitate intubation and prolonged mechanical ventilation.

14 Advances in Airway Management

Geetanjali S Verma

WHAT IS NEW IN ASA GUIDELINES FOR DIFFICULT AIRWAY

1993 (original)	*2013 changes*	*Recent (2015)*
Recommendations: 1. Perform airway history and assessment 2. A portable cart with airway equipment should be "readily available" 3. Create a strategy for airway management 4. Create a strategy for extubation of a difficult airway Also included: 1. Difficult airway definitions in appendix 2. Recommended equipment for a specialized cart 3. Recommended techniques for difficult mask ventilation and intubation	1. Addition of LMA as rescue ventilation device or intubating conduit 2. Rigid bronchoscopy added as an emergency non-invasive option 3. Assessment for difficult tracheostomy added	1. LMA changed to SGA 2. Assessment of difficult SGA placement added to step #1 3. Video-assisted laryngoscopy as an initial approach to intubation was added to step #3 4. Expanded difficult airway definition: Definition includes: • Difficult face mask or SGA ventilation • Difficult SGA placement • Difficult laryngoscopy • Difficult tracheal intubation • Failed intubation

Role of Videolaryngoscopy

- As an initial approach to intubation
- As an alternate approach after failed direct laryngoscopy
- Also added to list of suggested items to be included on a difficult airway cart
- Provides an indirect view of larynx

- Evidence of higher success rates, improved laryngeal view in the difficult airway
- Less neck movement compared to direct laryngoscopy.

Standardization of Airway Equipment

- *ASA difficult airway guidelines 2013*: Recommend "at least one portable storage unit that contains specialized equipment for difficult airway management should be readily available."
- *NAP4 report*: "The contents of difficult airway trolleys should be the same throughout the hospital including those used in the ICU and ED.

Recommended Extubation Strategies

- Create a preformulated strategy
- Consider merits of awake versus deep extubation
- Consider factors that may affect ventilation postextubation
- Consider use of a device as a bridge to extubation.

Options for Bridging Extubation

- *Supraglottic airway devices*: Placed before or after removal of endotracheal tube.
- *Airway exchange catheters*: Placed through *in situ* endotracheal tube - Left in place after extubation in a monitored setting until airway no longer at risk.

Airway Exchange Catheters for Extubation

- Placed prior to extubation through tube
- Allows ventilation and oxygenation via catheter
- Can be used as a guide for reintubation
- Left in place postoperatively in a monitored setting until airway no longer at risk
- Well-tolerated, patients able to phonate and cough.

What are Your Airway Resources?

- Do you have an airway cart?
- If you need a surgical airway, who do you call?
- How long will it take for additional resources to arrive?
- Do you have resources to manage an intubated patient in the PACU?

Airway Considerations in the Ambulatory Setting

- What type of center do you work in?
  - Are alternate airway devices immediately available?
  - Is additional back-up, including personnel to perform a surgical airway, immediately available?
  - Are there resources to manage failed extubation of the difficult airway patient?

If the answer to any of the previous questions is NO...

- Consider if known or suspected difficult airway patients should be moved to another setting
- Prescreening of patients may help identify patients not appropriate for your center.

Role of Simulation

1. Simulation of rare events has been proven to be useful
2. Clarifies provider roles in an emergency
3. Can identify resource needs and limitations: Time needed to obtain additional personnel and equipment—Is needed equipment immediately available?
4. Allows for immediate debriefing
5. Opportunity to learn and practice airway devices on mannequin models
6. Can be used for team training and communication skills
7. Providers learn from experience.

OTHER INSTRUMENTATIONS

Indirect Rigid Fiberoptic Bronchoscopes

Bullard Laryngoscope

- Rigid metal blade of shape to follow contour of oropharynx
- Fiberoptic bundles placed in a sheath posteriorly on the blade
- A viewing arm with eyepiece present which extends 45° from the handle
- Snap on diopter also available (uncorrected vision users)
- Video camera may also be attached for viewing
- *Power*: Battery
- Bulb: Halogen - in handle or adaptor
- *Working channel*: Extends from scope body to tip—suction, oxygen insufflation, LA administration, jet ventilation may be done
- *Sizes*: Pediatric (infants), pediatric long (8–10-year-old), adult (>10-year-old)

- Extensor (plastic) available for tall patients
- *Stylet*: Intubating (curved at 20° to left near tip, attached near base of viewing arm), multifunctional (long, hollow tube curved at tip, attaches to viewing arm with screw clamp; can be used for guiding flexible fiberscope, tracheal tube exchanger or small catheter).

WU Scope

- Rigid tubular blade and flexible fiberscope
- *Flexible fiberscope*: It has short light and image transmitting fiberoptic bundles and tip deflection control
- *Blade*: 3 parts—handle, main blade, bivalve element
  Handle: Cone-shaped, receives fiberscope at the top, connects main blade at base. Handle to blade angle is 110°
  Main blade and bivalve element: When positioned together, form a passageway for suction catheter/tracheal tube and fiberscope separately. Oxygen channel is present alongside slot for fiberscope.
  Adult blade accommodates tracheal tube up to 8.5 mm.
  Large adult blade can accommodate up to 9 mm.

Upsher Scope

- C-shaped metal blade, ends 1 inch from end of blade
- Distal part of blade has upward curve
- Two tubes carry fiberoptic bundles to the left, end in semicircular channels
- *Eyepiece*: It has focusing ring
- Upsher handle to be used with it
- Camera may be attached to it.

Video Laryngoscopes

Glidescope

- Available in pediatric and adult sizes
- Made of palstic
- Has a miniature digital camera under the blade
- Blade is 60° bent at midpoint (specialty: as antifogging system)
- LED mounted besides the camera provides illumination.

Video Macintosh Intubation Laryngoscope

- Macintosh blade attached to handle
- Image light bundle threaded through a metal guide in the blade; advanced 2/3rd of length of blade

- Also available with angulated blade—tip angulated at 25° and vertical flange flattened (especially useful in children requiring manual in line neck stabilization).

Optical Intubating Stylets

Shikani Optical Stylet

- Made of stainless steel
- Malleable
- Has a preformed J shape but a bendable tip
- *Parts*: Handle, eyepiece, adjustable tube stop, port for insufflating oxygen
- *Sizes*: Adult (fits tracheal tube of 5.5 mm), pediatric (fits tube of 3–5 mm).

Bonfils Retromolar Intubation Fiberscope

- Nonmalleable
- Distal curve 40°
- Length 40 cm, OD 5 mm (accommodates 6–7 mm ETT)
- Adapter has a connector for oxygen administration during intubation.

Lighted Intubation Stylets

- Uses transillumination of soft tissues in anterior neck to guide and determine position of the tip of ETT
- *Handle*: Reusable, with power source
- Malleable wand with light at end (detachable)
- Available in adult and pediatric sizes (accommodates up to 2.5 mm smallest ETT).

Introduction of Newer Supraglottic Devices

- Intubating LMA
- C - TRACH
- I-Gel
- SLIPA.

(discussed in airway equipments).

AIRWAY ULTRASONOGRAPHY (US)

Advantages of US: Safe, quick, repeatable, portable, widely available and gives real-time dynamic images relevant for several aspects of management of the airway.

- US must be used dynamically for maximum benefit in airway management and in direct conjunction with the airway management: immediately before, during and after, airway interventions.

Limitations

US may be limited due to a variety of factors such as patient habitus (i.e. bariatric patients).

Therefore in some cases, it still may be necessary to supplement ultrasonography with other imaging modalities.

Structures that can be seen with US:

Mouth
Tongue
Oropharynx
Hypopharynx
Hyoid bone
Epiglottis
Larynx
Vocal cords
Cricothyroid membrane
Cricoid cartilage
Trachea
Esophagus
Stomach
Lungs
Pleurae

Clinical applications of airway ultrasonography	*Comment*
Prediction of difficult airway management	Only shown to be useful in smaller series in obese patients
Diagnosing pathology that can affect airway management	E.g. tumors in the neck, tongue, vallecula, pharynx or larynx or a Zenker diverticulum that can represent an increased risk of aspiration
Identification of the cricothyroid membrane	To be performed before managing a difficult airway, in case that identification by palpation is not possible. Allows preparation for emergency cricothyroidotomy, oxygen insufflation, and distribution of local anesthetics or retrograde intubation
Measuring gastric content prior to airway management	Best performed in the right lateral decubitus position
Airway-related nerve blocks	
Prediction of the appropriate diameter of endotracheal, endobronchial, or tracheostomy tubes	

Contd...

Contd...

Differentiating between tracheal and esophageal intubation	Detects esophageal intubation before ventilation is initiated and works when there is no circulation (e.g., cardiac arrest), as opposed to CO_2-detection
Differentiating between tracheal and endobronchial intubation	Useful in noisy environments where a stethoscope is useless
Confirmation of gastric tube placement	
Diagnosis of pneumothorax	The fastest way to rule out a suspicion of intraoperative pneumothorax
Differentiating between different causes of dyspnea/hypoxia and pulmonary edema	Diagnosing pulmonary edema and other types of lung and pleura pathology
Prediction of successful weaning from ventilator treatment	Obtained by measuring whether the respiratory forces of the patients, and/or the width of the airway, are large enough to allow extubation of the trachea
Localization of trachea and tracheal ring interspaces for tracheostomy and percutaneous dilatational tracheostomy	

AIRWAY ULTRASOUND VIEWS

(Discussed in Figs. 1 to 8)

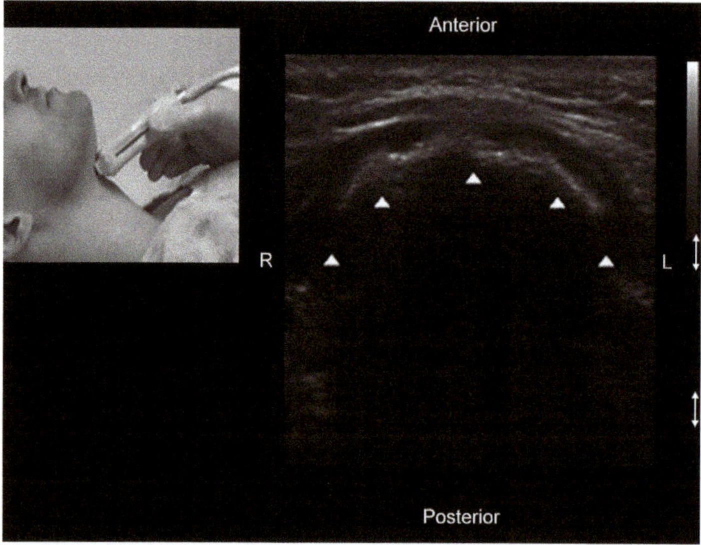

Fig. 1: Sonogram of the hyoid bone on a midline transverse view using a linear transducer. The hyoid bone is shown as an inverted U hyperechoic curvilinear line (arrowheads) with posterior acoustic shadowing. The inset shows the transducer position on the skin.

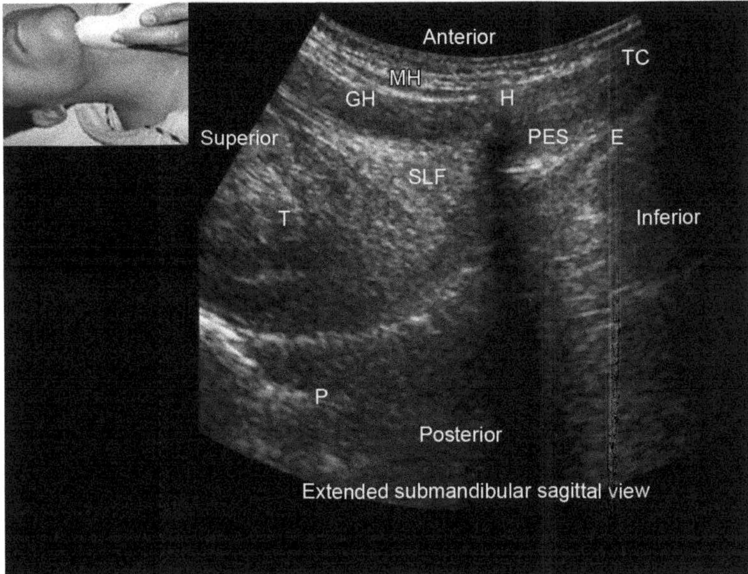

Fig. 2: Extended submandibular sagittal view using a curved transducer.
(T: Tongue; H: Hyoid bone; E: Epiglottis; GH: Geniohyoid; MH: Mylohyoid; PES: Pre-epiglottic space; P: Palate; TC: Thyroid cartilage).

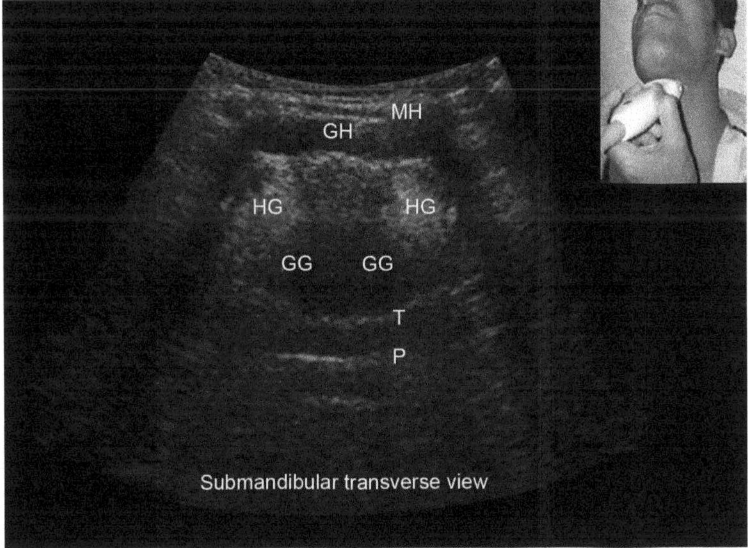

Fig. 3: Transverse views at the submandibular position.
(GG: Genioglossus; GH: Geniohyoid; MH: Mylohyoid; HG: Hyoglossus; T: Tongue; P: Palate).

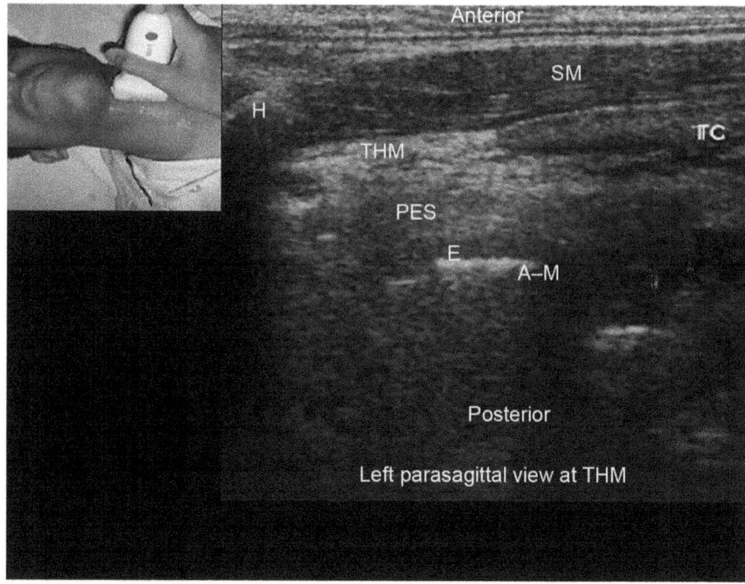

Fig. 4: Left parasagittal view at thyrohyoid membrane (THM).
(H: Hyoid bone; SM: Strap muscles; THM: Thyrohyoid membrane; TC: Thyroid cartilage; PES: Pre-epiglottic space; E: Epiglottis; A-M: Air mucosal interface).

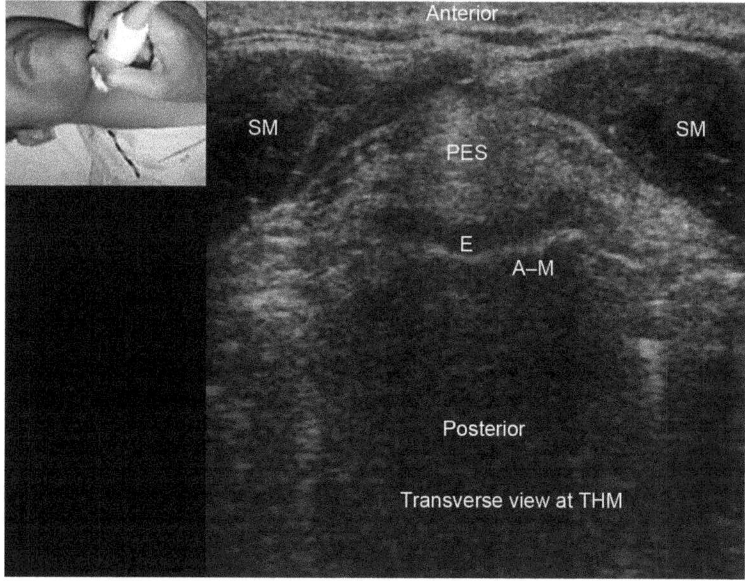

Fig. 5: Transverse view at thyrohyoid membrane (THM).
(E: Epiglottis; A-M: Air-mucosal interface; PES: Pre-epiglottic space; SM: Strap muscles).

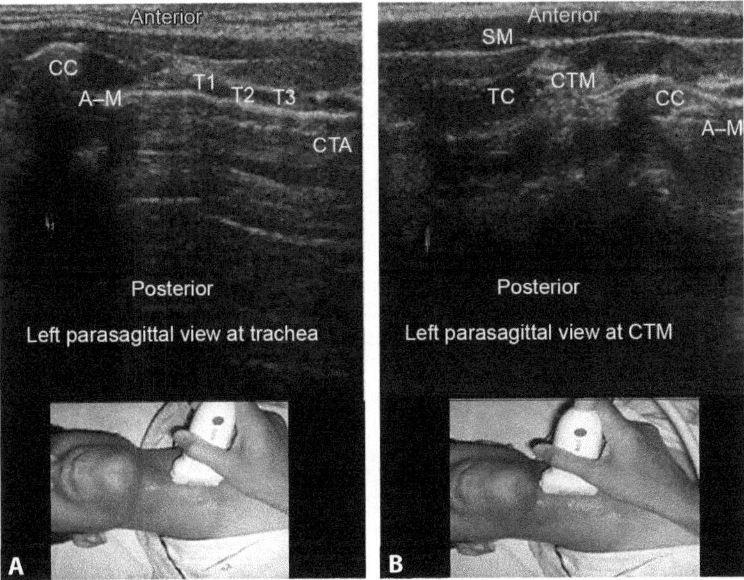

Figs. 6A and B: (A) Left parasagittal view at trachea; (B) Left parasagittal view at cricothyroid membrane.
(CC: Cricoid cartilage; T1-T3: Tracheal cartilages; A-M: Air-mucosal interface; CTA: Comet tail artefact).

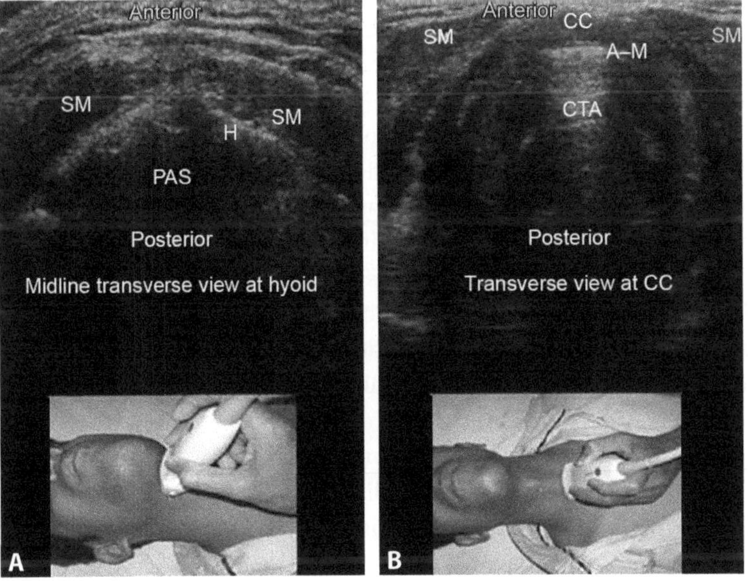

Figs. 7A and B: Transverse view at hyoid and cricoid cartilage.
(SM: Strap muscles; H: Hyoid; CC: Cricoid cartilage; A-M: Air mucosal interface; CTA: Comet tail artefact).

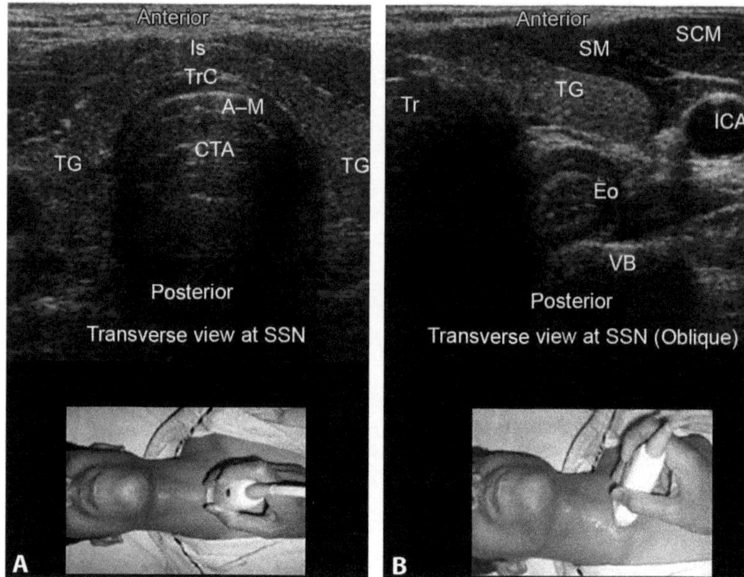

Figs. 8A and B: (A) Transverse and (B) Oblique transverse view at the level of the suprasternal notch (SSN) showing trachea, thyroid gland, and esophagus.
(TG: Thyroid gland; Tr: Trachea; TrC: Tracheal cartilage; A-M: Air-mucosal interface; CTA: Comet tail artefact; ICA: Internal carotid artery; Eo: Esophagus; SCM: Sternocleidomastoid muscle; SM: Strap muscle; VB: Vertebral body).

Real-time visualization of the endotracheal tube insertion, looking for lung-sliding and diaphragmatic movement bilaterally can help confirm the endotracheal intubation. Esophageal intubation can be reliably detected as a bright hyperechoic curved line on one side of and deeper to trachea.

Similarly, endobronchial intubation can be diagnosed by unilateral pleural and diaphragmatic movement. Filling the ETT cuff with fluid can help in locating its position. In children, during real-time visualization of ETT with US, widening of vocal cords is seen as the ETT crosses them.

US can also be used to confirm correct laryngeal mask airway (LMA) placement and rule out causes of inadequate ventilation. LMA cuff (inflated with fluid) should be visualized equally on both sides of larynx for proper seal. Grading of LMA placement thus obtained using US is more convenient as compared to fiberoptic examination with good correlation of the results.

Postextubation stridor can be reliably predicted in intubated patients by measuring the width of air column after deflating the ETT cuff. An air column width of less than 4.5 ± 0.8 mm was found to be associated with stridor.

Also, US can be used in diagnosis of various conditions that can have implication for airway management, e.g. vocal cord malfunction, swallowing abnormalities, sialolithiasis, supraglottic hemangiomas, respiratory papillomatosis, laryngeal stenosis, Zenker's diverticulum, maxillary sinusitis, etc.

LUNG ULTRASONOGRAPHY (LUS)

Pneumothorax

Suggestive findings: The visceral and parietal pleura will not be in contact with each other, and lung sliding will be absent. The absence of lung sliding is not pathognomonic of a pneumothorax as lung sliding can also be absent when pleural adhesions, lung bullae, apnea, or inadvertent intubation of the opposite mainstem bronchus.

Diagnostic findings: When patients are in the supine position, any air in the pleural cavity will tend rise to just below the anterior surface of the chest. Depending on the size of the pneumothorax, there might be no air between the two pleural blades more laterally or posteriorly; and in these areas, lung sliding will be present. The boundary between an area where the pleura blades are in contact and an area with air in between the blades will move in conjunction with the patients breathing. With LUS, the change from no-air to air between the pleural blades can be directly visualized. If the transducer is placed in such a transition zone during the patient's respiratory cycle, the US image will change from lung sliding to no lung sliding. The visualization of such a transition is known as "lung point"= confirmatory of pneumothorax.

Interstitial Syndrome (IS)

By systematically scanning two anterior, two lateral and three posterior zones, IS is defined by the presence of both of the following criteria:

1. A positive scanning zone, defined by the presence of three or more B-lines in a longitudinal plane between two ribs.
2. At least two zones have to be positive on each side when scanning the anterior and lateral zones.

Any findings on the posterior surface are not included in the definition of IS.

Cardiogenic IS

Typically, the location of the B-lines follows the effects of gravity and is therefore often more pronounced in the posterior and lateral scanning zones, rather than the anterior zones. The pleura line should appear normal and intact. B-lines are highly dynamic in cardiogenic pulmonary edema.

Due to its high sensitivity in detecting IS, the absence of IS on LUS can be used as a pivotal diagnostic tool in ruling out cardiogenic pulmonary edema.

Noncardiogenic IS

The pleural line may appear thickened and fragmented, some spared areas may be devoid of B-lines, and subpleural consolidations may be seen. In other cases of pulmonary edema from fluid overload and renal failure, the LUS findings will be similar to those of cardiogenic pulmonary edema. Hence, when IS is detected, supplementary focused echocardiography can be employed in order to establish whether the IS is of cardiogenic origin or not.

Focal B-lines

Occurrence of multiple, isolated, B-lines can both be a normal and pathological sign. Of patients with normal chest imaging, 21–28% have multiple B-lines in the lower lateral intercostal space. Focal areas with multiple B-lines can also be seen in any disease with localized increased density of the lung tissue, e.g. lower lobe pneumonia. If the density increases and

Common sonomorphological appearance of atelectasis and common causes for lung contusion.

Condition	*Echogenicity*	*Demarcation*	*Bronchograms*	*Miscellaneous*
Pneumonia	Hyperechoic	Diffuse		Air bronchograms present
Pulmonary embolism	Hypoechoic	Sharp	Absent	Triangular/rounded shape multiple lesions may be present Often minor pleural effusion present
Tumor	Hypoechoic	Diffuse/ sharp	Absent	Abnormal vessel supply may be present Visible growth into or destruction of organs and anatomical structures may be present
Lung contusion	Hyperechoic	Diffuse		Air bronchograms may be present

Contd...

Contd...

Condition	*Echogenicity*	*Demarcation*	*Bronchograms*	*Miscellaneous*
Compres-sion atelectasis	Hyperechoic	Sharp	Absent	Wedge shape Adjoining pleural effusion present "Jelly fish" sign Reventilation during inspiration may be present
Obstruction atelectasis	Hyperechoic	Diffuse	Fluid broncho-grams present	No or minimal pleural effusion present No reventilation during inspiration present

the lung tissue becomes filled with fluid, the pattern will change to that of lung consolidation. Other causes of focal B-lines are pneumonitis, atelectasis, pulmonary contusion, pulmonary embolism, pleural disease and malignancy.

Pulmonary Embolism

Confirmed pulmonary embolism: Two or more characteristic triangular or rounded pleura-based lesions.

Probable pulmonary embolism: One typical lesion with a corresponding low-grade pleural effusion.

Possible pulmonary embolism: Nonspecific subpleural lesions <5 mm in size or a single pleural effusion alone.

Algorithms

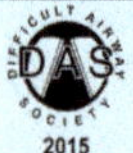

DAS Difficult Intubation Guidelines—Overview

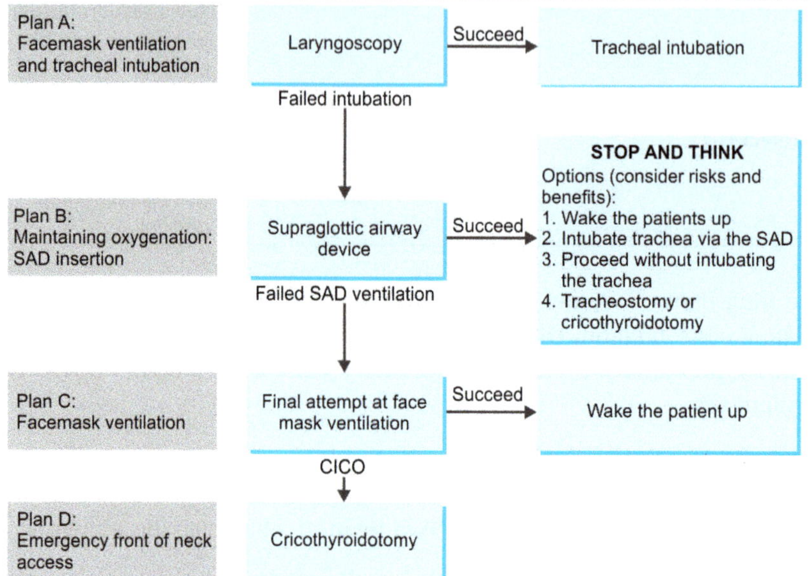

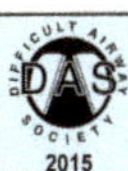

Management of Unanticipated Difficult Tracheal Intubation in Adults

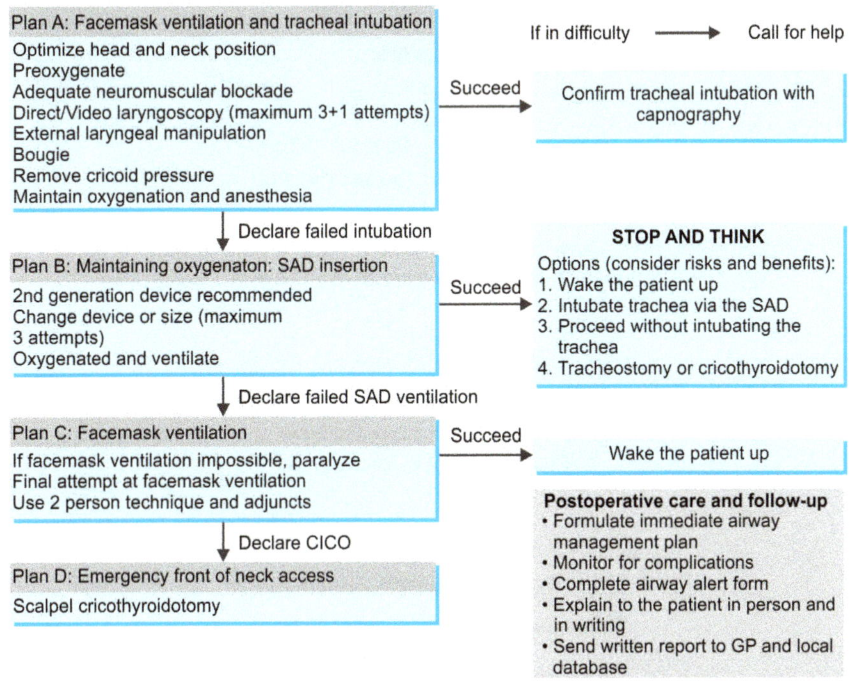

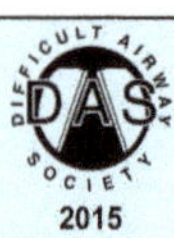

Failed intubation, Failed Oxygenation in the Paralyzed, Anesthetized Patient

Call for help

Continue 100% O_2

Declare CICO

Plan D: Emergency front of neck access

Continue to give oxygen via upper airway
Ensure neuromuscular blockade
Position patient to extend neck

Scalpel cricothyroidotomy

Equipment: 1. Scalpel (number 10 blade)
2. Bougie
3. Tube (cuffed 6.0 mm ID)

Laryngeal handshake to identify cricothyroid membrane

Palpable cricothyroid membrane

Transverse stab incision through cricothyroid membrane
Turn blade through 90° (sharp edge caudally)
Slide coude tip of bougie along blade into trachea
Railroad lubricated 6.0 mm cuffed tracheal tube into trachea
Ventilate, inflate cuff and confirm position with capnography
Secure tube

Impalpable cricothyroid membrane

Make an 8–10 cm vertical skin incision, caudad to cephalad
Use blunt dissection with fingers of both hands to separate tissues
Identify and stabilize the larynx
Proceed with technique for palpable cricothyroid membrane as above

Postoperative care and follow-up

- Postpone surgery unless immediately life threatening
- Urgent surgical review of cricothyroidotomy site
- Document and follow-up as in main flowchart

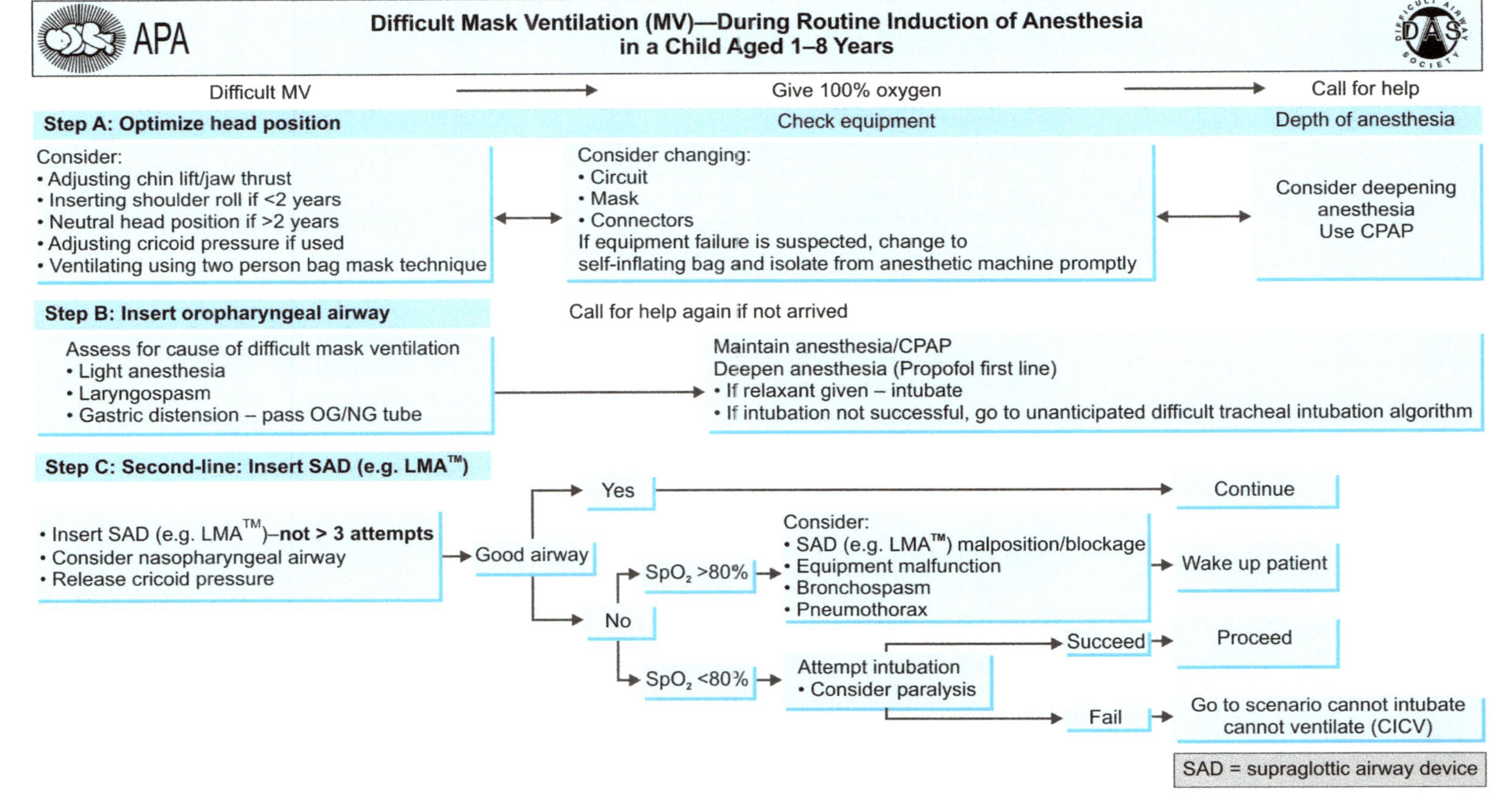
APA
Difficult Mask Ventilation (MV)—During Routine Induction of Anesthesia in a Child Aged 1–8 Years
DAS
Difficult MV
Give 100% oxygen
Call for help
Step A: Optimize head position
Check equipment
Depth of anesthesia
Consider:
• Adjusting chin lift/jaw thrust
• Inserting shoulder roll if <2 years
• Neutral head position if >2 years
• Adjusting cricoid pressure if used
• Ventilating using two person bag mask technique
Consider changing:
• Circuit
• Mask
• Connectors
If equipment failure is suspected, change to self-inflating bag and isolate from anesthetic machine promptly
Consider deepening anesthesia
Use CPAP
Step B: Insert oropharyngeal airway
Call for help again if not arrived
Assess for cause of difficult mask ventilation
• Light anesthesia
• Laryngospasm
• Gastric distension – pass OG/NG tube
Maintain anesthesia/CPAP
Deepen anesthesia (Propofol first line)
• If relaxant given – intubate
• If intubation not successful, go to unanticipated difficult tracheal intubation algorithm
Step C: Second-line: Insert SAD (e.g. LMA™)
• Insert SAD (e.g. LMA™)–not > 3 attempts
• Consider nasopharyngeal airway
• Release cricoid pressure
Good airway
Yes
Continue
No
SpO2 >80%
Consider:
• SAD (e.g. LMA™) malposition/blockage
• Equipment malfunction
• Bronchospasm
• Pneumothorax
Wake up patient
SpO2 <80%
Attempt intubation
• Consider paralysis
Succeed
Proceed
Fail
Go to scenario cannot intubate cannot ventilate (CICV)
SAD = supraglottic airway device

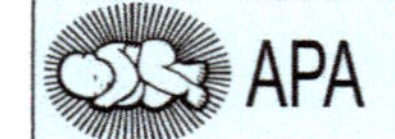

Unanticipated Difficult Tracheal Intubation—During Routine Induction of Anesthesia in a Child Aged 1–8 Years

DAS (Difficult Airway Society)

Difficult direct laryngoscopy → Give 100% oxygen and maintain anesthesia → Call for help

Step A: Initial tracheal intubation plan when mask ventilation is satisfaction

Ensure: Oxygenation, anesthesia, CPAP, management of gastric distension with OG/NG tube

Direct laryngoscopy – **not > 4 attempts**
Check:
- Neck flexion and head extension
- Laryngoscopy technique
- External laryngeal manipulation – remove or adjust
- Vocal cords open and immobile (adequate paralysis)

If poor view – consider bougie, straight blade laryngoscope* and/or smaller ETT

→ Succeed → Tracheal intubation → Verify ETT position
- Capnography
- Visual if possible
- Auscultation

If ETT too small consider using throat pack and tie to ETT
If in doubt, take ETT out

↓ Failed intubation with good oxygenation

Step B: Secondary tracheal intubation plan

Call for help again if not arrived

- Insert SAD (e.g. LMA™) – **not > 3 attempts**
- Oxygenate and ventilate
- Consider increasing size of SAD (e.g. LMA™) once if ventilation inadequate

→ Succeed →
- Consider modifying anesthesia and surgery plan
- Assess safety of proceeding with surgery using a SAD (e.g. LMA™)

→ Unsafe → **Postpone surgery wake up patient**
→ Safe → **Proceed with surgery**

↓ Safe ↓

- **Consider 1 attempt at FOI via SAD (e.g. LMA™)**
- Verify intubation, leave SAD (e.g. LMA™) in place and proceed with surgery

→ Succeed → **Proceed with surgery**

↓ Failed intubation via SAD (e.g. LMA™) → **Postpone surgery Wake up patient**

↓ Failed oxygenation e.g. SpO_2 <90% with FiO_2 1.0

- Convert to face mask
- Optimize head position
- Oxygenate and ventilate
- Ventilate using two person bag mask technique, CPAP and oro/nasopharyngeal airway
- Manage gastric distension with OG/NG tube
- Reverse non-depolarizing relaxant

→ Succeed → **Postpone surgery Wake up patient**
→ Failed ventilation and oxygenation → Go to scenario cannot intubate cannot ventilate (CICV)

Following intubation attempts, consider • Trauma to the airway • Extubation in a controlled setting
*Consider using indirect laryngoscope if experienced in their use

SAD = supraglottic airway device

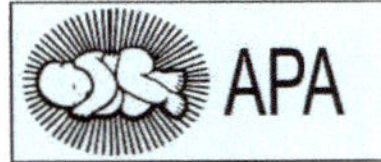 APA

Cannot Intubate and Cannot Ventilate (CICV) in a Paralyzed Anesthetized Child Aged 1–8 Years

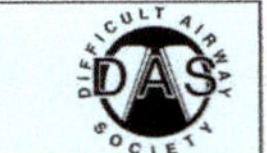

Failed intubation inadequate ventilation → Give 100% oxygen → Call for help

Step A: Continue to attempt oxygenation and ventilation — Check equipment — Depth of anesthesia

- FiO_2 1.0
- Optimize head position and chin lift/jaw thrust
- Insert oropharyngeal airway or SAD (e.g. LMA™)
- Ventilate using two person bag mask technique
- Manage gastric distension with an OG/NG tube

Step B: Attempt wake up if maintaining SpO_2 >80%

If rocuronium or vecuronium used, consider sugammadex (16 mg/kg) for full reversal

Prepare for rescue techniques in case child deteriorates

Step C: Airway rescue techniques for CICV (SpO_2 <80% and falling) and/or heart rate decreasing

Call for help again if not arrived

Call for specialist ENT assistance

- ENT available → Consider:
  - Sugical tracheostomy
  - Rigid bronchoscopy + ventilate/ jet ventilation (pressure limited)
- ENT not available → Percutaneous cannula cricothyroidotomy/transtracheal jet ventilation (pressure limited)
  - Succeed → Continue jet ventilation set to lowest delivery pressure until wake up or definitive airway established
  - Fail →
    - Perform surgical cricothyroidotomy/transtracheal and insertion of ETT/tracheostomy tube*
    - Consider passive O_2 insufflation while preparing

Cannula cricothyroidotomy

- Extend the neck (shoulder roll)
- Stabilize larynx with non-dominant hand
- Access the cricothyroidotomy membrane with a dedicated 14/16 gauge cannula
- Aim in a caudad direction
- Confirm position by air aspiration using a syringe with saline
- Connect to either:
  - Adjustable pressure limiting device, set to lowest delivery pressure

  or

  - 4Bar O_2 source with a flowmeter (match flow l/min to child's age) and Y connector
- Cautiously increase inflation pressure/ flow rate to achieve adequate chest expansion
  Wait for full expiration before next inflation
- Maintain upper airway patency to aid expiration

*Note: Cricothyroidotomy techniques can have serious complications and training is required—only use in life-threatening situations and convert to a definitive airway as soon as possible

SAD = supraglottic airway device

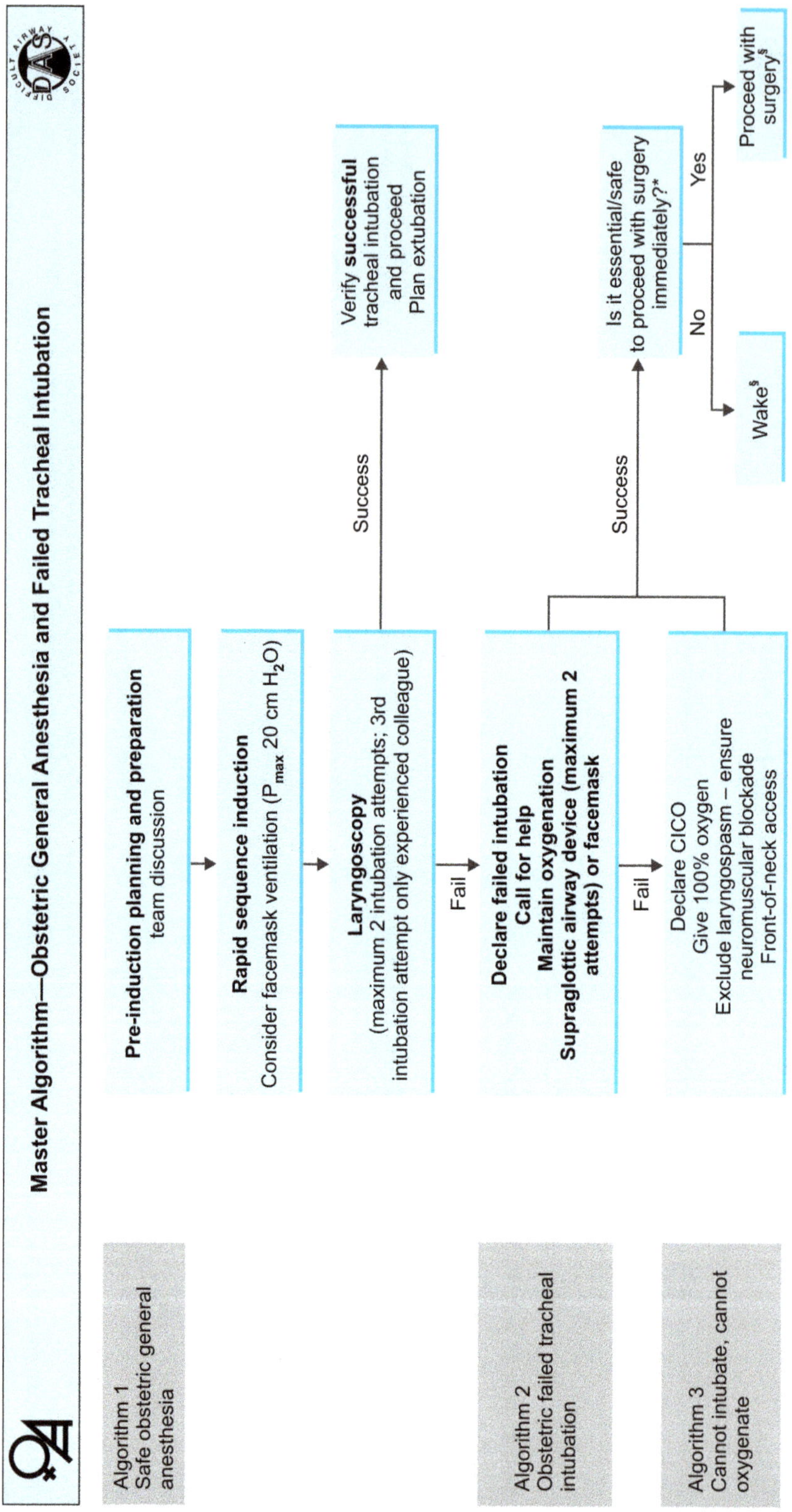

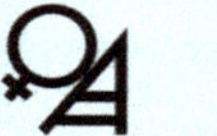

Master Algorithm—Obstetric General Anesthesia and Failed Tracheal Intubation

Algorithm 1
Safe obstetric general anesthesia

Pre-induction planning and preparation
team discussion

↓

Rapid sequence induction
Consider facemask ventilation (P_{max} 20 cm H_2O)

↓

Laryngoscopy
(maximum 2 intubation attempts; 3rd intubation attempt only experienced colleague)

→ Success → Verify **successful** tracheal intubation and proceed
Plan extubation

↓ Fail

Algorithm 2
Obstetric failed tracheal intubation

Declare failed intubation
Call for help
Maintain oxygenation
Supraglottic airway device (maximum 2 attempts) or facemask

↓ Fail

Algorithm 3
Cannot intubate, cannot oxygenate

Declare CICO
Give 100% oxygen
Exclude laryngospasm – ensure neuromuscular blockade
Front-of-neck access

→ Success (from Algorithm 2 or Algorithm 3) → Is it essential/safe to proceed with surgery immediately?*
- No → Wake§
- Yes → Proceed with surgery§

*See Table 1 , §See Table 2

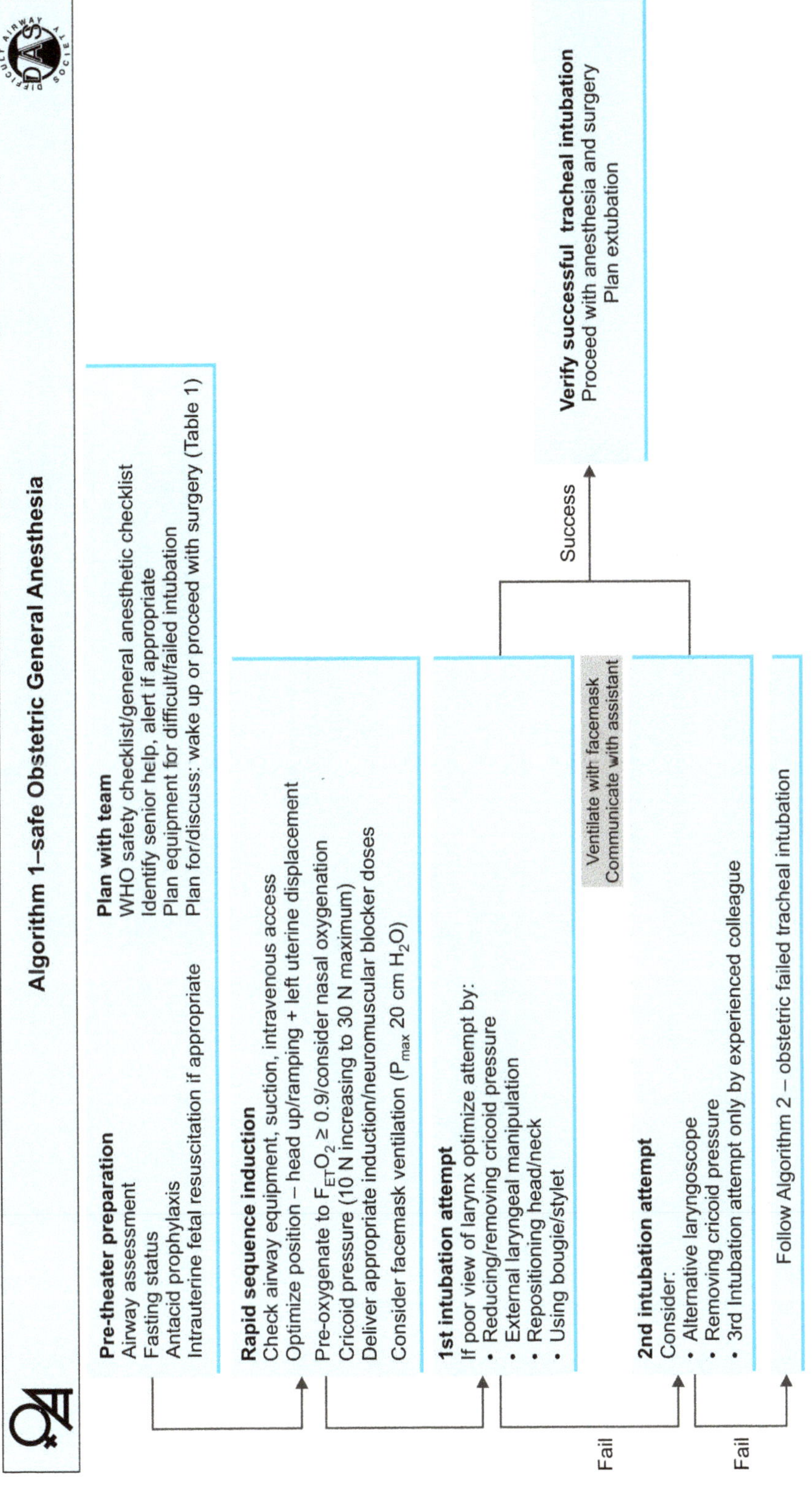
Algorithm 1–safe Obstetric General Anesthesia
DIFFICULT AIRWAY SOCIETY
DAS
Pre-theater preparation
Airway assessment
Fasting status
Antacid prophylaxis
Intrauterine fetal resuscitation if appropriate
Plan with team
WHO safety checklist/general anesthetic checklist
Identify senior help, alert if appropriate
Plan equipment for difficult/failed intubation
Plan for/discuss: wake up or proceed with surgery (Table 1)
Rapid sequence induction
Check airway equipment, suction, intravenous access
Optimize position – head up/ramping + left uterine displacement
Pre-oxygenate to $F_{ET}O_2 \geq 0.9$/consider nasal oxygenation
Cricoid pressure (10 N increasing to 30 N maximum)
Deliver appropriate induction/neuromuscular blocker doses
Consider facemask ventilation (P_{max} 20 cm H_2O)
1st intubation attempt
If poor view of larynx optimize attempt by:
• Reducing/removing cricoid pressure
• External laryngeal manipulation
• Repositioning head/neck
• Using bougie/stylet
Success
Verify successful tracheal intubation
Proceed with anesthesia and surgery
Plan extubation
Fail
Ventilate with facemask
Communicate with assistant
2nd intubation attempt
Consider:
• Alternative laryngoscope
• Removing cricoid pressure
• 3rd Intubation attempt only by experienced colleague
Fail
Follow Algorithm 2 – obstetric failed tracheal intubation

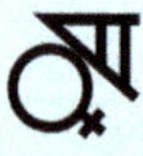

Algorithm 2–Obstetric Failed Tracheal Intubation

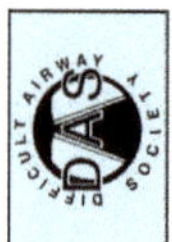

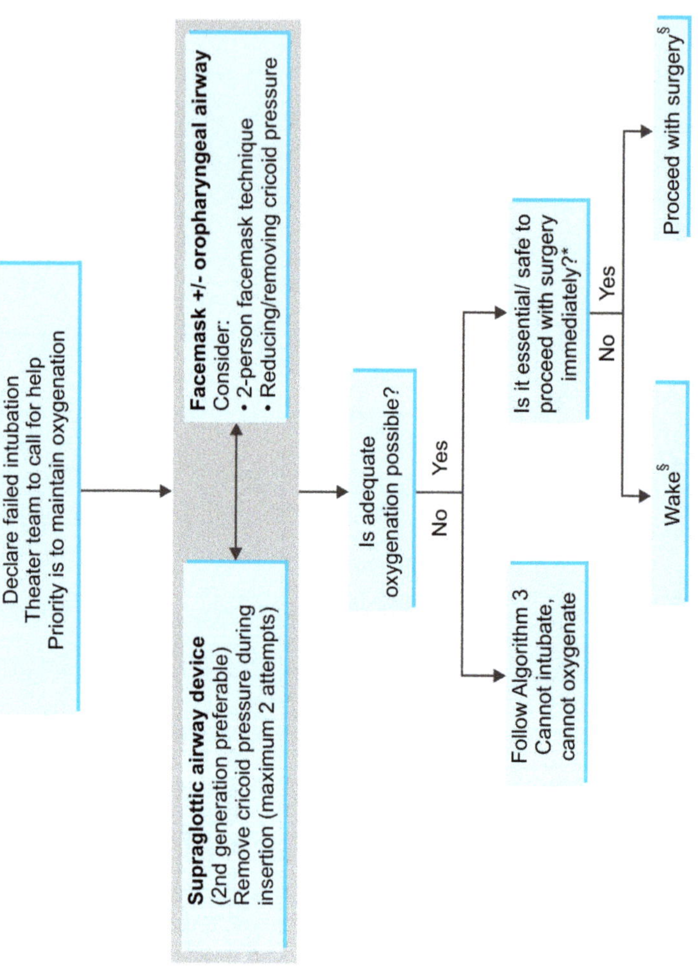

*See Table 1 , $See Table 2

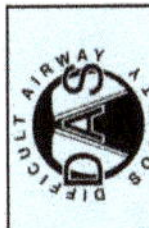

Algorithm 3–Cannot Intubate, Cannot Oxygenate

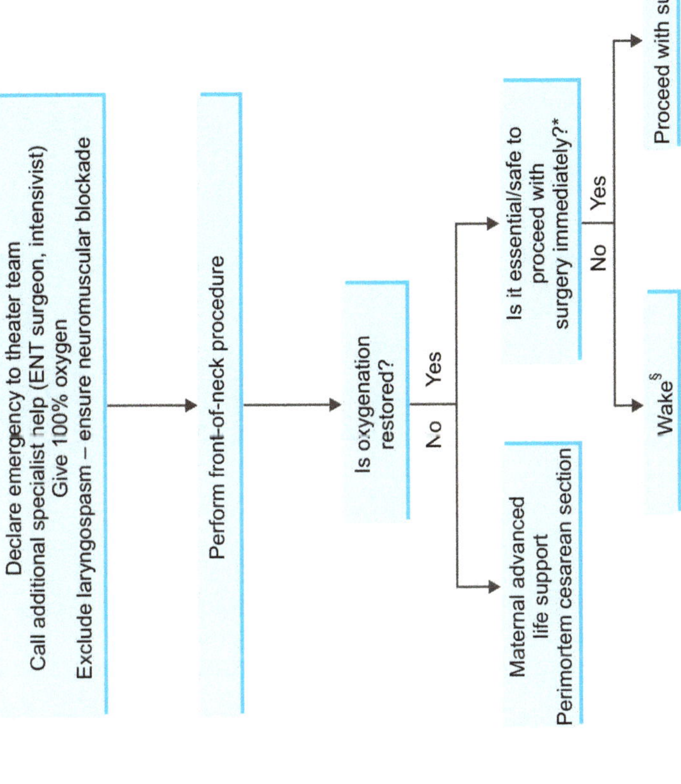

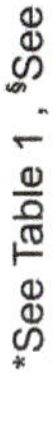

Table 1: Proceed with surgery?

	Factors to consider	*Wake* ←		→	*Proceed*
Before induction	Maternal condition	• No compromise	• Mild acute compromise	• Hemorrhage responsive to resuscitation	• Hypovolemia requiring corrective surgery • Critical cardiac or respiratory compromise, cardiac arrest
	Fetal condition	• No compromise	• Compromise corrected with intrauterine resuscitation, pH < 7.2 but > 7.15	• Continuing fetal heart rate abnormality despite intrauterine resuscitation, pH < 7.15	• Sustained bradycardia • Fetal hemorrhage • Suspected uterine rupture
	Anesthetist	• Novice	• Junior trainee	• Senior trainee	• Consultant/specialist
	Obesity	• Supermorbid	• Morbid	• Obese	• Normal
	Surgical factors	• Complex surgery or major hemorrhage anticipated	• Multiple uterine scars • Some surgical difficulties expected	• Single uterine scar	• No risk factors
	Aspiration risk	• Recent food	• No recent food • In labor • Opioids given • Antacids not given	• No recent food • In labor • Opioids not given • Antacids given	• Fasted • Not in labor • Antacids given
	Alternative anesthesia • regional • securing airway awake	• No anticipated difficulty	• Predicted difficulty	• Relatively contraindicated	• Absolutely contraindicated or has failed • Surgery started

Contd...

Contd...

	Factors to consider	*Wake* ←		→	*Proceed*
After failed intubation	Airway device/ventilation	• Difficult facemask ventilation • Front-of-neck	• Adequate facemask ventilation	• First generation supraglottic airway device	• Second generation supraglottic airway device
	Airway hazards	• Laryngeal edema • Stridor	• Bleeding • Trauma	• Secretions	• None evident

Criteria to be used in the decision to wake or proceed following failed tracheal intubation. In any individual patient, some factors may suggest waking and others proceeding. The final decision will depend on the anesthetist's clinical judgment.

Table 2: Management after failed tracheal intubation.

Wake	*Proceed with surgery*

• Maintain oxygenation
• Maintain cricoid pressure if not impeding ventilation
• Either maintain head-up position or turn left lateral recumbent
• If rocuronium used, reverse with sugammadex
• Assess neuromuscular blockade and manage awareness if paralysis is prolonged
• Anticipate laryngospasm/can't intubate, can't oxygenate
 	
After waking
 	
• Review urgency of surgery with obstetric team
• Intrauterine fetal resuscitation as appropriate
• For repeat anaesthesia, manage with two anaesthetists
• Anaesthetic options:
  ▪ Regional anaesthesia preferably inserted in lateral position
• Secure airway awake before repeat general anaesthesia
	• Maintain anesthesia
	• Maintain ventilation - consider merits of:
	  ▪ Controlled or spontaneous ventilation
	  ▪ Paralysis with rocuronium if sugammadex available
	• Anticipate laryngospasm/cannot intubate, cannot oxygenate
	• Minimise aspiration risk:
	  ▪ Maintain cricoid pressure until delivery (if not impeding ventilation)
	  ▪ After delivery maintain vigilance and reapply cricoid pressure if signs of regurgitation
	  ▪ Empty stomach with gastric drain tube if using second-generation supraglottic airway device
	  ▪ Minimise fundal pressure
	  ▪ Administer H_2 receptor blocker IV if not already given
	• Senior obstetrician to operate
	• Inform neonatal team about failed intubation
	• Consider total intravenous anesthesia

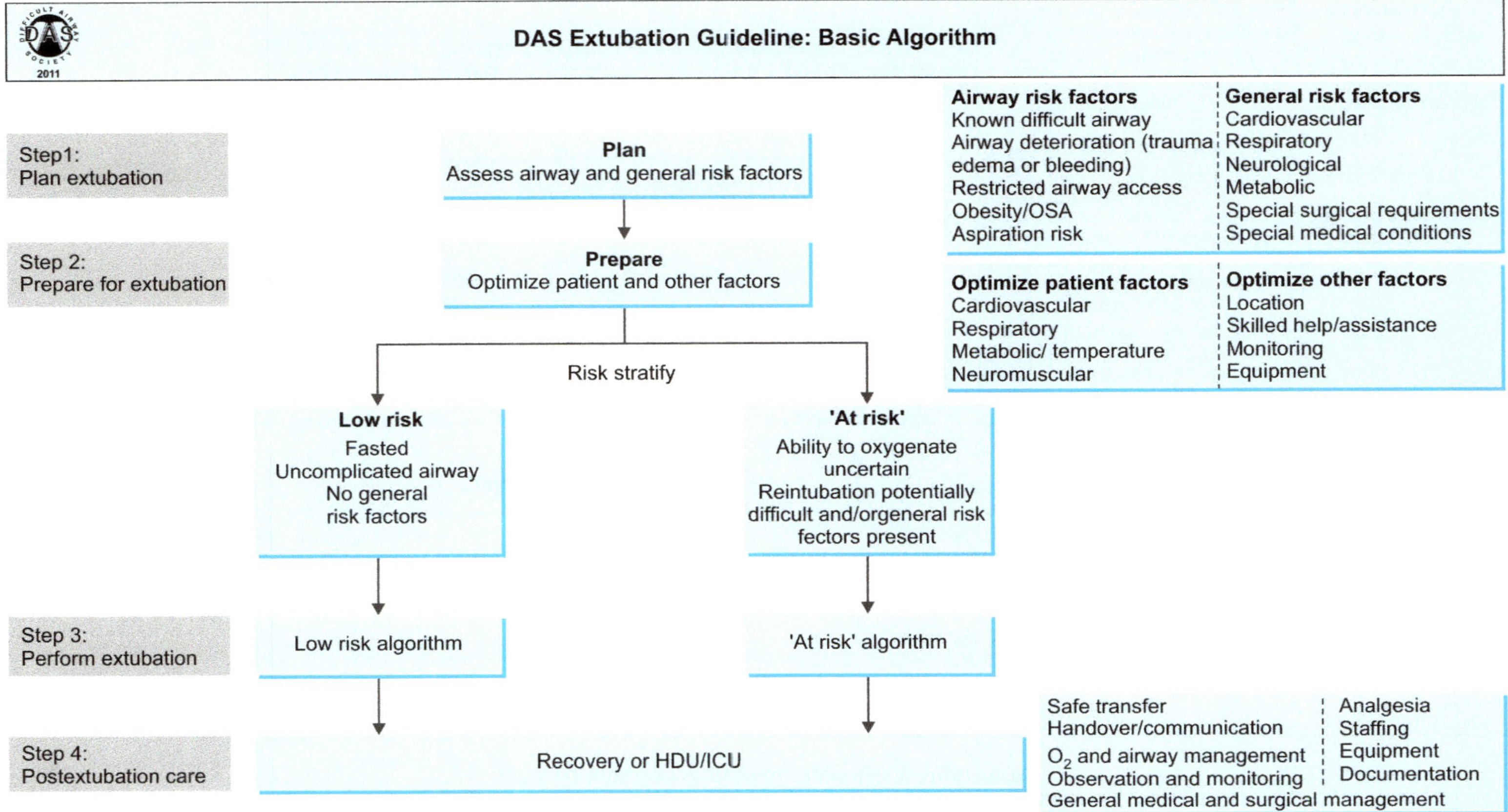
DAS Extubation Guideline: Basic Algorithm
DAS 2011
Step1:
Plan extubation
Step 2:
Prepare for extubation
Step 3:
Perform extubation
Step 4:
Postextubation care
Plan
Assess airway and general risk factors
Prepare
Optimize patient and other factors
Risk stratify
Low risk
Fasted
Uncomplicated airway
No general
risk factors
'At risk'
Ability to oxygenate
uncertain
Reintubation potentially
difficult and/orgeneral risk
factors present
Low risk algorithm
'At risk' algorithm
Recovery or HDU/ICU
Airway risk factors
Known difficult airway
Airway deterioration (trauma
edema or bleeding)
Restricted airway access
Obesity/OSA
Aspiration risk
General risk factors
Cardiovascular
Respiratory
Neurological
Metabolic
Special surgical requirements
Special medical conditions
Optimize patient factors
Cardiovascular
Respiratory
Metabolic/ temperature
Neuromuscular
Optimize other factors
Location
Skilled help/assistance
Monitoring
Equipment
Safe transfer
Handover/communication
O_2 and airway management
Observation and monitoring
General medical and surgical management
Analgesia
Staffing
Equipment
Documentation

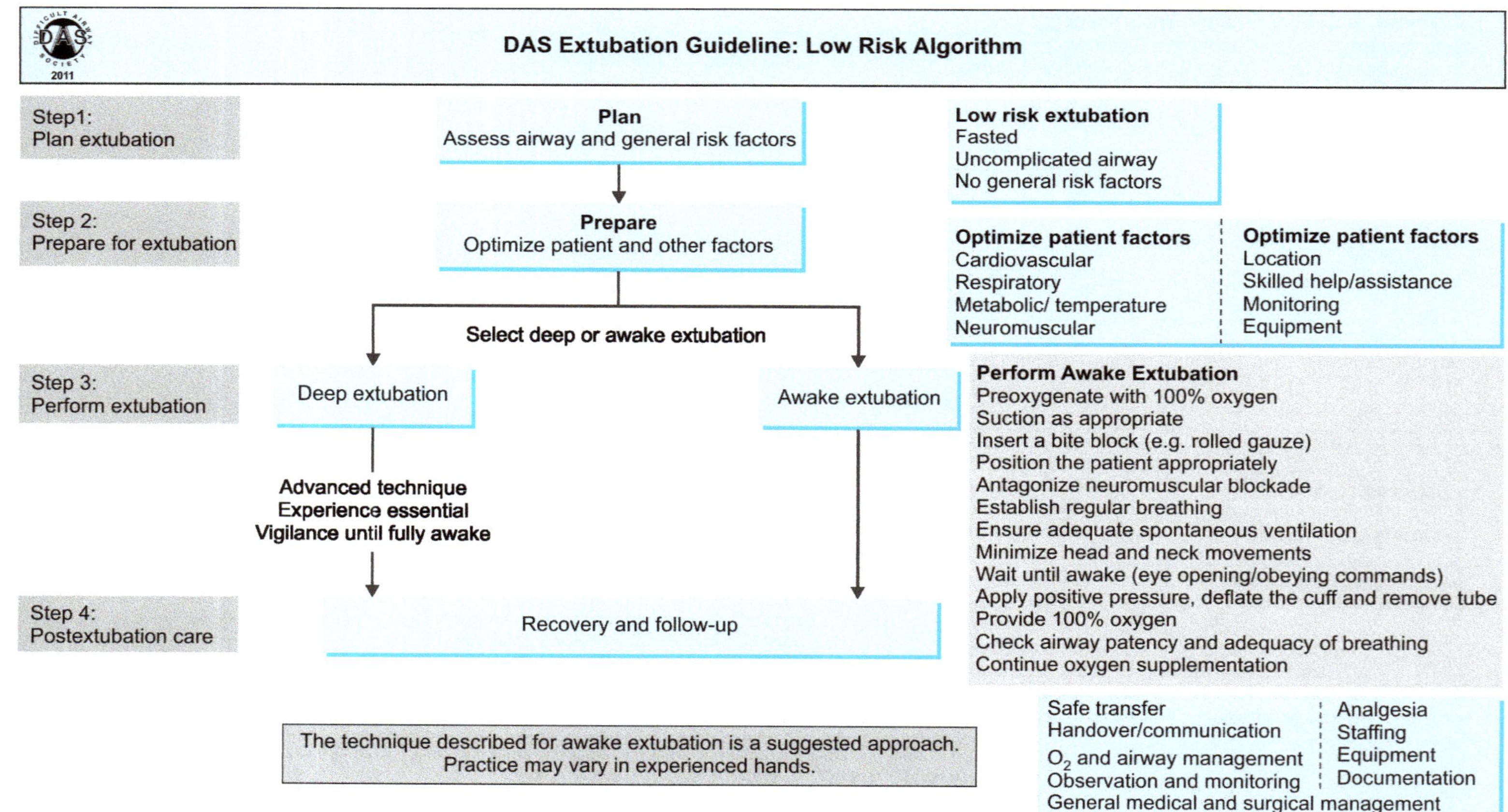

DAS Extubation Guideline: Low Risk Algorithm
DAS
2011
Step1:
Plan extubation
Plan
Assess airway and general risk factors
Low risk extubation
Fasted
Uncomplicated airway
No general risk factors
Step 2:
Prepare for extubation
Prepare
Optimize patient and other factors
Optimize patient factors
Cardiovascular
Respiratory
Metabolic/ temperature
Neuromuscular
Optimize patient factors
Location
Skilled help/assistance
Monitoring
Equipment
Select deep or awake extubation
Step 3:
Perform extubation
Deep extubation
Awake extubation
Advanced technique
Experience essential
Vigilance until fully awake
Perform Awake Extubation
Preoxygenate with 100% oxygen
Suction as appropriate
Insert a bite block (e.g. rolled gauze)
Position the patient appropriately
Antagonize neuromuscular blockade
Establish regular breathing
Ensure adequate spontaneous ventilation
Minimize head and neck movements
Wait until awake (eye opening/obeying commands)
Apply positive pressure, deflate the cuff and remove tube
Provide 100% oxygen
Check airway patency and adequacy of breathing
Continue oxygen supplementation
Step 4:
Postextubation care
Recovery and follow-up
Safe transfer
Handover/communication
O_2 and airway management
Observation and monitoring
General medical and surgical management
Analgesia
Staffing
Equipment
Documentation
The technique described for awake extubation is a suggested approach.
Practice may vary in experienced hands.

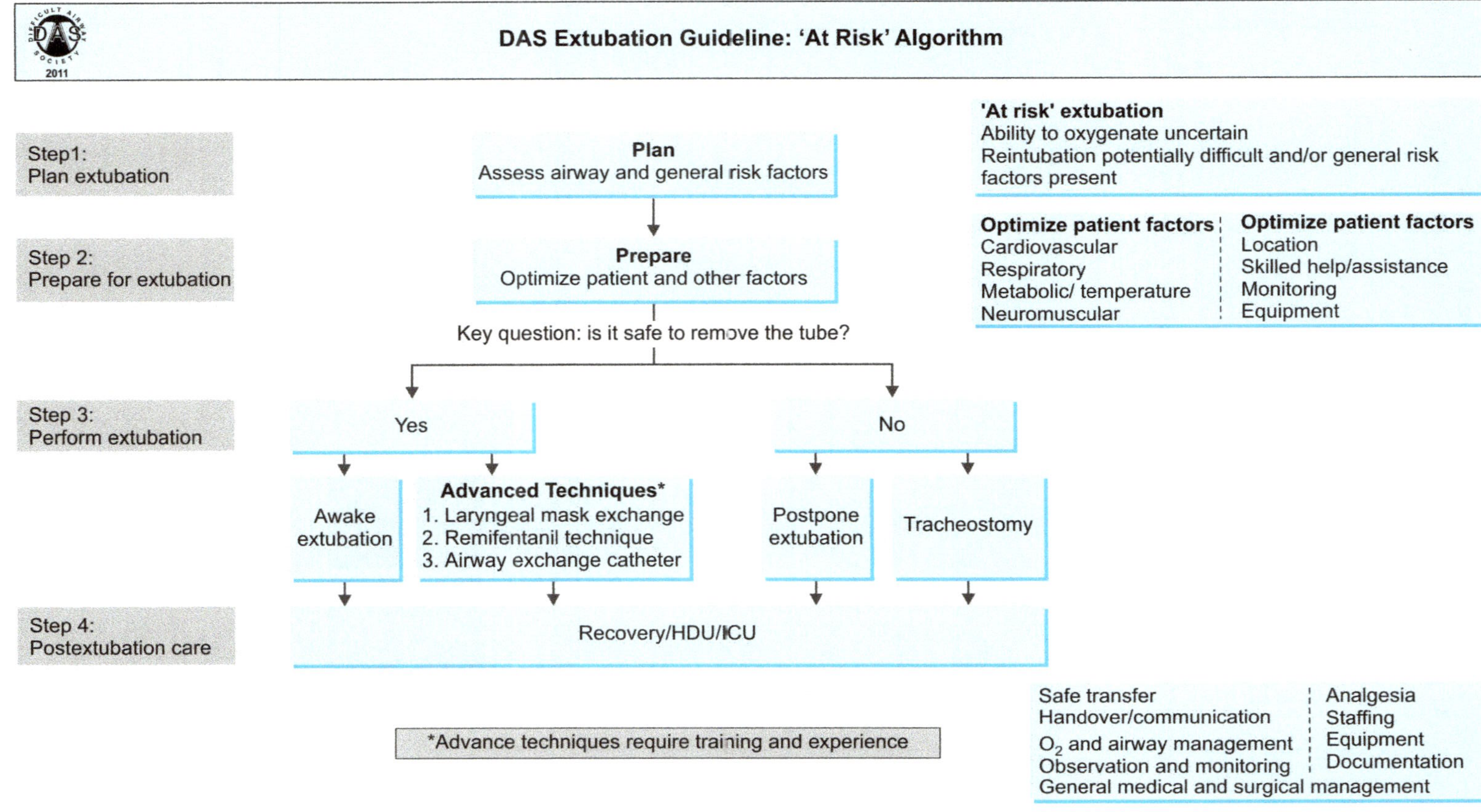
DIFFICULT AIRWAY SOCIETY 2011
DAS Extubation Guideline: 'At Risk' Algorithm
Step1:
Plan extubation
Plan
Assess airway and general risk factors
'At risk' extubation
Ability to oxygenate uncertain
Reintubation potentially difficult and/or general risk factors present
Step 2:
Prepare for extubation
Prepare
Optimize patient and other factors
Optimize patient factors
Cardiovascular
Respiratory
Metabolic/ temperature
Neuromuscular
Optimize patient factors
Location
Skilled help/assistance
Monitoring
Equipment
Key question: is it safe to remove the tube?
Step 3:
Perform extubation
Yes
No
Awake extubation
Advanced Techniques*
1. Laryngeal mask exchange
2. Remifentanil technique
3. Airway exchange catheter
Postpone extubation
Tracheostomy
Step 4:
Postextubation care
Recovery/HDU/ICU
*Advance techniques require training and experience
Safe transfer
Handover/communication
O_2 and airway management
Observation and monitoring
General medical and surgical management
Analgesia
Staffing
Equipment
Documentation

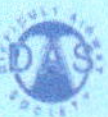

FIBEROPTIC GUIDED TRACHEAL INTUBATION THROUGH SUPRAGLOTTIC AIRWAY DEVICE (SAD) USING AINTREE INTUBATION CATHETER

NHS Lanarkshire

Please ensure the SAD is in place; give 100% oxygen; confirm adequate sedation/anesthesia, ventilation and paralysis

Aintree catheter
- 56 cm long hollow catheter
- 6.5 mm outer diameter; 4.7 mm inner diameter
- Easily preloaded onto an appropriately sized intubating fiberscope (maximum insetion cord diameter—4.2 mm)
- Flexible enough for loading over fiberscope
- Stiff enough to facilitate railroading of tracheal tube
- Comes with 2 rapifit adaptors (please refer to manufacturer's guidelines)
- Used for SAD assisted orotracheal fiberoptic intubation

1

Having prepared the fiberscope (FS) and camera system, lubricate the outer surfaces of both the Aintree Intubation Catheter (AIC) and FS. Preload AIC onto FS and secure with tape Attach a 15 mm bronchoscopic swivel connector (with port) to SAD and attach the anesthetic circuit to the swivel connector. Confirm adequate anesthesia, muscle relaxation and assisted ventilation.

2

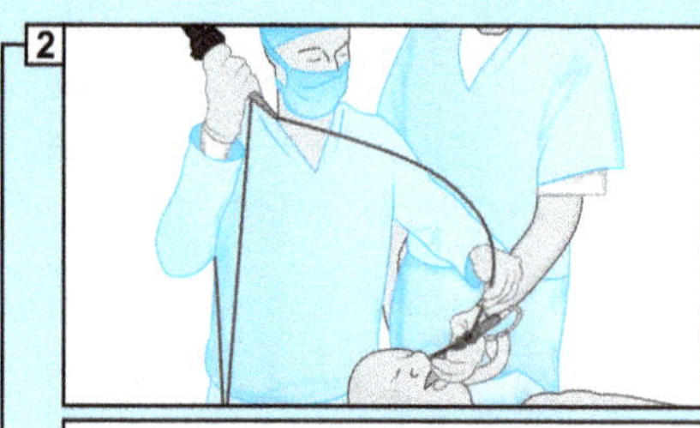

The SAD should be immobilized by an assistant. Introduce FS with loaded AIC through top port of swivel connector into the SAD lumen.

3

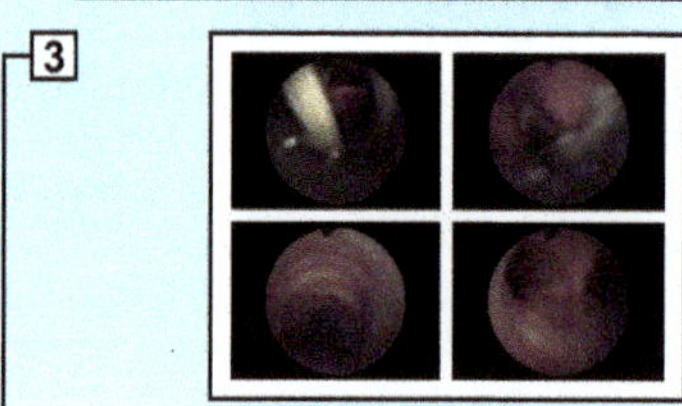

Sequentially visualize SAD aperture bars (if present), glottis, tracheal rings and finally carina as the FS passes caudally. **Never advance beyond carina.**

Permission for use granted by Cook Medical incorporated, Bloomington, Indians.
Authors: Dr Rajmohan Padmanabhan, Consultant Anesthetist, NHS Lanarkshire
Dr Barry McCuire, Consulant Anesthetist, NHS Tayside
Illustrations produced by Andy Morris, Medical Illustration Department, NHS Lanarkshire. 26/01/2011

The AIC was invented in Liverpool, UK;
Reference: Anasthesia, 1996, volume 51, pages 1123-1126

4

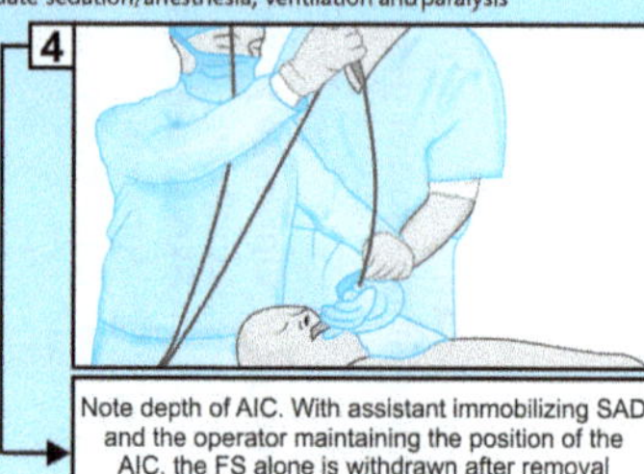

Note depth of AIC. With assistant immobilizing SAD and the operator maintaining the position of the AIC, the FS alone is withdrawn after removal of securing tape.

5

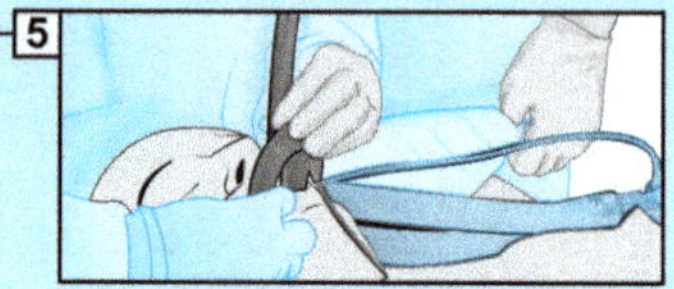

Briefly disconnect SAD (along with swivel connector) from anesthetic circuit deflate cuff (if present) and start withdrawing SAD (along with swivel connector), applying counter pressure on AIC to prevent movement. Once the SAD cuff becomes visible, grasp AIC in the mouth and fully remove SAD with swivel connector. The process should be done with care. Again note the depth of AIC at lips, ensuring that it **never exceeds 26 cm**.

6

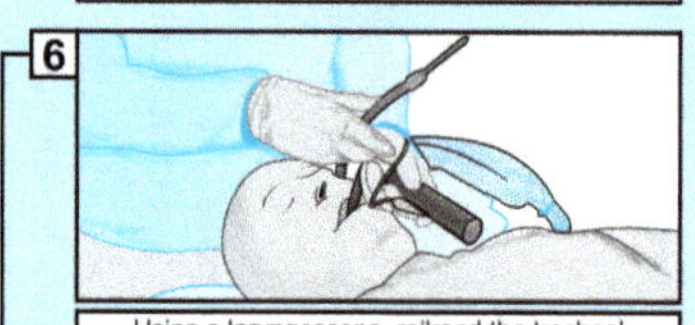

Using a laryngoscope, railroad the tracheal tube (ETT) over AIC ensuring a 'tip anterior' orientation. Use a conventional ETT-minimum size is 7.0 and pre cut to appropriate length.

7

Reconnect circuit and re-establish anesthesia and ventilation.

Confirm end-tidal CO_2.
Consider FS confirmation of ETT position.

- This is not an airway rescue technique
- It should be performed in a controlled stepwise process
- The process is designed to provide continued ventilation/oxygenation via the SAD swivel connector until the SAD is removed and tracheal tube is railroaded in place
- Oxygen can be delivered via the AIC in situations where railroading of tracheal tube is prolonged; assisting ventilation via this route is often suboptimal (narrow diameter/lack of cuff)-
Refer to manufacturer's guidelines for methods of oxygen delivery.

Recommendations
1. Consider a second anesthetist in addition to a trained assistant.
2. Use a camera system for fiberscope.

Caution
The aintree catheter is not recommended with the LMA Superme.

AIRWAY ALERT FORM

Name ....

Date of Birth ....

Hospital Number ....

Home Address ....

Telephone ....

Fax ....

Email ....

To the Patient

Please keep this letter safe and show it to your doctor if you are admitted to hospital.

Please show this letter to the anesthetic doctor if you need an operation.

This letter explains the difficulties that were found during your recent anesthetic and the information may be useful to doctors treating you in the future.

To the GP

Please copy this letter with any future referral.

Summary of Airway Management

Date of operation:

Type of operation:

		Reasons/comments
Difficult mask ventilation?	Yes/No	
Difficult direct laryngoscopy?	Yes/No	
Difficult tracheal intubation?	Yes/No	
Laryngoscopy grade	1/2/3/4	

Equipment used:

Other information:

Is awake intubation necessary in the future?

Follow-up care (tick when completed)

- Copies of letter
- One copy to patient
- One copy to GP
- One copy in case notes
- One copy in anesthetic department
- Spoken to patient
- Anesthetic chart complete
- Information on front of case notes
- Medic alert or difficult airway Society referral (specify)

Name of anesthetist: Grade: Date:

If you require further information please contact the Anesthetic department.

American Society of Anesthesiologists®

DIFFICULT AIRWAY ALGORITHM

1. Assess the likelihood and clinical impact of basic management problems:
   - Difficulty with patient cooperation or consent
   - Difficult mask ventilation
   - Difficult supraglottic airway placement
   - Difficult laryngoscopy
   - Difficult intubation
   - Difficult surgical airway access.
2. Actively pursue opportunities to deliver supplemental oxygen throughout the process of difficult airway management.
3. Consider the relative merits and feasibility of basic management choices:
   - Awake intubation *vs.* intubation after induction of general anesthesia
   - Non-invasive technique *vs.* invasive techniques for the initial approach to intubation
   - Video-assisted laryngoscopy as an initial approach to intubation
   - Preservation vs. ablation of spontaneous ventilation.
4. Develop primary and alternative strategies:

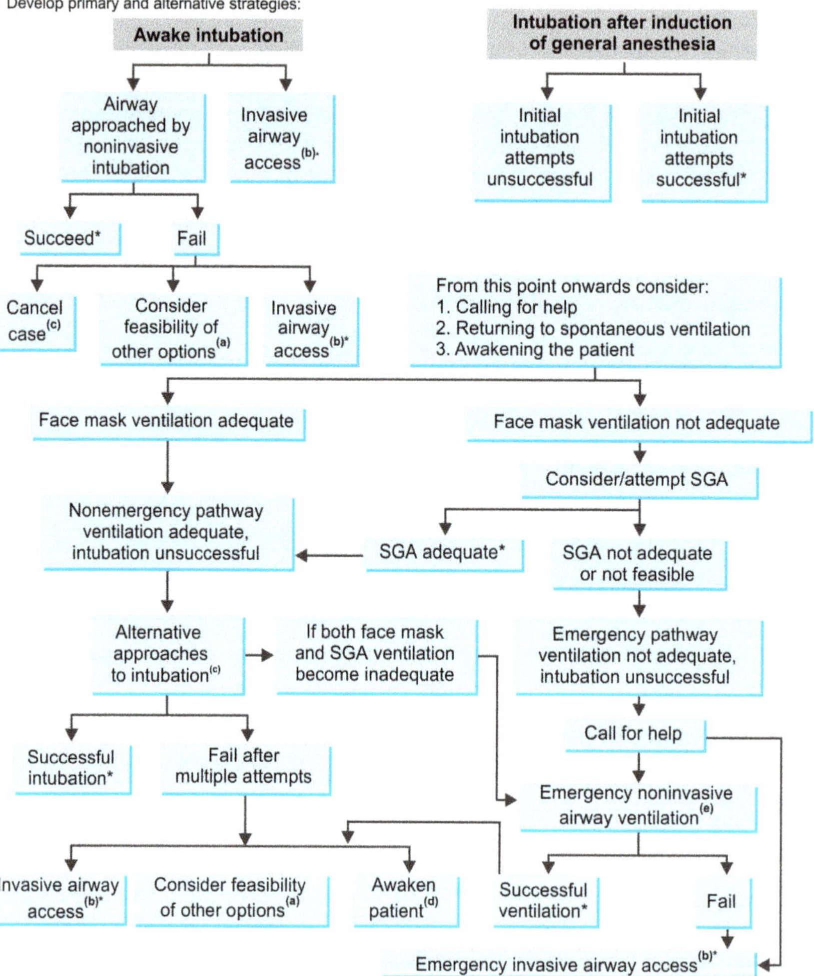

***Confirm ventilation, tracheal intubation, or SGA placement with exhaled CO_2.**

a. Other options include (but are not limited to): surgery utilizing face mask or supraglottic airway (SGA) anesthesia (e.g., LMA, ILMA, laryngeal tube), local anesthesia infiltration or regional nerve blockade. Pursuit of these options usually implies that mask ventilation will not be problematic. Therefore, these options may be of limited value if this step in the algorithm has been reached via the emergency pathway.

b. Invasive airway access includes surgical or percutaneous airway, jet ventilation, and retrograde intubation.

c. Alternative difficult intubation approaches include (but are not limited to): video-assisted laryngoscopy, alternative laryngoscope blades, SGA (e.g., LMA or ILMA) as an intubation conduit (with or without fiberoptic guidance), fiberoptic intubation, intubating stylet or tube changer, light wand, and blind oral or nasal intubation.

d. Consider repreparation of the perfect for awake intubation or cancelling surgery.

e. Emergency non-invasive airway ventilation consists of a SGA.

Index

Page numbers followed by *f* refer to figure, *fc* refer to flowchart, and *t* refer to table.

A

B

C

D

E

F

O

P

R

S

T

U

V

W

Z

EU GSPR Authorised Reprsentative
Logos Europe, 9 rue Nicolas Poussin
1700, La Rochelle, France
Phone: +33 (0) 6 67 93 73 78
E-mail: contact@logoseurope.eu

www.ingramcontent.com/pod-product-compliance
Ingram Content Group UK Ltd.
Pitfield, Milton Keynes, MK11 3LW, UK
UKHW050923290726
14058UKWH00011B/682

* 9 7 8 9 3 5 2 7 0 1 7 0 4 *